OXFORD MEDICAL PUBLICATIONS

Gastric and Oesophageal Surgery

T0177557

Oxford Specialist Handbooks published and forthcoming

General Oxford Specialist Handbooks

A Resuscitation Room Guide
Addiction Medicine
Day Case Surgery
Perioperative Medicine, 2e
Pharmaceutical Medicine
Postoperative Complications, 2e
Renal Transplantation

Oxford Specialist Handbooks in Anaesthesia

Anaesthesia for Medical and Surgical
Emergencies
Cardiac Anaesthesia
Cardiothoracic Critical Care
Neuroanaethesia
Obstetric Anaesthesia
Ophthalmic Anaesthesia
Paediatric Anaesthesia
Regional Anaesthesia, Stimulation and
Ultrasound Techniques
Thoracic Anaesthesia

Oxford Specialist Handbooks in Cardiology

Adult Congenital Heart Disease
Cardiac Catheterization and Coronary
Intervention
Cardiac Electrophysiology and Catheter
Ablation
Cardiothoracic Critical Care
Cardiovascular Computed Tomography
Cardiovascular Magnetic Resonance
Echocardiography, 2e
Fetal Cardiology
Heart Failure
Hypertension
Inherited Cardiac Disease
Nuclear Cardiology
Pacemakers and ICDs
Pulmonary Hypertension
Valvular Heart Disease

Oxford Specialist Handbooks in Critical Care

Advanced Respiratory Critical Care

Oxford Specialist Handbooks in End of Life Care

End of Life Care in Cardiology
End of Life Care in Dementia
End of Life Care in Nephrology
End of Life Care in Respiratory Disease
End of Life in the Intensive Care Unit

Oxford Specialist Handbooks in Neurology

Epilepsy
Parkinson's Disease and Other
Movement Disorders
Stroke Medicine

Oxford Specialist Handbooks in Oncology

Practical Management of Complex
Cancer Pain

Oxford Specialist Handbooks in Paediatrics

Paediatric Dermatology
Paediatric Endocrinology
and Diabetes
Paediatric Gastroenterology,
Hepatology, and Nutrition
Paediatric Haematology
and Oncology
Paediatric Intensive Care
Paediatric Nephrology, 2e
Paediatric Neurology, 2e
Paediatric Radiology
Paediatric Respiratory Medicine
Paediatric Rheumatology

Oxford Specialist Handbooks in Pain Medicine

Spinal Interventions in Pain
Management

Oxford Specialist Handbooks in Psychiatry

Child and Adolescent Psychiatry
Forensic Psychiatry
Old Age Psychiatry

Oxford Specialist Handbooks in Radiology

Interventional Radiology
Musculoskeletal Imaging
Pulmonary Imaging
Thoracic Imaging

Oxford Specialist Handbooks in Surgery

Cardiothoracic Surgery, 2e
Colorectal Surgery
Gastric and Oesophageal Surgery
Hand Surgery
Hepatopancreatobiliary Surgery
Neurosurgery
Operative Surgery, 2e
Oral Maxillofacial Surgery
Otolaryngology and Head and
Neck Surgery
Paediatric Surgery
Plastic and Reconstructive Surgery
Surgical Oncology
Urological Surgery
Vascular Surgery

Oxford Specialist Handbooks in Surgery
Gastric and Oesophageal Surgery

Edited by

M. Asif Chaudry
Upper Gastrointestinal Surgeon,
St Thomas' Hospital, London, UK

Sri G. Thrumurthy
Core Surgical Trainee, Kingston Hospital,
Kingston-upon-Thames, UK

Muntzer Mughal
Honorary Clinical Professor and Head of Upper
Gastrointestinal Services, University College Hospitals,
London, UK

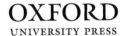

OXFORD
UNIVERSITY PRESS

OXFORD
UNIVERSITY PRESS

Great Clarendon Street, Oxford, OX2 6DP,
United Kingdom

Oxford University Press is a department of the University of Oxford.
It furthers the University's objective of excellence in research, scholarship,
and education by publishing worldwide. Oxford is a registered trade mark of
Oxford University Press in the UK and in certain other countries

© Oxford University Press 2014

The moral rights of the authors have been asserted

Impression: 3

Published in the United States of America by Oxford University Press
198 Madison Avenue, New York, NY 10016, United States of America

British Library Cataloguing in Publication Data
Data available

Library of Congress Control Number: 2013945735

ISBN 978–0–19–966320–0

Printed in Great Britain by
Ashford Colour Press Ltd.

Contents

Acknowledgements

For our teachers, from cradle to clinic—MAC

To my parents and greatest role models, Thrumurthy and Sobanah; to my outstanding wife and best friend, Ayishwarriyah; and to my baby sister, Sasha. To Asif, for standing steadfast against adversity. To Professor Mughal, my mentor and ambition—SGT

To John Bancewicz, for stimulating my interest in oesophago-gastric disease and for setting an example through his caring, compassionate and patient centred approach in delivering clinical care—MM

Contributors

Professor Stephen E A Attwood, Consultant Surgeon and Honorary Professor, Durham University, Northumbria Healthcare Foundation Trust, North Shields, UK

Dr M Adil Butt, Senior Research Associate, Gastroenterology and Laser Medicine, National Medical Laser Centre, University College London; Specialist Registrar in Gastroenterology, University College Hospital, UK

Mr M Asif Chaudry, Upper Gastrointestinal Surgeon, St Thomas' Hospital, London, UK

Dr Jason Dunn, Consultant Gastroenterologist, Guy's and St Thomas' Hospital, UK

Professor Alastair Forbes, Professor of Gastroenterology and Clinical Nutrition, University College London Hospitals NHS Foundation Trust, London, UK

Dr Rehan Haidry, Consultant Gastroenterologist, University College London Hospitals NHS Foundation Trust, London, UK

Mr Christopher J Lewis, Consultant Upper Gastrointestinal and General Surgeon, Wrightington Wigan and Leigh NHS Foundation Trust, UK

Dr Laurence B Lovat, Reader in Gastroenterology and Laser Medicine and Head of Research Department of Tissue and Energy, University College London; Consultant Gastroenterologist, University College Hospital, UK

Professor Muntzer Mughal, Honorary Clinical Professor and Head of Upper Gastrointestinal Services, University College Hospitals, London, UK

Mr James S Pollard, Specialist Registrar, University Hospital of South Manchester, NHS Foundation Trust, Manchester, UK

Mr Kishore G Pursnani, Consultant Upper GI Surgeon, Lancashire Teaching Hospitals NHS Foundation Trust, Preston, UK

Dr Sangeeta Sharma, Consultant Anaesthetist, Lancashire Teaching Hospitals NHS Foundation Trust, Preston, UK

Professor Daniel Sifrim, Professor of Gastrointestinal Physiology, Barts and the London School of Medicine and Dentistry, Queen Mary University of London, London, UK

Miss Tania S de Silva, Specialist Registrar in General Surgery, Kent Surrey and Sussex Deanery, UK

Mr Sri G Thrumurthy, Core Surgical Trainee, Kingston Hospital, Kingston-upon-Thames, UK

Mr Paul D Turner, Consultant Upper GI Surgeon, Lancashire Teaching Hospitals NHS Foundation Trust, Preston, UK

Mr Jeremy B Ward, Consultant Upper GI Surgeon, Lancashire Teaching Hospitals NHS Foundation Trust, Preston, UK

Mr Sean Woodcock, Consultant Bariatric Surgeon, Northumbria Healthcare NHS Foundation Trust, North Shields, UK

Dr Elaine Young, Consultant Clinical Oncologist, Rosemere Cancer Centre, Lancashire Teaching Hospitals NHS Foundation Trust, Preston, UK

Abbreviations

ABC	airway, breathing, and circulation
ABG	arterial blood gas analysis
ACTS-GC	Adjuvant Chemotherapy Trial of TS-1for Gastric Cancer
AF	atrial fibrillation
AJCC	American Joint Committee on Cancer
ALA	aminolevulinic acid
APUD	amine precursor uptake and decarboxylation
ARS	anti-reflux surgery
ASA	American Society of Anesthesiologists
AspECT	Aspirin Esomeprazole Chemoprevention Trial
AT	anaerobic threshold
bd	twice daily
BE	Barrett's epithelium
BEST2	Barrett's oesophagus screening trial
BICAP	bipolar circumactive probe
BMI	body mass index
BOLD	Bariatric Outcomes Longitudinal Database
BOMSS	British Obesity and Metabolic Surgical Society
BOSPA	British Obesity Surgical Patients Association
BOSS	Barrett's oesophagus surveillance study
BP	blood pressure
BPD	biliopancreatic diversion
BSC	Best Supportive Care
BSG	British Society of Gastroenterology
Bv	bevacizumab
cagA	cytotoxin-associated gene A
CBE	complete Barrett's eradication
CBET	Chemoprevention for Barrett's Esophagus Trial
CF	cisplatin and fluorouracil
CHAOS	coronary artery disease, hypertension, atherosclerosis, obesity, and stroke

CLO	Campylobacter-like organism
CML	chronic myeloid leukaemia
COG	Clinical Outcomes Group
COPD	chronic obstructive pulmonary disease
COX-1	cyclo-oxygenase enzyme
CPAP	continuous positive airway pressure
CR-D	complete reversal of dysplasia
CR-HGD	complete reversal of HGD
CT	computed tomography
CVA	cerebrovascular accident
CVP	central venous pressure
DCF	docetaxel, cisplatin and fluorouracil combination chemotherapy regimen
DCI	distal contractile integral
DFS	disease-free survival
DL	distal latency
DLT	double lumen endobronchial tube
DM	diabetes mellitus
DOS	diffuse oesophageal spasm
DU	duodenal ulcer
DVT	deep vein thrombosis
DXT	deep X-ray therapy
ECF	epirubicin, cisplatin and infusional fluorouracil
ECHO	echocardiography
ECX	epirubicin, cisplatin and capecitabine
EGC	early gastric cancer
EMR	endoscopic mucosal resection
EOX	epirubicin, oxaliplatin and capecitabine
ESD	endoscopic submucosal dissection
EUS	endoscopic ultrasound scan
FA	folinic acid
FBC	full blood count
FC	flow cytometry
FDA	Food and Drug Administration

FDG	18-fluorodeoxyglucose
FEV	forced expiratory volume
FFCD	Fédération Francophone de Cancérologie Digestive
FISH	fluorescent in situ hybridization
FLIP	functional lumen imaging probe
FNA	fine needle aspiration
FNCLCC	Fédération Nationale des Centres de Lutte Contre le Cancer
FPG	fasting plasma glucose
FU	fluorouracil
FVC	forced vital capacity
GA	general anaesthetic
GCS	Glasgow Coma Score
GDT	goal-directed therapy
GFR	glomerular filtration rate
GH	growth hormone
GI	gastrointestinal
GIP	gastric inhibiting peptide
GIST	gastrointestinal stromal tumour
GOJ	gastro-oesophageal junction
GORD	gastro-oesophageal reflux disease
Hb	haemoglobin
HDCG	hereditary diffuse gastric cancer
HDU	high dependency unit
HFIUS	high-frequency intraluminal ultrasound
HGD	high grade dysplasia
HH	hiatus hernia
HPV	human papillomavirus
HR	hazard ratio
HRM	high-resolution manometry
HRQL	health-related quality of life
HU	Hounsfield unit
IARC	International Agency for Research on Cancer
IBS	irritable bowel syndrome
ICDA	image cytometry DNA ploidy analysis

ICU	intensive care unit
IGRT	image-guided radiotherapy
IHD	ischaemic heart disease
IM	intestinal metaplasia
IMC	intramucosal cancer
IMRT	intensity-modulated radiotherapy
IRP	integrated relaxation pressure
ITU	intensive therapy unit
IV	intravenous
IWGCO	International Working Group for Classification of Oesophagitis
LA	local anaesthetic
LADG	laparoscopic-assisted distal gastrectomy
LAO	laparoscopically-assisted oesophagectomy
LARS	laparoscopic anti-reflux surgery
LATG	laparoscopy-assisted total gastrectomy
LDH	lactate dehydrogenase
LFT	liver function test
LGD	low grade dysplasia
LMWH	low molecular weight heparin
LN	lymph node
LOH	loss of heterozygosity
LOS	lower oesophageal sphincter
LSG	laparoscopic sleeve gastrectomy
LTA	left thoraco-abdominal oesophagectomy
LU	laparoscopic gastrectomy
LUQ	left upper quadrant
LV	left ventricle
LVEF	left ventricular ejection fraction
MAGIC	Medical Research Council Adjuvant Gastric Infusional Chemotherapy
MALT	mucosa-associated lymphoid tissue
MAOI	mono-amine oxidase inhibitors
MDT	multi-disciplinary meeting
MET	metabolic equivalent

MI	myocardial infarction
MII	multichannel intraluminal impedance
MIO	minimally invasive oesophagectomy
MODS	multiple organ dysfunction syndrome
MRC	Medical Research Council
MRI	magnetic resonance imaging
MUGA	multigated acquisition scan
MZL	marginal zone lymphomas
NASH	non-alcoholic steatosis hepatitis
NBM	nil by mouth
NBSR	National Bariatric Surgery Registry
NCCN	National Comprehensive Cancer Network
NERD	non-erosive reflux disease
NGT	nasogastric tube
NHL	non-Hodgkin's lymphoma
NJ	nasojejunal
NO	nitrous oxide
NSAID	non-steroidal anti-inflammatory drug
OAC	oesophageal adenocarcinoma
OCP	oral contraceptive pill
OG	oesophagogastric
OGD	oesophagogastroduodenoscopy
OHS	obesity hypoventilation syndrome
OLV	one-lung ventilation
OSA	obstructive sleep apnoea
OTG	open total gastrectomy
PAC	pulmonary artery catheter
PAND	para-aortic lymphadenectomy
PCA	patient-controlled analgesia
PCR	polymerase chain reaction
PDGRFA	platelet-derived growth factor-alpha
PDS	polydioxanone suture
PDT	photodynamic therapy
PE	pulmonary embolism

PEFR	peak expiratory flow rate
PEG	percutaneous endoscopic gastrostomy
PET	positron emission tomography
PMN	polymorphonuclear leukocyte
POEM	peroral endoscopic myotomy
PONV	post-operative nausea and vomiting
POSSUM	Physiological and Operative Severity Score for the enumeration of Mortality and Morbidity
PPI	proton-pump inhibitor
PS	photosensitizer
PUD	peptic ulcer disease
QALY	quality-adjusted life year
qds	four times daily
QoL	quality of life
R0	resection rates
RCT	randomized controlled trial
RECIST	Response Evaluation Criteria In Solid Tumors
RFA	radiofrequency ablation
ROS	reactive oxygen species
RR	relative risk
RSI	rapid sequence induction
Rx	'recipe' (treatment)
SAGES	Society of American Gastrointestinal and Endoscopic Surgeons
SAP	symptom-associated probability
SCC	squamous cell carcinoma
SCE	string-capsule endoscopy
SEMS	self-expanding metal stents
SER	stepwise endoscopic resection
SI	symptom index
SIM	specialized intestinal metaplasia
SIRS	systemic inflammatory response syndrome
SOS	Swedish Obesity Study
SPG	swallowing pattern generator
SpO_2	pulse oximeter oxygen saturation

SSBO	short-segment Barrett's oesophagus
STD	sodium tetradecyl sulphate
SWT	shuttle walk testing
T2DM	type 2 diabetes mellitus
TAO	thoracoscopically-assisted oesophagectomy
tds	three times daily
TEN	total enteral nutrition
TFF3	trefoil factor 3
TG	triglyceride
TLOSR	transient lower oesophageal sphincter relaxations
TNM	tumour, node, and metastasis
TPN	total parenteral nutrition
TSH	thyroid-stimulating hormone
U&E	urea and electrolytes
UBT	urea breath test
UGI	upper gastrointestinal
UKBOR	UK Barrett's Oesophagus Registry
UOS	upper oesophageal sphincter
V/Q	ventilation/perfusion
vacA	vacuolating cytotoxin-associated gene
VBG	vertical banded gastroplasty
VIP	vasoactive intestinal peptide
VO_{2max}	maximum oxygen uptake
VP	ventriculoperitoneal
VTE	venous thrombo-embolic
WBC	white blood cell
WCE	wireless capsule endoscopy

Chapter 1

Gastric anatomy and physiology

Gross anatomy

The stomach is the most dilated part of the gut (adult capacity 1–1.5L), extending from the oesophagus to the duodenum and lying in the upper left quadrant of the abdomen behind the lower ribs and anterior abdominal wall. It is separated from the left lung and pleura by the dome of the diaphragm. It is a piriform organ that includes several sections.

Antero-superior surface

- Covered by peritoneum and in contact with diaphragm.
- Right half lies in relation to left and quadrate hepatic lobes, and anterior abdominal wall.
- Transverse colon may lie on anterior surface when stomach is collapsed.

Postero-inferior surface

- Covered by peritoneum (apart from a small area near cardiac orifice limited to attachment of gastrophrenic ligament) and in apposition with diaphragm (and often with upper part of the suprarenal gland).
- Forms anterior boundary of the lesser sac (omental bursa), containing common hepatic artery, common bile duct, and portal vein. Can be accessed via an opening on free border of lesser omentum (epiploic foramen of Winslow).

Lesser curvature (concave)

- Extends from cardiac to pyloric orifice (see Fig. 1.1).
- Incisura angularis at junction between body and antrum.
- Two layers of hepatogastric ligament (lesser omentum) attached (see 📖 Greater and lesser omenta, p. 3).

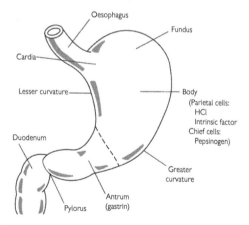

Fig. 1.1 Gross anatomy of the stomach (including the major secretory sites). Reproduced from *Upper Gastrointestinal Surgery*, Fielding et al., Springer, 2005, with permission of Springer Science and Business Media.

Greater curvature (convex)

- 4–5 times longer than lesser curvature.
- Extends from cardiac notch (angle of His) to pylorus.
- Sulcus intermedius (2.5cm from duodenopyloric constriction) lies opposite incisura.
- Two layers of greater omentum attached (see 📖 Greater and lesser omenta, p. 3).
- Oesophagus enters stomach on its right side about 2.5cm below its uppermost part.
- Right margin is continuous with lesser curvature; left margin joins greater curvature at an acute angle (cardiac notch).

The stomach comprises the following components:
- Cardiac orifice at the level of oesophageal opening (level of T10).
- Fundus proximal to oesophageal orifice.
- A body from fundus to pyloric antrum.
- Pyloric antrum is the dilated part between incisura angularis and sulcus intermedius.
- The pyloric[1] canal is 2.5cm long and passes from antrum to pyloric sphincter. The pylorus, which lies at the level of L1, is continuous with first part of the duodenum and features thickened muscle—the pyloric sphincter. Identified on gastric surface by a circular groove (duodeno-pyloric constriction).

Relations to the stomach

Anterior
Anterior abdominal wall:
- *Right anterior:* liver.
- *Left anterior:* diaphragm.

Posterior
- Body of pancreas.
- Part of left kidney.
- Left suprarenal gland.
- Splenic artery.
- Spleen.

These form the 'bed' of the stomach. The transverse mesocolon passes from the lower border of the pancreas to the transverse colon.

Greater and lesser omenta

Lesser omentum
- Extends from inferior and posterior hepatic surfaces to stomach and proximal 3cm of duodenum.
- Free border of lesser omentum contains hepatic artery, portal vein, common bile duct, lymphatics, and nerves. Behind free edge lies the epiploic foramen of Winslow.
- Remainder of lesser omentum (from left end of porta hepatis to lesser curvature) contains right and left gastric arteries, and accompanying veins, lymphatics, and anterior and posterior vagal branches.

[1] Greek *pylorus*, from *pyle* ('gate') and *ouros* ('guard').

Greater omentum

This is formed along the greater curvature by the union of peritoneal coats of antero-posterior gastric surfaces. It forms three ligaments:
- *Gastrophrenic ligament:* from fundus to diaphragm.
- *Gastrosplenic (lineal) ligament:* to spleen; contains short gastric branches of the splenic artery.
- *Gastrocolic ligament:* to transverse colon; contains right and left gastroepiploic vessels. Hangs down in front of intestines as a loose apron and extends as far as transverse colon, where its two layers separate to enclose that part of colon.

Layers of the gastric wall

The stomach and proximal 3cm of duodenum have walls comprising four layers: mucosa, submucosa, muscularis (externa), and adventitia (see Fig. 1.2).

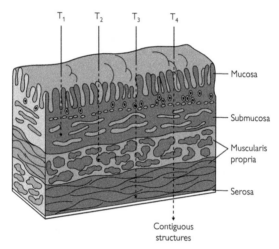

Fig. 1.2 Cross-section of the gastric wall including depth of tumour invasion by TNM classification.
Reproduced from *The Oxford Specialist Handbook of Surgical Oncology*, eds. Chaudry and Winslet, copyright Oxford University Press 2009, with permission of Oxford University Press.

Mucosa

This is subdivided into three layers—epithelium, lamina propria, and muscularis mucosae.

Epithelium

Simple columnar epithelium (surface mucus cells) lines the luminal surface and the numerous tubular invaginations (gastric pits or 'foveolae', into which the gastric glands open). These cells secrete mucus and are joined by tight junctions, protecting underlying layers from luminal acid. They are continuously desquamated into the lumen and are completely replaced every 3 days. Newly-formed cells appear in the deeper parts of the foveolae and the necks of glands, and are continually displaced upward to replace the lost surface cells.

Lamina propria
A delicate network of collagenous and reticular fibres, extending between necks of gastric glands to form a basement membrane. It contains plasma cells, mast cells, eosinophils, and lymphocytes, as well as blood and lymphatic capillaries, and nerve fibres, and is traversed by smooth muscle from the muscularis mucosae.

Muscularis mucosae
A thin layer of smooth muscle forming the border between the mucosa and submucosa. It has outer longitudinal and inner circular fibres, which extend from the inner layer through the lamina propria, around the gastric glands—these may aid glandular emptying via compression.

Submucosa
A layer of loose areolar tissue containing elastic fibres, lying between the muscularis mucosae and muscularis externa, containing many mast cells, macrophages, lymphocytes, eosinophils, and plasma cells, as well as arteries, veins, lymphatics and *Meissner's plexuses*. Gastric submucosa does not contain glands (unlike in the duodenum, i.e. Brunner's glands).

Muscularis externa
Comprises smooth muscle fibres forming three layers—external longitudinal, middle circular, and inner oblique layers. Inner oblique fibres extend from the fundus to the angular notch (i.e. from here to the pyloric region; themuscularis externa is composed only of outer longitudinal and inner circular layers).

Adventitia
This comprises the visceral peritoneum, a thin layer of loose connective tissue covered with mesothelium. Adventitia is attached to the muscularis externa (except at the greater and lesser curvatures, where it is continuous with the greater and lesser omentum, respectively). The pyloric region shares its peritoneal covering with the first part of the duodenum (i.e. mobile duodenal bulb), unlike the remainder of duodenum, which is retroperitoneal.

Mucosal zones
Gastric mucosa is lined by glands that open into gastric pits (Fig. 1.3). The blind ends of gastric glands extend deep into the mucosa, and are somewhat expanded and coiled, branching up to three times. Four major types of secretory epithelial cells line the mucosal surface, gastric pits and glands:
- *Mucous cells:* secrete alkaline mucus that protects epithelium against acid and shear stress.

- *Parietal (oxyntic[2]) cells*: secrete hydrochloric acid; may also contain intrinsic factor.
- *Chief cells[3]*: secrete pepsinogen (precursor of pepsin).
- *G cells*: secrete gastrin. Highest density of G cells occurs in distal 3 cm of stomach and first part of duodenum.

The mucosa itself can be broadly divided into three zones, based on predominant cell type within the gastric glands:

- *Oxyntic zone*: proximal two-thirds of stomach. Glands here ('fundic', 'proper gastric', or 'principle gastric' glands) secrete mucus, as well as nearly all enzymes and hydrochloric acid secreted by stomach.
- *Cardiac zone*: ring-shaped region around gastro-oesophageal junction (GOJ); glands secrete mucus.
- *Pyloric zone*: distal one-third of stomach; contains the deepest pits and the most extensive/coiled glands. The glands secrete mucus and produce endocrine, paracrine and neurocrine regulatory peptides (via amine precursor uptake and decarboxylation or amine precursor uptake and decarboxylation (APUD) cells).

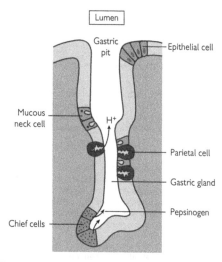

Fig. 1.3 Various cell types within a gastric pit.
Reproduced from *Training in Anaesthesia*, eds. Kiff and Spoors, copyright Oxford University Press 2009, with permission of Oxford University Press.

---

[1] Greek *oxyntic*: acid-forming.

[3] Chief cells are also known as 'zymogenic' or 'peptic' cells.

Blood supply

Arterial supply

The coeliac artery ('artery of the foregut') arises anteriorly from the aorta between the diaphragmatic crura, surrounded by coeliac lymph nodes and sympathetic coeliac ganglia. It supplies the stomach via three branches (Fig. 1.4).

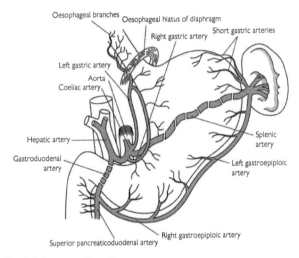

Fig. 1.4 Gastric arterial supply.
Reproduced from *Upper Gastrointestinal Surgery*, Fielding et al., Springer, 2005, with permission of Springer Science and Business Media.

Left gastric artery
- Runs to left, giving off an ascending oesophageal branch. Turning downwards between layers of lesser omentum, it runs right along lesser curvature before dividing into two parallel branches supplying anterior and posterior gastric walls. These vessels freely anastomose with arteries of greater curvature, and finally anastomose (around the angular notch) with two branches of right gastric artery.
- May arise directly from the aorta (5–7%), and may supply one or both inferior phrenic arteries. Duplicate arteries may exist, as can an enlarged (accessory) branch (8–25%), which may replace left hepatic artery (11–12%).

Common hepatic artery
- Second branch of coeliac trunk; extends to D1, then passes forward and below epiploic foramen to ascend between layers of lesser omentum (towards porta hepatis) to supply liver.
- Right gastric and gastroduodenal arteries are given off as it enters lesser omentum.

Right gastric artery
Runs along the lesser curvature and divides into two branches that anastomose with branches of the left gastric. Also gives off branches to the anterior and posterior gastric walls, and anastomosing branches to the right gastroepiploic artery.

Gastroduodenal artery
Descends behind and supplies the first part of the duodenum. Its terminal divisions are the *superior pancreaticoduodenal artery* (supplying the second part of the duodenum) and the right gastroepiploic artery.

Right gastroepiploic artery
- Passes along greater curvature between layers of greater omentum before anastomosing with left gastroepiploic artery.
- Common hepatic artery may arise directly from left gastric artery.

Splenic artery
Passes left retroperitoneally along the upper border of the pancreas to supply the spleen. Just before entering the hilum, it gives off the left gastro-epiploic artery and short gastric arteries, which supply the gastric fundus.

Left gastroepiploic artery
- Passes right/downward along greater curvature, between layers of the greater omentum, to anastomose with right gastroepiploic artery. Its branches supply anterior and posterior gastric walls, and anastomose with gastric arteries along lesser curvature.
- Division into terminal branches close to spleen (within 2cm from hilum) is termed 'magistral splenic'; earlier division is termed 'distributing splenic'.

Splenic artery
May divide into two branches that reunite (with the splenic vein passing through this loop), or form branches normally derived from other vessels (e.g. left gastric, middle colic, left hepatic). Short gastric arteries may arise from the gastroepiploic or splenic artery (proper), splenic branches, or any combination of these. In 30% of individuals, the dorsal pancreatic artery may also arise from the splenic artery. A 'posterior' gastric artery (branch of the splenic) may also be present in 50–70% of individuals and supplies the posterior gastric wall.

> **Note:** gastric blood flow increases simultaneously with acid secretion, and is reduced by aspirin and alcohol.

Venous drainage

Gastric veins are in a similar position to their corresponding arteries along the lesser and greater curvatures. They drain either directly or indirectly into the portal venous system:

- *Left gastric vein:* runs left along lesser curvature; receives oesophageal veins below diaphragmatic hiatus; drains directly into portal vein at superior pancreatic border.
- *Right gastric vein:* runs right along lesser curvature towards pylorus; joins portal vein behind first part of duodenum; also receives prepyloric vein (which drains first 2cm of duodenum).
- *Left gastroepiploic vein:* runs left along greater curvature; together with short gastric veins, it drains into splenic vein.
- *Right gastroepiploic vein:* runs right to head of pancreas and joins superior mesenteric vein to drain into portal vein. (*Note:* there is no gastroduodenal vein).
- *Splenic vein:* joined with tributaries from pancreas and inferior mesenteric vein; these join superior mesenteric vein to form portal vein.

Lymphatic drainage

- Gastric lymphatics originate in subepithelial interglandular mucosal tissue, extending outwards between glands to communicate with each other in periglandular plexus.
- Channels extend into subglandular plexus (between glands and muscularis mucosae).
- Short vessels, traversing muscularis mucosae, form submucous plexus, while larger vessels pass through muscular coats to reach networks among muscle fibres, opening into subserosal plexus. From here, valved collecting vessels radiate to gastric curvatures to enter omenta.
- Gastric lymphatics can be divided into three systems:
  - *Intramural:* three networks—*submucosal, intermuscular,* and *subserosal.* Submucosal channels communicate freely throughout gastric submucosa, and also with intermuscular and subserosal networks.
  - *Intermediary:* multiple small channels between subserosal network and extramural collecting systems.
  - *Extramural:* four major zones of lymphatic drainage corresponding to arterial supply. All zones ultimately drain into coeliac nodes (around coeliac arterial trunk of aorta).
- Divided into four zones (Fig. 1.5 and Fig. 1.6):
  - *Zone 1*—upper two-thirds of lesser curvature and majority of gastric body. Drains into left gastric nodes (along left gastric artery), which together with distal oesophageal lymphatics, drain into coeliac nodes.
  - *Zone 2*—distal aspect of lesser curvature and suprapyloric nodes (along right gastric artery). Drains into hepatic, then coeliac and aortic nodes.

- *Zone 3*—pyloric region and right half of greater curvature. Drains into right gastroepiploic nodes (in gastrocolic ligament, lying along right gastroepiploic vessels) and pyloric nodes (anterior to head of pancreas). From these 'subpyloric' nodes, drainage follows gastroduodenal artery to hepatic nodes (along hepatic artery) and thereafter to coeliac nodes.
- *Zone 4*—left half of greater curvature and gastric fundus. Drains into left gastroepiploic nodes (along left gastroepiploic artery), then into pancreaticolienal nodes (along splenic artery), and eventually into coeliac nodes.

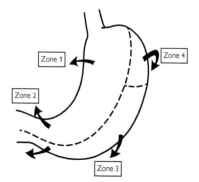

Fig. 1.5 Gastric lymphatic drainage zones.
Reproduced from *Upper Gastrointestinal Surgery*, Fielding et al., Springer, 2005, with permission of Springer Science and Business Media.

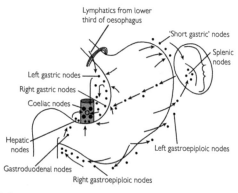

Fig. 1.6 Gastric lymph nodes.
Reproduced from *Upper Gastrointestinal Surgery*, Fielding et al., Springer, 2005, with permission of Springer Science and Business Media.

Nerve supply

Autonomic nerve supply to the stomach

Two main components—cholinergic (mainly parasympathetic) and adr-
energic (mainly sympathetic)—and a third component, the 'peptidergic'
system, comprising nerves that release an active purine nucleotide.

Parasympathetic supply

- *Anterior vagus:* derived mainly from left vagus, but also with fibres from
  right vagus and sympathetics from splanchnic nerves. After supplying
  distal oesophagus and gastric cardia, forms three main branches:
  - *Set 1*—4–5 direct branches (emanating in a stepwise fashion)
    supplying proximal part of lesser curvature. Most prominent branch
    innervates region from cardia to pylorus. It was termed 'principle
    anterior nerve of the lesser curvature' by Latarjet.[4]
  - *Set 2*—3–5 branches to liver. Descend in lesser omentum onto
    superior margin of pylorus and first part of duodenum.
  - *Set 3*—vagal filaments from hepatic branches. Accompany
    sympathetic nerves along right gastroepiploic artery, supplying
    inferior margin of pylorus.
  - Latarjet segregated nerves of the anterior vagus into two functional
    divisions: (i) direct branches supplying the fundus and body (i.e. the
    'reservoir' aspect); and (ii) supplying the pylorus and the first part
    of the duodenum (i.e. the 'sphincteric' aspect) via hepatic branches.
- *Posterior vagus:* derived mainly from right vagus. After entering
  abdomen posterior to the oesophagus, it divides into two main
  branches (coeliac and posterior gastric) before continuing along lesser
  curvature to innervate posterior gastric wall, up to angular notch.

Sympathetic supply

- Derived almost entirely from the coeliac plexus. These nerves pass
  from the coeliac plexus along:
  - *Left inferior phrenic artery*—nerves pass anterior to lower
    oesophagus, communicating with branches of anterior vagus, and
    supplying cardia and fundus.
  - *Left gastric artery*—nerve fibres follow this artery in three
    ways: (i) along the oesophageal and superior branches, towards
    the cardia and proximal gastric body (these communicate with
    both vagal trunks); (ii) along main artery, down lesser curvature to
    anterior and posterior surfaces the gastric body and antrum;
    (iii) through lesser omentum towards porta hepatis, communicating
    with hepatic branches of anterior vagal trunk.
- *Hepatic artery:* nerves reach pyloric region, together with right gastric
  and right gastroepiploic arteries.
- *Note:* preganglionic sympathetic fibres end in coeliac ganglia. Postganglionic
  fibres emerge as efferents from these ganglia to accompany arteries.
  Visceral afferents from stomach travel vice versa to ganglion cells in
  posterior spinal nerve roots, without synapsing in sympathetic ganglia.

---

[4] André Latarjet (1876–1947), Professor of Anatomy, Lyon, France.

Peptidergic system

The peptidergic system comprises embryologically-derived neuroendocrine cells, referred to as APUD cells. These cells produce peptides including gastrin, vasoactive intestinal peptide (VIP), somatostatin, enkephalin, neurotensin, and substance P. These peptides have various endocrine, paracrine, and neurocrine functions.

Gastric secretions

The gastric glands secrete about 2500mL of gastric juice daily. This contains various substances and gastric enzymes to kill ingested bacteria, digest proteins, and stimulate biliary and pancreatic juice flow.

Normal (fasting) gastric juice contains cations (Na^+, K^+, Mg^{2+}, H^+), anions (Cl^-, HPO_4^{2-}, SO_4^{2-}), pepsins (I–III), gelatinase, mucus, intrinsic factor, and water.

Mucous secretion

- *Mucus-secreting columnar cells* (the most abundant gastric epithelial cells): secrete bicarbonate-rich mucous that lubricates gastric surface and forms water insoluble gel impermeable to H^+ ions.
- Mucus production is stimulated by luminal acid and vagal activity, and is increased by prostaglandins.[5]

Pepsinogen secretion

- *Chief cells*: secrete pepsinogen I (stored within zymogen granules), converted to active pepsin by presence of gastric acid. Pepsin initiates protein digestion at pH 1.5–2.5 (it is inactivated above pH 5.4).
- Occurs mainly under vagal stimulation (but also via histamine and gastrin secretion; stimulation by alcohol, cortisol, caffeine, and acetazolamide; and prolonged periods of hypoglycaemia or raised intracranial pressure[6]).

Hormone secretion

Gastrin

- Secreted into bloodstream in response to luminal stimuli.
- Two main types (gastrin I and II) are produced mainly in pyloric mucosa, but also by duodenal G cells and D cells in the pancreatic islets of Langerhans.
- Fasting gastrin levels are increased by achlorhydria (i.e. in pernicious anaemia), surgical vagotomy, gastrinoma (e.g. in Zollinger–Ellison syndrome), chronic renal failure, and extensive small bowel resection.

---

[5] NSAIDs inflict gastric damage by inhibiting prostaglandin formation, as well as by crystallizing within gastric cells.

[6] Cushing's ulcer (or von Rokintasky–Cushing syndrome): gastric ulcer induced by increased acid secretion, from stimulation of vagal nuclei due to prolonged raised intracranial pressure.

Effects of gastrin

Secretory
- *Gastric*: increased secretion of acid, pepsinogen, and intrinsic factor.
- *Pancreatobiliary*: increased endocrine (insulin, glucagon, and calcitonin release) and exocrine activity (flow of pancreatic juices and bile).
- *Small bowel*: increased secretions.
- *Motility*: increased contraction of the lower oesophageal sphincter; increased gastric and small bowel motility; induction of the gastrocolic reflex.
- *Miscellaneous*: increased mitotic activity of gastric and small bowel mucosa.

Somatostatin
- Produced in pyloric and oxyntic zones, and pancreatic islet D cells.
- Suppresses release of:
  - Growth hormone (GH) and thyroid-stimulating hormone (TSH) from the pituitary gland.
  - Gastrin, gastric acid, and pepsin from the stomach.
  - Glucagon, insulin, and exocrine secretions from the pancreas.
  - Cholecystokinin, motilin, and secretin from the intestine.
- Suppresses gastric acid secretion by direct action on parietal cells and, indirectly, by suppressing gastrin secretion. Low gastric pH, by stimulating somatostatin release, ∴ corrects itself by negative feedback.

Vasoactive intestinal peptide

- *VIP*: central and peripheral neurotransmitter; its neurones are present in oxyntic and pyloric zones, and are under dual (vagal and splanchnic) control.
- VIP causes vasodilatation, increased cardiac output, glycogenolysis, and smooth muscle relaxation (i.e. particularly of the GOJ, pyloric sphincter, sphincter of Oddi, internal anal sphincter, and openings of ureters and urethra into bladder trigonum).
- Its release significantly decreases gastric secretion (probably via paracrine, rather than endocrine action).

Substance P

Neurones containing substance P are present mainly within the myenteric plexus and so heavily innervate circular musculature. Substance P causes contraction of the muscularis mucosae.

Miscellaneous gastric hormones

- *Encephalin*: endogenous opiate-like compound, mainly from pyloric antrum; its exact function is unclear.
- *Galanin*: may act as a regulatory factor in controlling gastrointestinal motility.
- *Neurotensin*: may inhibit post-prandial gastric acid and pepsin secretion, and delay gastric emptying, resulting in controlled release of chyme into duodenum.

Other secretions
- Acid-resistant lipase and gelatinase.
- Intrinsic factor produced by parietal cells (after vagal, gastrin, or histamine stimulation). This binds to vitamin B12 and is vital for its absorption in terminal ileum. Lack of intrinsic factor due to reduction in parietal cell mass following gastric surgery, or production of auto-antibodies to parietal cells (i.e. in pernicious anaemia), leads to megaloblastic anaemia.
- 'Bariatric' hormones, e.g. ghrelins secreted by P/D1 cells of gastric fundus—28 amino acid hunger-stimulating peptide.
- Ghrelins increase preprandially and decrease post-prandially. Sleeve gastrectomies for obesity lead to a reduction in ghrelin secretion.

Gastric acid formation

Within each parietal cell, the H^+ obtained from the ionization of water is actively transported into the gastric lumen in exchange for K^+ (by membrane H^+–K^+ ATPase) (Fig. 1.7). Cl^- is also actively transported into the gastric lumen. The resulting OH^- ion is neutralized by the carbonic acid buffer system, forming a bicarbonate ion that diffuses into the interstitium to be replaced by a further Cl^- ion (by a HCO_3^-–Cl^- exchange mechanism within the interstitium). Carbonic acid is replenished by the hydration of CO_2, which is produced by cellular metabolism from the abundant mucosal carbonic anhydrase. Post-prandially, this produces a negative respiratory quotient (with arterial CO_2 being higher than venous) and a gastric venous return with a high HCO_3^- content. The resultant acid secretion is isotonic with a pH<1.

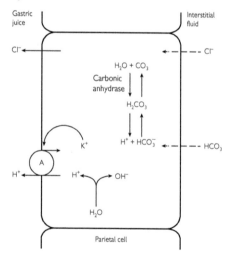

Fig. 1.7 Hydrochloric acid production within the gastric parietal cell.
Reproduced from *Upper Gastrointestinal Surgery*, Fielding et al., Springer, 2005, with permission of Springer Science and Business Media.

Gastric absorption

- Lipid-soluble compounds (e.g. ethyl alcohol, aspirin, and other non-steroidal anti-inflammatory drugs (NSAIDs)) are absorbed relatively rapidly—over-use of these particular substances is also known to cause gastric irritation, with subsequent development of gastritis and ulceration.
- Sugars are absorbed to an extent. This varies with *type* (i.e. from most to least absorbed—galactose, glucose, lactose, fructose, sucrose) and *concentration* (which is proportionate to rate of absorption).
- Water is readily absorbed—half ingested volume is usually absorbed within 20min.
- Proteins are absorbed only slightly and fats are not absorbed.

Control of gastric secretion

Gastric secretion divided into two phases (Fig. 1.8)—*interprandial* (secretion rate 1–5mmol/h) and *stimulated* (20–35mmol/h). The latter is subdivided into *cephalic*, *gastric*, and *intestinal* phases. Healthy individuals maximally secrete 0.5mmol/h/kg (of body weight).

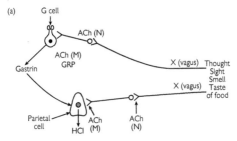

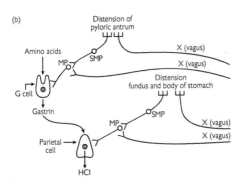

Fig. 1.8 (a) Cephalic and (b) gastric phases of acid secretion. X: vagus nerve. ACh(N): acetylcholine (nicotinic receptor). ACh(M): acetylcholine (mucarinic receptor). GRP: gastrin-releasing peptide. SMP: submucosal plexus. MP: myenteric plexus.

Reproduced from *Upper Gastrointestinal Surgery*, Fielding et al., Springer, 2005, with permission of Springer Science and Business Media.

Interprandial secretion

Resting secretion occurs in the absence of all gut stimulation. Note that a bilateral truncal vagotomy and pyloric antrum excision would be necessary to completely abolish all gastric acid secretion.

Stimulated secretion

Cephalic phase

- Sight, smell, and anticipation of food cause limbic system and hypothalamus to stimulate dorsal motor nuclei of vagus. The vagus transmits this stimulus to enteric nervous system, resulting in acetylcholine release to G cells and parietal cells.
- Vagal ACh causes G cells to secrete gastrin, which enters portal circulation to stimulate parietal cells. ACh also directly stimulates parietal cells to secrete small amounts of acid.
- Simultaneously, histamine (from adjacent mast cells) sensitizes parietal cells to action of gastrin and acetylcholine by acting on their H2 receptors. H2 receptor blockers (e.g. cimetidine, ranitidine), thus reduce, but do not prevent acid secretion.
- A low-level of gastric motility is also induced.

Gastric phase

- Food entering stomach causes gastric distension and mucosal irritation, activating stretch receptors and chemoreceptors, respectively. Consequently, enteric neurones secrete acetylcholine to further stimulate parietal and G cells. Gastrin from G cells further stimulates parietal cells (mediated by vagovagal reflexes through dorsal motor nucleus).
- Activation of enteric nervous system and gastrin release also cause vigorous smooth muscle contractions: results in maximal motor function, with mixing of secreted acid and pepsinogen (and pepsinogen conversion to pepsin).
- Gastric phase acid secretion limited locally once antral pH<1.5 as luminal acid directly inhibits gastrin release from G cells; and somatostatin from antral D cells inhibits parietal and G cells via paracrine effect.

Intestinal phase

As chyme leaves stomach, gastric emptying is limited to allow time for acid neutralization and nutrient absorption by duodenum. This occurs via nervous and endocrine pathways:

- Bowel distension and chemical (and osmotic) irritation of the mucosa induces gastro-inhibitory impulses in the enteric nervous system–the enterogastric reflex.
- Carbohydrate and fat within chyme cause the release of gastric inhibiting peptide (GIP) to inhibit gastrin secretion. Enteric hormones (e.g. cholecystokinin and secretin) from small intestinal cells also suppress gastric activity. Gastrin within the circulation also stimulates calcitonin release from thyroid C cells, which inhibits further gastrin release by negative feedback.
- As chyme is digested, these stimuli diminish, allowing gastric secretion and motor activity to resume.

Control of gastric motility

Resting gastric motility

Resting gastric electrical activity

Gastric pacemaker

- Longitudinal muscle (near greater curve of cardia) controls contraction frequency.
- Depolarizes at a rate of 3/min—forms basal electrical rhythm and each 'slow wave' spreads through longitudinal and circular muscles, increasing cell membrane sodium permeability.
- In empty stomach (volume ~50mL), the low resting potential (–50mV) and unequal wave amplitudes do not set off action potentials. Only when critical threshold is passed, does the resulting action potential set off an excitation-contraction coupling, causing a contraction to spread throughout stomach.

Intra-gastric pressure

- Intra-gastric pressure relatively constant (5mmHg or 0.7kPa) due to *receptive relaxation* (i.e. relaxation of the musculature of fundus and body as food enters stomach).
- Although gastric radius increases with wall tension (i.e. keeping intra-luminal pressure constant—Laplace's law), radius cannot increase above 1000 mL, so wall tension and intra-gastric pressures rise above this capacity.

Gastric tone

- Gastroparesis is usually idiopathic and of little clinical significance. However, if severe may progress to acute gastric dilatation in some instances (e.g. post-operatively, post-traumatically, and in electrolyte disturbances).
- Gastric hypertonia may cause a 'steerhorn' (short, transversely situated) stomach. In such cases, immediate emptying of liquid barium usually occurs in erect posture before onset of peristalsis or cyclical contractions of pyloric sphincteric cylinder.

Hunger contractions

Several hours post-prandially, hypothalamic stimulation leads to a feeling of hunger. Vagal stimulation causes increased gastric motility—contraction of the empty stomach raises the intra-gastric pressure, stimulating tension and pain receptors within the gastric wall and leading to mild abdominal discomfort.

Feeding gastric motility

- An increase of gastric volume over 1000mL stimulates stretch receptors within gastric wall through a vagovagal reflex arc, causing depolarization in longitudinal and circular muscles, and a contraction wave passing from fundus to antrum. Force of contraction increases along stomach. Intragastric pressure is initially low at fundus (where muscular layer is thinnest), but may reach 50mmHg at pylorus.

- Contraction wave causes pyloric sphincter to contract (*the sphincter is otherwise open at rest and is not a high-pressure zone*), but some chyme (5–15mL) will bypass pylorus before gastric slow wave reaches it. Antrum and pylorus contract together ('terminal contraction'), acting to recirculate or 'churn' the gastric contents. When duodenal pressure drops due to relaxation, the pyloric pressure *also* drops.

Factors influencing gastric motility
- Vagal stimuli and gastrin both increase antral motility and emptying. Although now seldom practiced, truncal vagotomies reduce force of antral pump and prolong gastric emptying, thereby necessitating a drainage procedure afterwards.
- Antral pump force is also moderated by chyme volume and composition.
- Gastric emptying regulated by duodenal distension (via vagal feedback), increased duodenal osmolarity (via osmoreceptors), duodenal acidity (via local enteric neurones), and duodenal fat content (via release of GIP and cholecystokinin).
- Sympathetic stimuli reduce gastric emptying (via limbic and hypothalamic nuclei).

Nausea, retching, and vomiting
- Vomiting sequence involves three successive phases:
  - Initial nausea.
  - Subsequent retching.
  - Forcible expulsion of gastric contents orally (vomiting)— coordinated effort between the upper small bowel, stomach, oesophagus, diaphragm, voluntary abdominal muscles, and glottis.
- Sequence controlled by vomiting centre (bilateral medulla oblongata at level of olivary nuclei, near tractus solitarius at level of dorsal vagal nuclei).
- Complex efferent pathway involving cranial nerves V, VII, IX, X (vagus), and XII contracts intercostal muscles, diaphragm, and abdominal musculature.
- Afferent impulses from gut to vomiting centre pass via vagus and sympathetic pathways. Other afferent impulses may originate from labyrinth, limbic system, and chemoreceptor trigger zone (medulla– bilaterally in wall of 4th ventricle).

Nausea
- This is conscious perception of subconscious excitation of vomiting centre.
- Initiated by gastrointestinal impulses, lower brain (e.g. in response to motion sickness), or cortical impulses.
- Physiologically associated with decreased gastric motility and increased small bowel tone. Often also reverse peristalsis in proximal small intestine.

Initiation of vomiting

- Excessive irritation, distension, or stimulation of the upper gastrointestinal tract may induce anti-peristaltic waves, which may occur as distally as the ileum.
- Waves travel at 2–3cm/s, potentially shifting large volumes of intestinal content into the duodenum and stomach, causing distension in minutes and resulting in retching.

Retching phase

- 'Dry heaves', characterized by series of violent, spasmodic abdomino-thoracic contractions with closed glottis. Inspiratory movements of chest wall and diaphragm oppose expiratory contractions of abdominal musculature.
- Simultaneously, gastric antrum contracts, and fundus and cardia relax.

The act of vomiting

- Following retching, a deep inspiratory movement occurs with elevation of the hyoid bone (opening upper oesophageal sphincter and closing glottis). Soft palate rises to close posterior nares.
- Downward contraction of diaphragm with simultaneous contraction of abdominal wall raises intra-gastric pressure. Sudden relaxation of lower oesophageal sphincter then allows for expulsion to occur.

Vomiting vs. regurgitation

Regurgitation is distinct from vomiting, as it involves the *passive* oral expulsion of ingested material; often occurs even before this has reached the stomach and usually results from oesophageal disease.

Oesophageal anatomy and basic physiology

Gross anatomy

- The oesophagus is a hollow viscus approximately 25cm (10 inches) long and 2cm in diameter with a sphincter at each end.
- Length depends on individual height–particularly suprasternal-xiphoid distance (Fig. 2.1).
- Extends from the cricopharyngeal sphincter at the level of the 6th cervical vertebra to the cardia of the stomach. Comprises:
  - *Cervical oesophagus:* from level of lower border of cricoid cartilage (C6) to jugular notch (thoracic inlet, T1); 18cm from incisors.
  - *Upper oesophagus:* from level of jugular notch to level of carina (T5), within *superior mediastinum*; 18–23cm from incisors.
  - *Middle oesophagus:* from carina to midpoint between carina and oesophagogastric junction, within *posterior mediastinum*; 24–32cm from incisors.
  - *Lower oesophagus:* includes lower thoracic oesophagus (within *posterior mediastinum*) and hiatal segment of oesophagus (or *abdominal oesophagus*); 32–40cm from incisors.
- Passes through lower part of neck, superior, and then posterior mediastinum, and traverses diaphragm at T10. Lowermost part lies below level of diaphragm.

Cervical segment (C6–T1)

- *Anterior:* trachea.
- *Posterior:* prevertebral layer of cervical fascia.
- *Bilaterally:* carotid sheath (common carotid artery, internal jugular vein, vagus nerve). Dorsal parts of thyroid lie bilaterally between oesophagus and carotid arteries. Recurrent laryngeal nerves run caudally and bilaterally within tracheo-oesophageal groove.

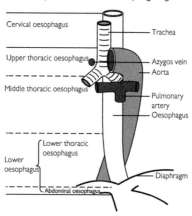

Fig. 2.1 Segmental divisions and anatomical relations of the oesophagus.
Reproduced from *Upper Gastrointestinal Surgery*, Fielding et al., Springer, 2005, with permission of Springer Science and Business Media.

Relations to the oesophagus

See Fig. 2.2.

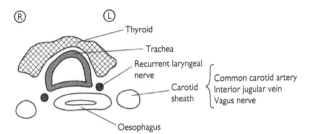

Fig. 2.2 Cross-sectional view of oesophagus (lower neck, as viewed from below).
Reproduced from *Upper Gastrointestinal Surgery*, Fielding et al., Springer, 2005, with permission of Springer Science and Business Media.

Thoracic segment (T1–T10)

- *Upper thoracic oesophagus:*
  - *Anterior*—trachea.
  - *Posterior*—prevertebral fascia.
  - *Left*—aortic arch.
  - *Right*—azygos vein. Descending posteriorly, it is crossed anteriorly by left main bronchus and right pulmonary artery.
- *Middle thoracic oesophagus:*
  - *Anterior*—left main bronchus.
  - *Posterior and right*—right mediastinal pleura. As it descends, azygos vein, thoracic duct, right upper five intercostal arteries, and descending aorta all pass posteriorly.
- *Lower thoracic oesophagus:*
  - *Anterior*—pericardium and left atrium.
  - *Posterior*—vertebral column, azygos vein, thoracic duct, thoracic aorta (left posterior).
  - *Bilaterally*—mediastinal pleura. Directly above diaphragm, the last part of the thoracic aorta crosses behind the oesophagus.

Abdominal segment (T10–T11)

- *Anterior and posterior:* anterior and posterior vagal trunks, respectively.
- *Right anterior:*
  - Left hepatic lobe.
  - Intra-abdominal oesophagus covered by peritoneum (gastrophrenic ligament) and accompanied by oesophageal branches of left gastric artery, associated veins, and lymphatics phreno-oesophageal membrane attaches to oesophagus while it passes through diaphragm: consists of peritoneum and transversalis fascia, and blends into adventitial layer, giving elastic mobility to distal oesophagus.

- *Oesophagus is essentially a midline structure*: various deviations (left in neck, right in posterior mediastinum, and left and anteriorly towards diaphragmatic hiatus) are of surgical significance as they determine operative approach to oesophagus.
- *Optimum exposure*: cervical oesophagus approached from left, thoracic oesophagus from right of the thorax; and lower oesophagus (and gastro-oesophageal junction) from abdomen, or by a left thoraco-abdominal approach.

Layers of the oesophageal wall

The oesophageal wall comprises of four layers (Fig. 2.3). The submucosa is the most robust as there is no serosal layer.
- *Mucosa*: surface epithelium (non-keratinized stratified squamous) with a basement membrane separating it from underlying *lamina propria* and *muscularis mucosa*.
- *Submucosa*: connective tissue, blood, and lymphatic vessels, *submucosal nerve plexus* and glands.
- *Muscularis*: inner circular and outer longitudinal muscle layers between which lies the *myenteric nerve plexus*. Muscle type within this layer varies cranially to caudally:
  - Upper third (striated muscle).
  - Middle third (striated and smooth muscle).
  - Lower third (smooth muscle).
- *Adventitia*: loose connective tissue that merges with connective tissue of surrounding structures. Longitudinal muscle fibres split above gastro-oesophageal junction, creating a potential vertical weakness on the left posterolateral aspect. Commonest site of tear in spontaneous oesophageal rupture (Boerhaave's syndrome).

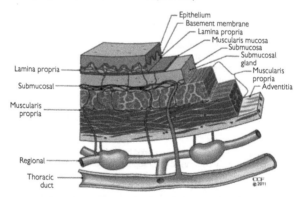

Fig. 2.3 Layers of the oesophageal wall.
Reproduced from 'Esophageal submucosa: The watershed for esophageal cancer', Siva Raja, Thomas W Rice, John R Goldblum, et al., *The Journal of Thoracic and Cardiovascular Surgery* 2011; **142**(6): 1403–11.

Blood supply

Arterial supply

See Fig. 2.4.

- Principle oesophageal arterial branches follow longitudinal course of oesophagus on entering submucosal layer.
- Form a longitudinal network, giving minute perpendicular branches: surround circumference to communicate with opposite side.
- Cervical, thoracic, and abdominal oesophageal arterial branches connected by a dense anastomosing submucosal network of small vessels: provides adequate circulation during mobilization.

Cervical oesophagus

- *Inferior thyroid artery* of thyrocervical trunk + branches from superior thyroid artery and trachea-oesophageal artery.
- Multiple anastomoses formed on anterior and posterior walls.
- Rarely, subclavian artery produces an oesophageal branch.

Thoracic oesophagus

- *Proximally:* 2–3 bronchial arteries from *descending thoracic aorta.*
- *Distally:* 1–2 direct aortic branches.

Abdominal oesophagus

- Ascending branches of *left gastric artery* (from the coeliac axis) and the *inferior phrenic artery.*
- Dorsal wall of distal oesophagus is supplied by branches of both inferior phrenic and splenic arteries.

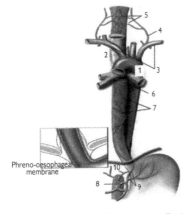

Fig. 2.4 Arterial supply of the oesophagus. 1, Thoracic aorta. 2, Trachea. 3, Brachiocephalic and left subclavian arteries. 4, Inferior thyroid artery. 5, Oesophageal branches. 6, Bronchial artery. 7, Aortic oesophageal arteries. 8, Left gastric artery. 9, Ascending branches of left gastric artery. 10, Ascending branch of left inferior phrenic artery.
Reproduced from *Surgery of the Esophagus: Textbook and Atlas of Surgical Practice*, Izbicki et al., Springer 2009, with permission of Springer Science and Business Media.

Venous drainage

- Commences with submucosal venous plexus, which drains into an extrinsic plexus on oesophageal surface.
- As with arterial supply, precise drainage variable.
- *Upper oesophagus:* drains via *inferior thyroid veins* into brachiocephalic vein.
- *Middle oesophagus:* drains via *azygos, hemiazygous* and *accessory hemiazygous veins* into superior vena cava.
- *Lower oesophagus:* drains via *left gastric vein* into portal vein, thus forming a portosystemic anastomosis.

Lymphatic drainage

- The presence of lymphatics within oesophageal mucosa is unique within gastrointestinal (GI) tract (Table 2.1 and Fig. 2.5).
- Complex interconnecting networks of mucosal and submucosal lymphatics extend length of oesophagus, piercing muscular layers to drain into *para-oesophageal plexus.*
- Para-oesophageal nodes lie along the oesophageal wall, draining into *peri-oesophageal* and more distant *lateral oesophageal nodes.* These eventually empty into thoracic duct (although direct drainage from the oesophageal plexus may occur).
- Lymph node (LN) arrangement allows for early and widespread lymphatic dissemination of oesophageal carcinoma once basement membrane has been breached.
- *Lymphatic drainage largely mirrors arterial blood supply:*
  - *Cervical oesophagus*—drains cranially to cervical lymph nodes (via para-oesophageal nodes and retropharyngeal nodes).
  - *Upper thoracic oesophagus*—drains to superior para-oesophageal nodes and prevertebral nodes.
  - *Middle thoracic oesophagus*—drains via medial para-oesophageal nodes into paratracheal, tracheobronchial, and bronchopulmonary nodes (can drain directly into thoracic duct on rare occasions).
  - *Lower thoracic oesophagus:* inferior para-oesophageal and prevertebral nodes.
  - *Abdominal oesophagus*—drains into left and right gastric lymph nodes along lesser curvature into gastro-omental, pyloric, and/or coeliac lymph nodes along greater curvature.

Table 2.1 Lymph nodes of the oesophagus: data from UICC classification

Drainage region	UICC LN group	Anatomical classification	Location
Cervical compartment	100	Superficial lateral cervical	Along external jugular vein
	102	Deep lateral cervical	Along internal jugular vein
	101	Cervical para-oesophageal nodes	Beside oesophagus
	103	Retropharyngeal nodes	Between dorsal aspect of pharynx and prevertebral fascia
	104	Supraclavicular nodes	Lowest of deep cervical nodes
Mediastinal compartment	105,108,110	Prevertebral nodes	Beside (and)
	105	Upper para-oesophageal nodes	Above
	108	Middle para-oesophageal nodes	Beside/behind middle oesophagus
	110	Lower para-oesophageal nodes	Beside/behind lower oesophagus
	106	Paratracheal nodes	Along trachea
	107	Tracheobronchial (carinal) nodes	Between carina along main bronchi
	109	Pulmonary hilar nodes	At pulmonary hilum
	111	Diaphragmatic nodes	Along attachment of pericardium with diaphragm
	112	Posterior mediastinal nodes	Along distal thoracic aorta
Perigastric compartment	1 & 2	Right and left cardiac nodes	Right and left of cardia
	3	Lesser curvature nodes	Along lesser curvature
	4	Greater curvature nodes	Along greater curvature
	5 & 6	Supra- and sub-pyloric nodes	Above and below pylorus
	7	Left gastric artery nodes	Along left gastric artery

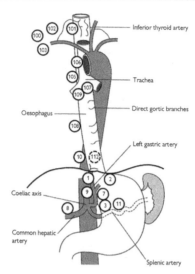

Fig. 2.5 Oesophageal lymphatic drainage. *Cervical lymph nodes*—100, lateral cervical. 101, Cervical para-oesophageal. 102, Deep cervical. 103, Supraclavicular. *Mediastinal lymph nodes*—105, upper para-oesophageal. 106, Paratracheal. 107, Carinal. 108, Middle para-oesophageal. 109, Left and right bronchial. 110, Lower para-oesophageal. 112, Posterior mediastinal. *Abdominal lymph nodes*—1, Right paracardial. 2, Left paracardial. 3, Lesser curve. 7, Left gastric. 8, Common hepatic. 9, Coeliac axis. 11, Splenic artery.
Reproduced from *Upper Gastrointestinal Surgery*, Fielding et al., Springer, 2005, with permission of Springer Science and Business Media.

Endoscopic anatomy

There are four main sites of constriction to note at endoscopy (variable with patient height).

Measured from the incisor teeth, they are at:
- *15cm (narrowest point):* cricopharyngeal sphincter.
- *22cm:* aortic arch.
- *27cm:* left main bronchus.
- *38cm:* diaphragmatic hiatus.
- These are commonest levels for foreign bodies to arrest at.
- GOJ is defined endoscopically as upper margin of the proximal gastric folds (~37cm in females and 40cm in males).
- GOJ migrates proximally in the case of a sliding hiatus hernia.
- Squamocolumnar junction is visible endoscopically as the Z-line—this usually coincides with GOJ, but will be more proximal in Barrett's oesophagus.

Nerve supply, sensation, and motility

Oesophageal innervation

Parasympathetic supply
Primarily through the *recurrent laryngeal* nerve and the *oesophageal plexus* arising from the *vagus nerve*. The vagus nerve is in close relationship with the oesophagus throughout its length.

Sympathetic supply
Cervical and thoracic sympathetic chain—plays only a minor role in oesophageal function.

Intramural plexi
- Myenteric (Auerbach's) plexus lies between circular and longitudinal muscle layers and is more prominent in smooth muscle portion of oesophagus.
- Submucosal (Meissner's) plexus is sparser, containing fibres, but no ganglia.

Oesophageal sensation
- Oesophageal myenteric ganglia contain mechanoreceptors that activate subconscious reflexes and also transduce painful sensations (as demonstrated by progressive oesophageal balloon distension which initially stimulates $2°$ peristalsis, but causes pain at higher pressures).
- Low-threshold receptors mediate involuntary reflexes via vagal pathways.
- Higher-threshold receptors mediate nociception via splanchnic sympathetic pathways (under vagal modulation).
- Oesophageal intraepithelial nerve endings act as thermo-, chemo-, and osmoreceptors.
- Myenteric plexus degeneration around lower oesophageal sphincter results in achalasia of cardia.

Fasting state
- Oesophageal body relaxed.
- *Intraluminal pressure*: atmospheric in cervical portion, but becomes negative distally (approximating with intrapleural pressure; -5 to -10mmHg on inspiration, 0 to $+5$mmHg on expiration).
- Upper and lower sphincters tonically contracted to prevent aerophagia, gastro-oesophageal reflux, and aspiration.
- Unlike stomach and small bowel, oesophageal smooth muscle has no spontaneous phasic slow wave activity, depending instead on its intrinsic and extrinsic nerve supply.

Swallowing
- Healthy individuals swallow approximately 70 times per hour whilst awake and 7 times per hour during sleep (increasing to 200 times per hour during eating).
- Swallowing mechanism can be described in three phases.

Buccal phase
Initiation is voluntary. The tongue propels the food bolus into the posterior oropharynx.

Pharyngeal phase
- Switch occurs from respiratory to swallowing pathway (including pharyngeal filling, passive emptying, and active peristalsis).
- Elevation of hyoid bone allows epiglottis to cover larynx.
- Simultaneous relaxation of upper oesophageal sphincter (UOS) and pharyngeal.
- Contraction propels bolus into oesophagus.

Oesophageal phase
Once the bolus has passed into the oesophagus, the UOS exhibits rebound hypertension coinciding with the initiation of oesophageal peristalsis to prevent pharyngeal reflux.

Primary peristalsis
- Triggered by swallowing; regulated by deglutition centre in medulla oblongata and mediated by vagus.
- Commences in proximal oesophagus following pharyngeal contraction and UOS relaxation.
- Longitudinal muscle layer contracts first to shorten and fix oesophagus.
- Progressive lumen-occluding circular muscle contraction (preceded by a wave of inhibition).
- LOS relaxes, then closes after bolus passes, with a prolonged contraction.
- Normally, only one 1° peristaltic wave per swallow, but during rapid, repeated swallowing, oesophageal activity is inhibited and so only final swallow is followed by an inhibitory wave. This deglutitive inhibition is vital for swallowed food to pass through to the stomach.

Secondary peristalsis
- Localized to the oesophagus and not preceded by pharyngeal contraction or UOS relaxation.
- Intrinsic system is triggered by oesophageal distension by bolus following ineffective peristalsis or by refluxed gastric contents.
- Accounts for about 10% of oesophageal motor activity.

Tertiary contractions
- *Simultaneous:* unrelated to swallowing or oesophageal distension.
- Non-peristaltic contractions do not propel a bolus; if multiple, may be considered pathological.

Control of peristalsis
- *Proximal oesophagus (striated):* directed by brainstem (medulla) by sequential vagal excitation via recurrent laryngeal branches.
- *Middle/distal oesophagus (smooth):* more complex; requires integration of central and peripheral innervations.
- Swallow-induced 1° peristalsis is dependent on activation of the swallowing centre and vagal pathways (and is abolished by bilateral cervical vagotomy).

- Peristaltic propagation in smooth muscle segment involves two peripheral vagal pathways mediating:
  - *Cholinergic excitation (depolarization)* of both longitudinal and circular muscle.
  - *Non-adrenergic, non-cholinergic inhibition of circular muscle (hyperpolarization)* via nitrous oxide (NO; inhibitory neurotransmitter).
- Upon swallowing, near simultaneous activation of inhibitory pathway followed by delayed sequential activation of excitatory pathway creates a wave of mechanical inhibition (latency) followed by contraction—this constitutes peristalsis.
- *Cholinergic excitation* occurs mainly proximally whilst inhibition increases distally—these neural gradients slow velocity of propagation distally.
- Once adequate cholinergic excitation is reached, a local myogenic control system is stimulated: slow-wave type action potentials and coupling of smooth muscle cells allow for whole tissue to function as a unit. Peristalsis can thus progress at a myogenic level once adequate neural excitation is present.

Lower oesophageal sphincter function

- LOS enables a 2–4cm high-pressure zone at GOJ and a resting pressure of 10–25mmHg that is greatest distally and to left side.
- Both the intra-abdominal and intrathoracic components (when no hiatus hernia is present) are directly influenced by contraction of crural diaphragm.
- Three major factors controlling LOS pressure are its *myogenic properties*, *inhibitory* and *excitatory neural influences*. Basal pressure is due to the myogenic properties of muscle fibres involving continuous electrical spike activity, stimulating Ca^{2+} influx and maintaining a depolarized resting state.
- *Neural activity modulates sphincter pressure*: the myenteric plexus here is innervated by both vagal preganglionic and sympathetic postganglionic fibres. 1° neurotransmitters are *NO (inhibitory)* and *acetylcholine (excitatory)*.
- LOS relaxation (towards intra-gastric pressure) is vagally-mediated; it occurs within 2s of deglutition and is initiated by peristaltic contractions in the cervical oesophagus. Relaxation lasts 8–10s and is followed by after-contraction in proximal portion of sphincter. During repeated swallowing, the LOS remains relaxed until after final swallow.
- LOS relaxation occurs without oesophageal contraction during belching and vomiting, but during rumination, it occurs together with reverse oesophageal peristalsis.
- *Transient LOS relaxation*: responsible for most episodes of gastro-oesophageal reflux (GORD and physiological): relaxation unrelated to swallowing and augmented by pharyngeal stimulation and gastric distension (particularly after fatty meals and in the upright posture). It is a vagally-mediated reflex involving NO.

Oesophageal physiology, clinical evaluation of oesophageal motility disorders, and gastro-oesophageal reflux disease

Normal oesophageal motility and physiology

Anatomy
The normal adult human oesophagus is 18–26cm long and contains both striated and smooth muscle. Sphincters at each end act as valves preventing reflux of gastric contents into the oesophagus, and oesophageal contents into the pharynx. The sphincters must also open temporarily to allow passage of food during swallowing, and venting of air during belching.

The oesophageal wall is composed of:
- Mucosa (comprising stratified squamous epithelial cells, lamina propria, and muscularis mucosae).
- Submucosa (containing connective tissue and submucosal glands).
- Muscularis propria (a circular muscle layer surrounded by a longitudinal muscle layer).

The muscularis propria in the proximal one-third of the oesophagus (cervical oesophagus) is composed of striated muscle. This is followed distally by a 4–6-cm mixed segment of 'transition zone' from striated to smooth muscle. Below this, the muscularis propria is composed solely of smooth muscle.

Control of swallowing
- Initiation of swallowing is voluntary.
- Coordinated control of muscle contraction in oropharynx, upper oesophageal sphincter, and upper (striated muscle) oesophagus requires central control.
- Central control interacts and coordinates with intrinsic control mechanisms of more distal (smooth muscle) oesophagus and lower oesophageal sphincter.

Swallowing pattern generator
The swallowing pattern generator (SPG) is a series of neuronal networks in the brainstem medulla that coordinate the swallow from oropharynx to LOS, such that there is efficient bolus transit and protection of the airway. It can be activated voluntarily via the cortex (i.e. 1° peristalsis), or involuntarily via reflex activity (i.e. 2° peristalsis).

Each network of the SPG consists of:
- Dorsal neuronal group in nucleus of solitary tract and reticular formation. Control timing and sequencing of swallowing events.
- Ventral neuronal group in ventrolateral medulla that serves as switching station for signals to cranial nerves controlling swallowing muscles.

Sensory signals involved in swallowing
- Sensory feedback for oropharyngeal stage carried by cranial nerves V (trigeminal), VII (facial), IX (glossopharyngeal) and X (vagus).
- Pharyngeal stage of swallowing primarily initiated via sensory input from superior largyngeal nerve branch of vagus nerve.
- Oesophageal sensory feedback occurs via vagus nerve.

Motor signals involved in swallowing
- Motor function in oropharyngeal phase is mediated by cranial nerves V (trigeminal), VII (facial), XII (hypoglossal), and nucleus ambiguous portion of vagus.
- Striated segment of oesophagus receives motor innervation from nucleus ambiguous portion of vagus.
- Smooth muscle segment of oesophagus receives motor innervation from dorsal motor nucleus of vagus.

Oesophageal peristalsis
- Sequential timing of peristalsis in the thoracic oesophagus depends on progressively increasing depolarization latency of vagal fibres from proximal to distal oesophagus.
- Propagation of the intraluminal pressure wave takes 2–7s from proximal to distal oesophagus.
- 1° peristalsis is initiated by swallowing.
- 2° peristalsis is independent of swallowing and initiated by sensory signals from mechanoceptors in oesophageal body (from retained food bolus, or gastro-oesophageal reflux event).

Mean peak intraluminal pressures are:
- Proximal oesophagus: 53 ± 9mmHg.
- Mid-oesophagus 35 ± 6mmHg.
- Distal oesophagus 70 ± 12mmHg.

Deglutative inhibition
See Fig. 3.1.
- The act of swallowing is able to inhibit propagation of an impending peristaltic contraction—essential to efficient and coordinated bolus passage.
- Can be demonstrated on repetitive rapid swallows (e.g. drinking a cup of water very fast)—only final swallow will normally result in oesophageal peristalsis.

The 1° peristaltic wave travels fastest in the mid-oesophagus and slowest immediately above the LOS (average velocity 4cm/s) (Fig. 3.2). The muscular contraction itself is most prolonged in the distal oesophagus and lasts 2–7s. The mean peak amplitude of contraction ranges from 35 to 70mmHg, and is lowest at the junction of striated and smooth muscle (mid-oesophagus), increasing progressively towards the distal end. Hypotensive (<30mmHg) peristaltic waves are associated with retrograde escape of liquid and incomplete oesophageal clearance. Hypertensive (>200mmHg) contractions in the distal segment ('nutcracker oesophagus') often cause chest pain and dysphagia. Warm boluses enhance peristalsis, while cold boluses inhibit it. The velocity and amplitude of 2° peristalsis resemble 1° peristalsis.

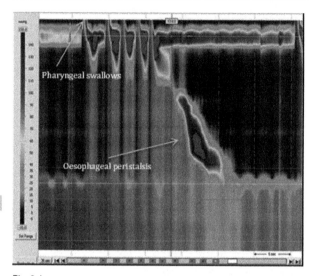

Fig. 3.1 High resolution oesophageal manometry study demonstrating deglutative inhibition. Five pharyngeal swallows are seen, but only final swallow results in peristalsis. See also Plate 1, colour plate section.

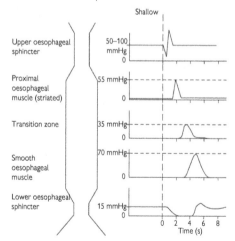

Fig. 3.2 Manometric properties of the 1° peristaltic wave.
Reproduced from *Upper Gastrointestinal Surgery*, Fielding et al., Springer, 2005, with permission of Springer Science and Business Media.

The gastro-oesophageal junction

This is a 3–4cm high-pressure zone at the distal oesophagus that acts as an anti-reflux barrier. There are usually two components to this high-pressure zone:
- A smooth muscle sphincter (LOS).
- The diaphragmatic crura.

The LOS receives preganglionic vagal fibres from the dorsal motor nucleus of the vagus nerve. These synapse on excitatory and inhibitory neurons.

A tonically active vagal excitatory pathway appears to effect a resting LOS tone. During swallowing the tonic excitation ceases, and an inhibitory vagal pathway is activated, so causing sphincter relaxation. Factors influencing contraction and relaxation of the LOS are shown in Table 3.2.

Separation of the LOS from the crura (as in hiatus hernia) results in reduction in efficacy of the anti-reflux barrier.

Transient lower oesophageal sphincter relaxations (TLOSRs)
- Spontaneous relaxations of LOS, independent of swallowing.
- A vagal reflex initiated by gastric distension, resulting in belching and venting of pressure.
- In patients with normal LOS pressure this is the most common mechanism of gastro-oesophageal reflux.

Physiological barriers to reflux

In health, a number of protective mechanisms are in place to defend against the potentially damaging effects of gastro-oesophageal reflux (Table 3.1 and Table 3.2).

Table 3.1 Mechanisms of defence against oesophageal damage from gastric refluxate

Mechanical	Lower oesophageal sphincter
	Diaphragmatic crura
	$2°$ Oesophageal peristalsis (to clear refluxates)
Epithelial	Epithelial junctional complexes (e.g. tight junctions)
	Ion exchange mechanisms (e.g. Na^+/H^+ exchanger, Cl^-/HCO_3^- exchanger)
	Buffers (HCO_3^-, PO_4^-, basic proteins)
	Reparative processes (cell replication/regeneration)
	Mucous barrier
Salivary	Salivary HCO_3^- secretion

Table 3.2 Factors influencing contraction or relaxation of the LOS

Factor	Increases LOS pressure	Decreases LOS pressure
Hormones	Gastrin Histamine Motilin Pancreatic polypeptide	Glucagon Cholecystokinin Progesterone Oestrogens
Neurotransmitters	Acetylcholine Substance P Histamine	NO VIP Dopamine (D2)
Prostaglandins	F2	E1, E2, A2
Drugs	Metoclopramide Domperidone Cisapride Erythromycin Cholinergic drugs	Calcium antagonists Atropine Nitrates Tricyclic antidepressants
Foods	Protein meal Red pepper	Fats Chocolate Caffeine Alcohol
Miscellaneous		Cigarette smoking

Benign oesophageal pathology

Introduction

Benign oesophageal conditions can be broadly divided into motility disorders and gastro-oesophageal reflux disease (GORD). Motility disorders usually present as dysphagia, whilst GORD typically leads to symptoms of heartburn and regurgitation. Distinguishing between the two can be difficult, due to significant overlaps in symptomatology. Therefore, motility and reflux testing are often performed together, especially when at least a standard pull-through manometry is required to locate LOS prior to insertion of the pH probe.

Approach to patients with dysphagia

Dysphagia is common and can be due to either mechanical obstruction or dysmotility. Careful history-taking is the first important step in determining the likely cause and guide subsequent management (Box 3.1).

> **Box 3.1 Ten essential questions during symptom evaluation of dysphagia**
> 1. Presence of symptom when not swallowing (e.g. in globus)?
> 2. Is swallowing of solids/liquids or both affected (solids only suggest mechanical obstruction, both solids/liquids affected suggests dysmotility)?
> 3. Localization of symptom (throat suggests oropharyngeal cause, and lower sternum suggests oesophageal cause)?
> 4. Duration and progression of symptom (long duration of symptom suggests benign disease)?
> 5. Presence of regurgitation between meals (e.g. in Zenker's diverticulum)?
> 6. Presence of reflux symptoms (e.g. in reflux-related dysmotility)?
> 7. Other risk factors for carcinoma (smoking, alcohol)?
> 8. Presence of allergic conditions (asthma, hay fever, eczema) predisposes to eosinophilic oesophagitis?
> 9. Medical history (oropharyngeal surgery/radiotherapy, connective tissue diseases, stroke, and other neurological diseases)?
> 10. Medications (dopamine antagonists, anticholinergics, bisphosphonates)?

Available oesophageal motility tests

Once mechanical obstruction has been excluded, e.g. by way of gastroscopy, the next step is to perform dedicated motility testing. The choice of tests includes manometry, barium swallow, and scintigraphy, with newer tests such as functional lumen imaging probe (FLIP) and high-frequency intraluminal ultrasound (HFIUS) appearing promising.

Manometry
- Most sensitive technique for detecting oesophageal dysmotility.
- Gold-standard test for diagnosing achalasia and oesophageal spasm.
- Involves transnasal insertion of manometric catheter that detects pressures from within oesophageal lumen.
- Standard manometry is performed by water-perfused silicone catheters that contain a variable number (up to 8) of pressure channels distributed along length of catheter, covering at least lower oesophageal body and LOS. Some catheters also have a 6-cm sleeve sensor that sits across LOS that allows more accurate measurement of LOS pressure.
- High-resolution manometry (HRM) has now replaced standard manometry as the test of choice due to higher fidelity, and improved diagnostic accuracy for achalasia and spasm. It utilizes solid-state catheters that contain up to 36 circumferential electronic sensors, spaced 1cm apart, and covers entire oesophagus including upper and lower oesophageal sphincters.
- HRM is coupled with a topographical (or contour, or colour) plot that translates the amplitude of pressures detected into different colours (Fig. 3.3).
- Motility is assessed by peristaltic appearance after 10 swallows of 5mL of water, with patient lying supine.
- The Chicago classification was developed specifically to categorize motility disorders detected by HRM, and is currently the only classification available for such purpose (Table 3.3).

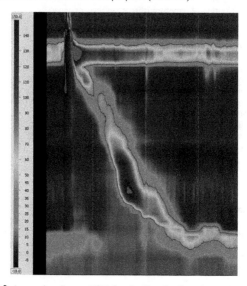

Fig. 3.3 A normal swallow on HRM. See also Plate 2, colour plate section.

Table 3.3 Chicago classification criteria of oesophageal motility disorders defined in high resolution oesophageal pressure topography

Diagnosis	Diagnostic criteria
Achalasia	
Type I achalasia	Classic achalasia: IRP > upper limit of normal, 100% failed peristalsis
Type II achalasia	Achalasia with oesophageal compression: mean IRP > upper limit of normal, no normal peristalsis, panoesophageal pressurization with ≥20% of swallows
Type III achalasia	Mean IRP > upper limit or normal, no normal peristalsis, preserved fragments of distal peristalsis or premature (spastic) contractions with ≥20% of swallows
GOJ outflow obstruction	Mean IRP > upper limit of normal, some instances of intact peristalsis or weak peristalsis with small breaks such that the criteria for achalasia are not met
Distal oesophageal spasm	Normal mean IRP, ≥20% premature contractions
Hypercontractile oesophagus	At least one swallow DCI >8000mmHg/s/cm with single-peaked or multi-peaked (jackhammer) contraction
Absent peristalsis	Normal mean IRP, 100% of swallows with failed peristalsis
Weak peristalsis with large peristaltic defects	Mean IRP <15mmHg and >20% swallows with large breaks in the 20mmHg isobaric contour (>5cm in length)
Weak peristalsis with small peristaltic defects	Mean IRP <15mmHg and >30% swallows with small breaks in the 20mmHg isobaric contour (2–5cm in length)
Rapid contractions with normal latency	Rapid contraction with ≥20% swallows, DL > 4.5s
Hypertensive peristalsis (nutcracker oesophagus)	Mean DCI > 5,000 mmHg-s-cm, but not meeting criteria for hypercontractile oesophagus
Frequent failed peristalsis	>30%, but <100% of swallows with failed peristalsis
Normal	Not achieving any of the diagnostic criteria listed here

IRP = integrated relaxation pressure; DCI = distal contractile integral; DL = distal latency.

Reproduced from 'Chicago classification criteria of esophageal motility disorders defined in high resolution esophageal pressure topography', A. J. Bredenoord, M. Fox, P. J. Kahrilas et al., *Neurogastroenterology & Motility*, Mar; **24** Suppl 1: 57–65, copyright 2012 with permission of Elsevier.

Barium swallow

- Offers real-time assessment of oropharyngeal coordination, oesophageal bolus transit, LOS opening, and pharyngo-oesophagogastric anatomy, as well as risk of aspiration.
- Barium liquid only standard.
- Solid swallows useful in patients experiencing dysphagia with solids, but not liquids.
- Often performed as an adjunct to gastroscopy and manometry, or as 1° investigation in those who cannot tolerate other procedures.
- Advantages of being non-invasive and lower cost.
- Quality and diagnostic accuracy is greatly influenced by local expertise: best performed at specialized centres.
- Diagnostic accuracy for achalasia 58–95%, less for oesophageal spasm and reflux, partly due to intermittent nature of these events.
- Timed barium oesophagogram measures height of barium column at 1, 2, and 5min post-contrast ingestion after treatment for achalasia. It has been advocated as a method to monitor success of treatment, and detect disease recurrence prior to symptom redevelopment. However, this method requires further validation.

Scintigraphy

- Superseded by other tests.
- Main role is as screening test for oesophageal transit problems and, possibly, to detect evidence of micro-aspirations.
- Involves ingestion of solids or liquids labelled with radionuclide such as 99mTc-DTPA.
- Disadvantages include handling of radioactive material, poor anatomical definition compared with barium swallow, and lack of well-defined diagnostic criteria.

Future and emerging tests

- *Multichannel intraluminal impedance monitoring (MII)*: used to measure oesophageal bolus transit in the experimental setting. One potential clinical use is in diagnosing rumination syndrome, in combination with HRM, where typical post-prandial abdominal straining is accompanied by retrograde flow in the oesophagus.
- *Functional lumen imaging probe (FLIP)*:
  - EndoFLIP® device (Fig. 3.4) utilizes impedance to measure luminal diameter and, together with pressure and volume, allows calculation of distensibility and compliance, respectively. Appears promising in evaluating LOS before and after achalasia treatment.
  - EndoFLIP® can be placed in GOJ act as a smart bougie during laparoscopic fundoplication surgery—allow measurement of distensibility/tightness at GOJ after crural repair, during and after fundoplication wrap fashioning.
  - Small hiatal hernias can be measured pre- and post-repair—spatial separation of crus, LOS, and wrap visualized by 8-cm long image field of EndoFLIP® catheter.

- Length of wrap may be measured.
- Can aid tailoring of wrap to desired narrowing or distensibility of LOS.
- Surgery for achalasia.
- EndoFLIP® placed in GOJ—as longitudinal and circular fibres cut, GOJ observed to open, increasing distensibility.
- Can be used performing a myotomy transorally, using endoscopic submucosal tunnelling/ peroral endoscopic myotomy (POEM).
- *HFIUS:* utilizes a catheter-based ultrasound probe with a diameter of 1–3mm, and is used to measure oesophageal longitudinal muscle contractions, as reflected by changes in oesophageal wall thickness. Its use is currently limited to the research setting.

The recommended approach to investigating dysphagia is shown in Fig. 3.5.

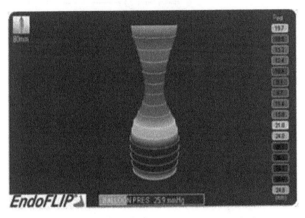

Fig. 3.4 EndoFLIP® device performing intraoperative pressure and volume measurements. See also Plate 3, colour plate section.

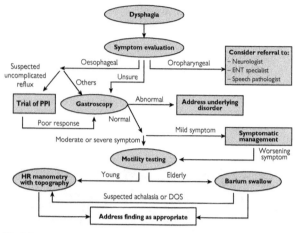

Fig. 3.5 Recommended approach to investigation of dysphagia. PPI, proton pump inhibitor. HR, high-resolution. DOS, diffuse oesophageal spasm.

Achalasia

Epidemiology

- *Incidence:* 1.6 per 100,000 and prevalence is 10.8 per 100,000 in the general population.
- *Mean age at diagnosis:* 53 years, without significant difference between males and females.
- Life expectancy generally regarded to be uncompromised, but there is evidence that, even after treatment, survival may be reduced.
- Risk for oesophageal cancer, especially squamous carcinoma cells (SCC), elevated 28-fold, and occurs typically over 10 years after diagnosis. Low absolute risk—routine cancer screening not indicated.

Pathogenesis

- Aetiology of 1° achalasia unknown.
- Disease results in loss of inhibitory neurons that are required for LOS relaxation and oesophageal peristalsis; consequently, LOS fails to relax with swallows, leading to dysphagia, and oesophageal body contraction becomes disorganized.
- Neurodegenerative process thought to be inflammatory in origin, with possible viral involvement.
- *2° achalasia:* cause for neurodegeneration known, most cases due to Chagas disease due to *Trypanozoma cruzi* infection.
- *Pseudoachalasia:*
  - Clinically and manometrically like achalasia.
  - Accounts for 2–4% of cases.
  - Caused most commonly by adenocarcinoma of lower oesophagus/gastro-oesophageal junction, and other conditions, such as lung and breast cancer, sarcoidosis, pancreatic cancer, histiocytosis x, and amyloidosis.
  - Post-operatively as a result of a tight fundoplication.

Symptoms

- Dysphagia, occurring in 90% of patients.
- Other symptoms, such as difficulty belching (80%), regurgitation (50%), chest pain (50%), heartburn (50%), and weight loss (50%) occurring at lesser frequencies.
- Weight loss is generally mild (5–10kg).
- Regurgitation, especially during recumbency at night, can result in aspiration.
- Rapid onset, particularly in older individuals, should raise suspicion of pseudoachalasia.

Diagnosis

- Manometry gold-standard test.
- High-resolution manometry with topography has been shown to greatly improve diagnostic sensitivity for achalasia over standard manometry (97% vs. 52%).

- Barium swallows typically shows bird's beak appearance with dilated oesophagus, tapering sharply distally, poor oesophageal emptying, and non-relaxing LOS.
- Endoscopy shows dilated immotile oesophagus, often with retained food and fluid, and a tight LOS sometimes preventing passage of endoscope.
- Due to high fidelity nature of HRM with topography, achalasia is further stratified into types I, II, and III, which carries prognostic implications (see Box 3.2).

Box 3.2 Classification of achalasia

- *Type I (classic):* oesophageal aperistalsis.
- *Type II (achalasia with oesophageal compression):* pan-oesophageal pressurization.
- *Type III:* spastic contractions or preserved fragments of distal peristalsis.

Management

The three main treatment options include:

- Surgical myotomy.
- Balloon dilatation.
- Botulinum toxin injection.

Pharmacological treatments that aim to relax the lower oesophageal sphincter, such as calcium channel blockers, nitrates, and phosphodiesterase inhibitors are not recommended due to poor quality of evidence to support their efficacy.

Surgical myotomy: general

- Most definitive treatment.
- Highest success rate of 95%.
- Low complication rate.
- Longest lasting symptomatic relief (~85% at 5 years).
- Traditionally performed as open procedure, with more recent publications recommending laparoscopic approach, which is associated with comparable efficacy and safety, while reducing perioperative morbidity.
- Myotomy generally extends several centimeters above and below lower oesophageal sphincter to ensure all sphincteric muscles are disrupted, including gastric sling fibres that form part of gastro-oesophageal junction.
- Most myotomies (Heller–Dor procedure) accompanied by anti-reflux procedure to reduce reflux (47 to 9%), but despite this, up to 30% of patients require proton-pump inhibitor (PPI) therapy post-operatively.
- Tends to be performed on younger patients who are better surgical candidates and have longer life expectancy.
- Best outcomes with type I and II achalasia.

The results of a 2008 retrospective study of the therapeutic responses of achalasia subtypes are demonstrated in Table 3.4.

Table 3.4 Response to therapeutic interventions among achalasia subtypes

Achalasia subtype	Type I ($n = 16$)	Type II ($n = 46$)	Type III ($n = 21$)	All ($n = 83$)
Number of interventions, mean (SD)	1.6 (SD, 1.5)	1.2a (SD, 0.4)	2.4a,b (SD, 1.0)	1.8 (SD, 0.7)
Success with Botox (first intervention) (%)	0 (0/2)	86 (6/7)	22 (2/9)	39 (7/18)
Success with dilation (first intervention with 30-mm balloon) (%)	38 (3/8)	73 (19/26)	0 (0/11)	53 (24/45)
Success with myotomy (first intervention) (%)	67 (4/6)	100 (13/13)	0 (0/1)	85 (17/20)
Success with first intervention (total) (%)	44 (7/16)	83 (38/46)	9 (2/21)	56 (47/83)
Success with last intervention (%) (last intervention type)	56 (B-0, P-10, M-6)	96a (B-6, P-25, M-15)	29a,b (B-8, P-8, M-5)	71 (B-14, P-43, M-26)

Pandolfino JE, Kwiatek MA, Nealis T, et al. Achalasia: a new clinically relevant classification by high-resolution manometry. *Gastroenterology* 2008; **135**(5): 1526–33.

Note: Pneumatic dilation initially performed with 30-mm microvasive balloon in all instances. If this failed, usually followed by 35-mm dilation accounting for difference in success rate for pneumatic dilation when applied as initial or last intervention. Botox (B), pneumatic dilation (P), surgical myotomy (M).

a, $P < 0.05$ vs. type I; b, $P < 0.05$ vs. type II.

Operative procedure: laparoscopic Heller's cardiomyotomy

See Fig. 3.6.

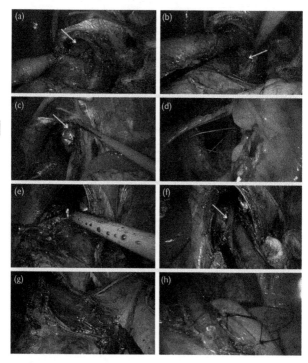

Fig. 3.6 Operative steps of laparoscopic Heller's cardiomyotomy for sigmoid oesophagus. (a) Widened hiatus with oesophageal axis deviation; arrow shows dilated part of oesophagus in mediastinum. (b) Circumferential mobilization of oesophagus exposing aorta posteriorly (arrow). (c) Extensive mediastinal dissection of oesophagus exposing pleura (arrow). (d) Crural repair using a 2-0 non-absorbable suture for widened hiatus. (e) Cardiomyotomy in progress on oesophageal side. (f) Cardiomyotomy completed on oesophageal side with mucosa pouting; arrow shows preserved anterior vagus nerve, it also shows relatively straightened oesophageal axis. (g) Cardiomyotomy in progress on gastric side. (h) Completed cardiomyotomy with angle of His accentuation as anti-reflux procedure.

- General anaesthetic (GA).
- French or reverse Trendelenburg position.
- Pneumoperitoneum established.
- Ports placed as for anti-reflux surgery (ARS).
- Liver retractor placed to expose GOJ adequately.
- Gastrohepatic ligament divided to reveal right pillar of crus, whilst preserving hepatic branch of the vagus.
- Peritoneum overlying right pillar of crus divided whilst preserving its epimysium.
- Mobilization extended to divide phreno-oesophageal ligament and along left pillar of crus.
- Passing a tape round GOJ and applying traction aids mobilization of adequate length of oesophagus.
- Dilated oesophagus mobilized gently by blunt mediastinal dissection 5–6cm drawn into the abdomen.
- Anterior vagus needs to be identified and safeguarded.
- Crural repair not required unless clear sizeable defect.
- Identify GOJ clearly by reflecting fat pad to right (thereby moving anterior vagus out of harm's way). There is a constant vein that crosses and marks GOJ. It is best formally divided.
- *Perform myotomy:* 6cm of oesophagus extending over 2cm of cardia. Outer longitudinal fibres divided with harmonic scalpel of bipolar scissors revealing thickened circular muscle that is carefully retracted from submucosa and teased apart. Submucosa should be seen to bulge, but should not be breached. A degree of bleeding is encountered when dividing circular muscle fibres at cardia due to abundant palisade vessels in a web-like configuration.
- An inadequate myotomy at the cardia may lead to failure, so care must be taken to extend myotomy distally
- Deal with bleeding from myotomy edges by pressure with a swab, which can be conveniently placed medial to spleen so that it can be applied quickly in event of bleeding.
- Common practice to perform a Dor partial anterior fundoplication:
  - Fundus mobilized drawn medially and sutured to two edges of myotomized segment in two longitudinal rows and then right crus effectively covering myotomy, but concurrently holding it open
  - *Post-operatively*—liquid diet for 1 week.

Balloon dilatation

- *Endoscopic or radiological:* larger balloons available for radiological dilatation under fluoroscopy.
- High success rate of 90%.
- Aims to stretch and rupture LOS muscle fibres.
- Symptomatic relief maintained in ~70% at 5 years.
- Low complication rate.
- Most serious complication oesophageal rupture that occurs in 2–3%.
- Repeat treatment(s) can be performed for 1° failure or recurrence.
- There is a probable increased long-term risk of gastro-oesophageal reflux compared with surgical myotomy.
- Tends to be performed on older patients who are either not fit for surgery or have shorter life expectancy.

Botulinum toxin injection
- Initial success rate of 80%.
- Paralyses LOS muscles with direct endoscopic injections of botulinum toxin.
- Short duration of symptomatic relief (~6 months).
- Lowest complication rate.
- Can be repeated easily.
- Tends to be reserved for those with very limited life expectancy, or as trial therapeutic procedure when diagnosis of achalasia is less certain, or acts as bridge, while waiting for more definitive treatment.

POEM procedure

- Per-oral endoscopic myotomy performed under GA.
- Used for non-sigmoid and sigmoid achalasia.
- First performed in 2008 by Haruhiro Inoue, Yokohama, Japan, evolution of tunnelled submucosal myotomy described by Pasricha.
- *Requires:* modified forward-viewing 9.8-mm endoscope with 1-cm transparent, oblique distal cap essential for entering and maintaining endoscopic visualization within submucosal space.

Procedure

See Fig. 3.7.

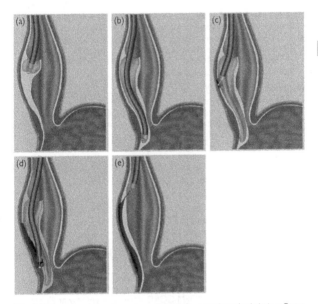

Fig. 3.7 Peroral endoscopic myotomy (POEM) for oesophageal achalasia. **a** Entry to submucosal space. After submucosal injection, a 2-cm longitudinal mucosal incision is made at approximately 13cm proximal to the gastroesophageal junction (GEJ). **b** Submucosal tunnelling. A long submucosal tunnel is created to 3cm distal to the GEJ. **c** Endoscopic myotomy is begun at 3cm distal to the mucosal entry point, and is carried out in a proximal to distal direction to a total length of 10cm. **d** Long endoscopic myotomy of inner circular muscle bundles is done, leaving the outer longitudinal muscle layer intact. The expected end point of myotomy is 2cm distal to the GEJ. **e** Closure of mucosal entry: the mucosal incision is closed using hemostatic clips.

Reproduced from 'Peroral endoscopic myotomy (POEM) for esophageal achalasia', H Inoue, H Minami, Y Kobayashi, et al., *Endoscopy* **42**(4): 265–71, copyright 2010 with permission from Thieme.

Mucosal entry

- Submucosal injection 10mL saline/0.3% indigo carmine.
- 2-cm anterior oesophageal longitudinal mucosal incision at 2'o'clock.
- Leads to lesser curve without injury to sling fibres.
- Submucosal injection at level of mid-oesophagus, 13cm proximal to GOJ. Length of tunnel 16cm (29–45cm).

Submucosal tunnel

- Submucosal tunnel created by endoscopic submucosal dissection (ESD) type approach using a 2.6-mm triangle-tip knife with spray diathermy used to dissect submucosal layer and to divide circular muscle bundles at GOJ. Insufflation with CO_2.
- Tunnel traverses GOJ and 3cm of gastric cardia, where lumen is entered. *Dissection plane* between submucosa and muscularis propria close to surface of muscularis. Dissection should never be performed directly adjacent to the mucosa to prevent mediastinal sepsis.
- Width of tunnel is one-third of circumference of oesophagus. Once tip of endoscope has reached the cardia, submucosal space is opened widely. Distal end of tunnel is verified by retroflexion. Large submucosal vessels coagulated using forceps.

Identification of the GOJ

- Distance from incisors.
- Marked increase in resistance when endoscope encounters GOJ, followed by prompt easing when endoscope passes through narrowed GOJ and enters gastric submucosal space.
- Endoscopic visualization of distal oesophageal submucosal palisade vessels.
- Few vessels in oesophageal submucosa, but vessels web-like and abundant once GOJ crossed.

Endoscopic myotomy

- Circular muscle dissection initiated 2cm distal to mucosal entry point, more than 10cm proximal to GOJ.
- Circular fibres divided using spray-coagulation (50W).
- Only circular muscle bundles lifted and cut while maintaining longitudinal muscle layer intact. Myotomy extended 2cm onto stomach.
- No anti-reflux procedure performed because endoscopist never touches the phreno-oesophageal membrane, Theoretically, hiatal attachments are left untouched and the flap-valve mechanism intact.
- To reduce risk of post-POEM GORD, anterior myotomy at 2'o'clock (supine) directs myotomy to lesser curve without disturbing angle of His, at 8'o'clock.

Myotomy length and myotomy direction

- Myotomy length routinely >10cm up to 25cm can be tailored.
- In patients with chest pain caused by abnormal contractions of hypertrophied muscle within oesophageal body, a long myotomy is

made. All abnormal contractions (endoscopically visible and measured with manometry) incorporated into site of circular muscle division.
- Mucosal entry site closed using haemostatic clips.

Outcomes
- *Intraoperative complications:* bleeding, pneumoperitoneum.
- *Post-operatively:* peritonitis, mediastinitis.
- *Average operative time:* 128min (95–310).
- *Hospital stay:* 1.4 days. 78% of patients receive no post-operative analgesia. 11% have a sore throat. 8% have left pleuritic chest pain. 3% left upper quadrant (LUQ) pain.
- *6/12 follow-up (F/U):* 90% require relief of dysphagia, 22% display occasional GORD symptoms.
- Reduction of Eckhardt dysphagia scores from 8.8 to 1.4.
- Eckardt score ≤ 3 is achieved in 94%.
- 70% drop in LOS pressure in patients with non-sigmoid oesophagi, and 50% drop in patients with sigmoid oesophagi.

Oesophageal spasm and nutcracker oesophagus

Diffuse oesophageal spasm (DOS) is a motility disorder characterized by simultaneous contractions, that can sometimes be prolonged, repetitive, or of high amplitude. However, the term diffuse oesophageal spasm (DOS) is considered somewhat a misnomer, as the contractile abnormality occurs typically in the distal oesophagus only. This fact has been recognized and in the current Chicago classification for oesophageal motility disorders, the term diffuse oesophageal spasm has been replaced by the term distal oesophageal spasm. As opposed to distal oesophageal spasm, nutcracker oesophagus is characterized by peristalsis that is coordinated, but of higher than normal amplitude. Both DOS and nutcracker oesophagus typically cause intermittent chest pain and/or dysphagia.

Epidemiology
- Diffuse oesophageal spasm (DOS) only present in small proportion of patients referred for motility testing, accounting for 0.6–2.8% of patients with non-cardiac chest pain, 3.3–5.3% of patients with dysphagia, and 4–4.5% of those with both chest pain and dysphagia.
- Nutcracker oesophagus occurs in 10% of patients with non-cardiac chest pain.
- Incidence does not appear to be affected by age, gender, or race.
- DOS associated with mitral valve prolapse, obesity, and psychiatric illness, but these only account for a small proportion of cases.
- Both DOS and nutcracker oesophagus have a relatively benign course and symptom tends to improve with time.

Pathogenesis
- Cause of DOS and nutcracker oesophagus is unknown.
- Loss of inhibitory neurons that leads to early and sometimes uncontrolled contractions in oesophagus, typically in distal oesophageal body.
- Oesophageal wall smooth muscle thickened on ultrasound.
- Mechanism of pain uncertain, due to:
  - High amplitude contractions (>300mmHg) leading to increased wall tension or
  - Prolonged contraction leading to ischaemia.
- Recent, evidence suggests pain may be caused by contraction of longitudinal muscles in oesophagus.

Symptoms
- DOS and nutcracker oesophagus.
- *Classic symptoms:* intermittent chest pain and/or dysphagia.
- Variable severity and duration, or even location. Can be provoked by consuming solids or liquids or independent of eating/drinking.
- Most commonly suspected with episodic non-cardiac chest pains, where cardiac cause excluded.
- Most cases of non-cardiac chest pain are due to GORD.

Diagnosis
Oesophageal spasm
See Fig. 3.8.
- The gold-standard diagnostic technique is manometry.
- Diagnosis on standard manometry requires at least 20% of swallows showing simultaneous contractions in the distal oesophagus (>8cm/s propagation) with a minimum amplitude of 30mmHg.
- Criteria lack specificity, high false positive rate. Other supportive features include high amplitude, spontaneous, repetitive, or multi-peaked contractions.
- HRM with topography has further refined diagnosis of spasm based on characteristic of premature contraction in distal oesophagus, whilst emphasis on speed of contraction has been removed.
- The change in HRM diagnostic criteria is based on loss of inhibitory neurons, leading to loss of refractoriness in distal oesophagus, and thus premature contractions.
- HRM improvement of diagnostic specificity from <5% to 25%, compared with standard manometry.
- *Provocative tests:* Tensilon and balloon distension may induce chest pain, utility controversial. Not routinely performed.
- 24-h ambulatory manometry may improve diagnostic accuracy over standard test.
- Barium swallow abnormal in 60% of patients, but only <5% show typical corkscrew appearance.

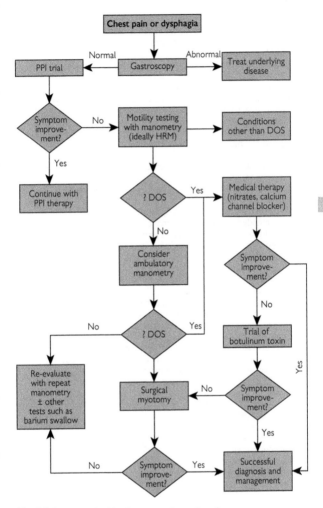

Fig. 3.8 Diagnostic algorithm for suspected oesophageal spasm.
Adapted from 'Diffuse esophageal spasm', Grubel C, J Borovicka, et al., *Am J Gastroenterol*
103(2): 450–7, copyright 2008 with permission from Elsevier.

Nutcracker oesophagus
- The gold-standard diagnostic technique is manometry.
- Unlike oesophageal spasm, in nutcracker oesophagus. Peristalsis intact, but of high amplitude.
- Characterized on standard manometry by high amplitude peristaltic contractions in distal 10cm of oesophagus, with average peristaltic pressure exceeding 220mmHg.
- Diagnosis of HRM based on measurement of DCI, which is product of amplitude × time × length and expressed as mmHg/s/cm. Mean DCI over 5000mmHg/s/cm is diagnostic of hypertensive peristalsis (nutcracker oesophagus), and a mean DCI of over 8000mmHg/s/cm is diagnostic of hypercontractile/jackhammer oesophagus, a more severe form of nutcracker oesophagus.
- Diagnostic accuracy on barium swallow is poor due to inability of technique to measure contractile strength.
- Oesophageal spasm and nutcracker oesophagus are managed in similar manner.
- Proportion felt to be triggered by GORD, ∴ acid suppressive therapy recommended as first-line treatment.
- Medical therapies centred around smooth muscle relaxants, e.g. calcium channel blockers (nifedipine, diltiazem, verapamil), nitric oxide donors (sildenafil, isosorbide mononitrate), and botulinum toxin that paralyses smooth muscle.
- Response to medical treatment generally disappointing, improvement in <25% of cases.
- Botulinum toxin injection (100U), either around squamocolumnar junction in distal oesophagus or into multiple sites along oesophageal wall, has been reported to achieve response rate of 50–90%, with beneficial effects lasting for ~6 months.
- Antidepressants with pain modulating effects, such as trazodone and imipramine, have been shown to improve symptoms in patients with chest pain and manometric abnormalities.
- Use of bougienage and pneumatic dilatation reported, but evidence lacking.
- Surgical oesophagomyotomy can be an option if medical therapy fails; associated with 70–80% success rate. Exact technique is controversial, but is likely to involve an incision extending above level of manometric abnormality and below lower oesophageal sphincter. Anti-reflux procedure often performed at same time. Open and minimally invasive (laparoscopic and thoracoscopic) methods described.
- Oesophagectomy an option in extreme cases.

Other oesophageal dysmotility disorders

Scleroderma with oesophageal involvement
- Connective tissue diseases, such as scleroderma typically affect smooth muscle in distal two-thirds of oesophagus, with sparing of skeletal component in proximal one-third.
- 50–90% of patients have oesophageal involvement.
- Disease in oesophagus tends to mimic severity of skin manifestation.
- Reflux very common. Can lead to dysphagia. First line treatment PPIs.
- Treat underlying disease, specific treatment options limited. Prokinetics unlikely to benefit.
- Anti-reflux surgery may be required in some, but dysmotility may increase risk of subsequent dysphagia.

Oesophageal hypomotility
- Umbrella term denoting reduced peristaltic vigour.
- Incorporates weak peristalsis with small or large defect, frequent failed peristalsis, and absent peristalsis in the Chicago classification of high resolution oesophageal manometry.
- Correlation to symptoms is variable, and ∴ is itself of uncertain clinical significance.
- May explain dysphagia only if symptom correlates well, with swallows showing at least large (>/= 5cm) peristaltic defect or failed peristalsis; small defect (2–5cm) insufficient to cause dysphagia.
- Response to prokinetic agents have been disappointing.

Gastro-oesophageal reflux disease

GORD is very common. 20% of adults complain of symptoms at least weekly. It is characterized by symptomatic or damaging reflux of gastric contents into the oesophagus.

Normal individuals have several physiological reflux events each day, and the lower oesophagus is acidified up to 5% of the time. This is not usually perceived and no mucosal injury results.

- Prevalence of 10–40% in developed countries.
- Incidence is rising.
- Many sufferers do not seek medical attention for their symptoms.
- *Pathological, GORD:* causes symptoms which affect lifestyle; or oesophageal pathology 2° to mucosal injury.
- Often an acquired condition, but congenital forms can significantly impact upon infant respiratory and nutritional status.

Symptoms of oesophageal reflux disease

Typical presentations are:

- *Heartburn:* retrosternal burning sensation.
- *Regurgitation:* unpleasant feeling of refluxed gastric content entering mouth or hypopharynx.

Symptoms often worse after eating, on bending or stooping, and on lying down at night.

'Atypical' manifestations are:

- *Epigastric pain.*
- *Chest pain:* similar to cardiac pain (GORD more common cause of this than oesophageal spasm).
- *Cough:* GORD has been considered 3rd most common cause of chronic cough, but true prevalence is difficult to assess. More likely to be due to an oesophago-bronchial reflex, rather than micro-aspiration. Frequently nocturnal.
- *Hoarseness/sore throat:* 50–60% of chronic laryngitis may be related to GORD. Laryngoscopy findings are neither sensitive nor specific.
- *Non-allergic asthma:* usually nocturnal.
- *Odynophagia, dysphagia.*
- *Asymptomatic:* 20%.

Differential diagnosis

- Great variability in presentation of GORD, ∴ wide differential must be considered.
- GORD may be present as synchronous pathology in addition to any others.
- Possible differential diagnoses include:
  - *Gastrointestinal*—upper gastrointestinal cancers, peptic ulcer disease, oesophageal motility disorders, oesophageal infection, gallstone disease, pancreatic disease, Crohn's disease, irritable bowel syndrome (IBS).
  - *Other*—ischaemic heart disease, aortic aneurysm, musculoskeletal disease, pneumonia, pulmonary embolus.

Complications of GORD

- Bleeding/anaemia from oesophageal erosions.
- Peptic stricture causing dysphagia occurs in 7–23% of patients with untreated erosive oesophagitis. Schatzki's ring (contains mucosal, submucosal, and smooth muscle elements)
- Barrett's oesophagus is estimated to be found in 5–15% of patients undergoing endoscopy for GORD symptoms.
- *Oesophageal adenocarcinoma:* progression from non-dysplastic Barrett's oesophagus is estimated at 0.5–1% per patient year.
- *Distant:* chronic pharyngitis, dental caries, aspiration pneumonitis.

Classification of GORD

GORD can be classified according to the findings of endoscopy and reflux monitoring, as well as into oesophageal and extra-oesophageal syndromes (Fig. 3.9). The severity of symptoms is a poor indicator as to the GORD phenotype (Fig. 3.10).

- *Non-erosive reflux disease (NERD):* up to 70% of patients with GORD have macroscopically normal mucosa on endoscopy (although will often have microscopic changes), despite pathological acid reflux.
- *Erosive oesophagitis:* minority (30–40%) of GORD patients have macroscopic erosions of oesophageal mucosa (classified by the Los Angeles classification, see Table 3.5).
- *Hypersensitive oesophagus:* patients with macroscopically normal mucosa, physiological oesophageal acid exposure on reflux studies, but association of symptoms with reflux events.
- *Functional heartburn:* typical symptoms, but normal mucosa, physiological oesophageal acid exposure, and no association of symptoms with reflux events (i.e. heartburn not caused by gastro-oesophageal reflux).

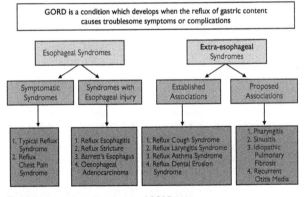

Fig. 3.9 The Montreal Classification of GORD 2006.
Reproduced from 'The Montreal definition and classification of gastroesophageal reflux disease: a global evidence-based consensus', Vakil N, van Zanten SV, Kahrilas P, et al., *Am J Gastroenterol* **101**: 1900–20, copyright 2006 with permission from Elsevier.

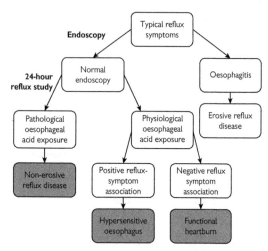

Fig. 3.10 GORD phenotypes according to endoscopy and 24-reflux study findings.

Table 3.5 The Los Angeles classification of erosive reflux disease	
Grade A	One or more mucosal breaks <5mm in maximal length
Grade B	One or more mucosal breaks >5mm, but without continuity across mucosal folds
Grade C	Mucosal breaks continuous between > 2 mucosal folds, but involving less than 75% of the oesophageal circumference
Grade D	Mucosal breaks involving more than 75% of oesophageal circumference

NERD

- Individuals satisfy definition of GORD, but no erosions, or Barrett's.
- Can have severe symptoms.
- *Specific features of NERD:*
  - *Aetiology*—higher prevalence in young females. Stress and psychological distress may have role in increasing oesophageal sensitivity. NERD may be misdiagnosed as functional pain.
  - *Investigation*—pH recording may be within normal limits and further investigation with more specialized techniques may be required. Oesophageal balloon distension may show a hypersensitive oesophagus.
  - *Treatment*—lower response rate to PPI than patients with oesophagitis. Surgery can present particular difficulties in symptomatic patients with normal oesophagogastroduodenoscopy (OGD) and pH studies with worse outcomes reported following fundoplication.

Aetiology of gastro-oesophageal reflux disease

It results from a failure of the anti-reflux mechanisms at the gastro-oesophageal junction which comprises:
- *LOS:* cannot be anatomically demonstrated. Formed by increased resting muscle tone in distal 5cm of the oesophagus (10–25mmHg).
- *Flap valve:* formed by a fold of gastric mucosa to occlude oesophageal lumen.
- *External components:* 'pinch-lock' by diaphragmatic crura and oblique muscular sling fibres, which maintain acute cardio-oesophageal angle of His. Relatively high intra-abdominal pressure, which surrounds the distal oesophagus helping to occlude the lumen.
  Any impairment of the components of the ARM can lead to GORD.

Decreased LOS tone
- *TLOSR:* inappropriate episodes of TLOSR unrelated to peristalsis, but linked to gastric distension.
- *Drugs:* nitrates, tricyclics, Ca^{2+} channel antagonists.
- *Hormones:* cholecystokinin, glucagon, progesterone, oestrogen.
- *Lifestyle:* smoking, alcohol, caffeine, fatty food.
- *Flap valve/external components:* disruption of Angle of His.
- *Hiatus hernia:* causes loss of acute angle of His and extrinsic compression by diaphragmatic crura. Can also lead to loss of higher, intra-abdominal pressure zone.[1]

Motility disorders
- *Oesophageal motility disorders associated with connective tissue disorders (e.g. scleroderma):* impaired ability of the oesophagus to clear reflux can lead to GORD.
- *Impaired gastric emptying:* obstruction to gastric outflow or impaired gastric motility.

Other factors
- Genetic predisposition.
- Increased abdominal pressure.
- Chronic cough.
- Constipation.
- Pregnancy.
- Obesity.

[1] Most patients with hiatus hernia do not have symptoms, but many GORD sufferers do have a hernia.

Investigations for gastro-oesophageal reflux disease

PPI trial

In most cases in general practice, this is the first and only test applied for GORD. In GORD, symptomatic response to PPI can be as high as 70–80%, and complete symptom resolution is highly suggestive of the diagnosis.

Further investigations indicated if there is concern about the accuracy of diagnosis, complications, treatment non-response, consideration of surgery, or patient choice.

In the UK, urgent referral criteria for upper GI endoscopy exist for patients with dyspepsia (Box 3.3).

Box 3.3 NICE criteria for urgent upper GI endoscopy in patients with dyspepsia in the UK
- Chronic gastrointestinal bleeding.
- Progressive dysphagia.
- Progressive unintentional weight loss.
- Persistent vomiting.
- Iron deficiency anaemia.
- Epigastric mass.
- >55 years with unexplained persistent or recent onset dyspepsia.

National Institute for Health and Clinical Excellence (2004). Adapted from 'CG 17 Dyspepsia: the management of dyspepsia in adults in primary care'. London: NICE. Available from http://www.nice.org.uk. Reproduced with permission.

Endoscopy

- *Evaluate:* presence of hiatus hernia, oesophagitis (Table 3.6), or complications such as Barrett's oesophagus or carcinoma.
- Oesophagitis is present in less than 50% of patients with GORD, and is very rare in those taking PPIs.
- Microscopic examination of oesophageal mucosal biopsy tissue can demonstrate microscopic oesophagitis and dilated intercellular spaces in NERD, but this is predominantly a research tool.

Table 3.6 Modified Savary–Miller classification of oesophagitis

Grade I	Single erosive lesion affecting only one longitudinal fold
Grade II	Multiple erosive lesions, non-circumferential, affecting more than one longitudinal fold, with or without confluence
Grade III	Circumferential erosive lesion
Grade IV	Chronic lesions—ulcer, stricture and/or short oesophagus
Grade V	Barrett's oesophagus with histologically confirmed intestinal differentiation within columnar epithelium

Reproduced from 'Norwendige Diagnostik: Endoskopie', Miller G, Savary M, Monnier P. In: *Reflux-therapie*, eds. Blum AL, Siewert JR, pp. 336–54. Copyright Berlin, 1981, with kind permission from Springer Science and Business Media.

Oesophageal manometry studies

- Although not a reflux study, this can demonstrate rare cases of regurgitation 2° to incomplete oesophageal emptying (e.g. in achalasia).
- Will demonstrate presence or absence of hiatal hernia, and show oesophageal motility patterns that may be consistent with reflux disease (e.g. hypomotility).
- Characterize oesophageal motility prior to consideration of anti-reflux surgery.

Ambulatory oesophageal pH monitoring

- Most commonly performed using transnasal catheter connected to data-logger.
- An integrated pH electrode sits 5cm above the manometrically-defined LOS, and recordings are made for 24h.
- Second sensor in upper oesophagus may be used to diagnose reflux-related throat symptoms.
- Study usually performed after witholding anti-secretory therapy for at least 5 days.
- Patient records symptom events, meal times and body position (upright/recumbent) on data-logger.
- Oesophageal acid exposure outside mealtimes is calculated.
- Normal ranges may be locally defined, but pathological acid (pH < 4) exposure is usually defined as greater than 4–5% of the study period (pathological nocturnal GORD usually defined as more than 2.5–3% acid exposure in the recumbent position).
- Reflux-symptom association is calculated by statistical means (usually symptom index and/or symptom-associated probability; Box 3.4).
- DeMeester score frequently reported (Box 3.5)
- Wireless pH monitoring (e.g. with the Bravo(R) capsule system) is increasing in popularity. A capsule anchored to oesophageal mucosa records oesophageal pH and transmits data wirelessly to data-logger, negating need for an unsightly and uncomfortable transnasal catheter.

Box 3.4 Testing of symptom-reflux association

Symptom index (SI)
- Percentage of symptom episodes preceded (within 2min) by reflux event.
- SI >50% is considered positive.

Symptom-associated probability (SAP)
- A statistical test of the probability that symptom episodes are truly related to preceding (within 2min) reflux events, not by chance alone.
- Uses a 2 × 2 contingency table method.
- An SAP >95% is considered positive.

Box 3.5 DeMeester Score

Components of 24-h oesophageal pH monitoring
- Percentage total time pH < 4.
- Percentage upright time pH < 4.
- Percentage supine time pH < 4.
- Number of reflux episodes.
- Number of reflux episodes ≥5min.
- Longest reflux episode (min).
- Composite score calculated.
- Score > 14.72 indicates reflux.

Ambulatory combined pH-impedance monitoring

- *Multichannel intraluminal impedance:* relatively new technique enabling detection of bolus movement up and down oesophagus.
- Liquid (low impedance) and air (high impedance) transit can be identified, and in conjunction with 24-h pH monitoring allows more accurate characterization of reflux events (Fig. 3.11).
- Allows detection of reflux events with pH greater than 4 (weakly acidic reflux) which can be a cause of PPI-refractory symptoms.

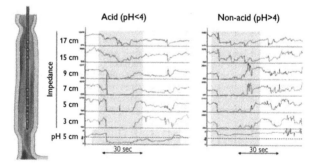

Fig. 3.11 Episodes of reflux identified by combined multichannel intraluminal impedance and pH monitoring.
Reproduced from 'Laboratory based investigations for diagnosing gastroesophageal reflux disease', Mathias Dolder, Radu Tutuian, *Best Practice & Research Clinical Gastroenterology*, **24**(6), 787–98, copyright 2012 with permission of Elsevier.

Ambulatory bilirubin monitoring (Bilitec)

- This is a tool to detect duodeno-gastro-oesophageal reflux (which contains noxious bile acids).
- Oesophageal bilirubin measured by way of spectrophotometric absorption measurement.
- Although correlates well with bile acid concentrations in oesophageal aspiration studies, there is potential for false positive reading with several foodstuffs (e.g. tomatoes, bananas, beets, beef, tea, coffee).
- Method has mostly been superceded by pH-impedance monitoring in clinical practice, since impedance can detect reflux irrespective of pH.

Physiological testing pre-fundoplication

- Prior to anti-reflux surgery most patients undergo oesophageal manometry and a 24-h reflux study.
- *Primary role of oesophageal manometry:* exclude serious motor abnormality (e.g. achalasia)—contra-indication to surgery.
- *High resolution oesophageal manometry:* additional benefit of characterizing severe oesophageal hypomotility. May be taken into account in tailoring surgery (although no studies have formally assessed this).
- *24-h reflux monitoring:* confirms diagnosis of GORD (thus, preventing surgery on patients with functional heartburn, which is unlikely to be successful).
- Useful in distinguishing which symptoms are attributable to reflux, and which are not (allowing a pre-operative discussion about realistic expectations of surgery outcome).

Physiological testing post-fundoplication

The most common indications for physiological testing post-fundoplication are dysphagia and persistent/recurrent reflux symptoms.

- *High resolution oesophageal manometry:* can demonstrate integrity the wrap in case of recurrent reflux symptoms (i.e. is there a single high pressure zone at the level of wrap, or a dual high pressure zone indicating slippage?). In case of dysphagia, it can demonstrate oesophageal outlet obstruction 2° to a tight wrap.
- *24-h reflux monitoring:* can demonstrate persistent gastro-oesophageal reflux in recurrent symptoms.

Medical management of gastro-oesophageal reflux disease

Lifestyle modifications

Little good outcome data available for efficacy of lifestyle modifications, but the following may be helpful:

- *Avoid eating 2–3h prior to bedtime:* may reduce TLOSRs in recumbent position.
- *Sleeping in left lateral position:* may reduce TLOSRs.
- Eat small meals.
- *Lose weight:* reduces proximal extent of reflux events, a factor that is important for reflux perception.

There is little/no evidence for alcohol and smoking avoidance (except for cancer reduction), or for sleeping with the head of the bed elevated.

Pharmacological therapies

Proton pump inhibitors (e.g. lansoprazole, omeprazole, pantoprazole)

- Achieve gastric acid control by inhibiting gastric parietal cell H^+/K^+-ATPase, the final common pathway of acid secretion.
- They bind to actively secreting pumps (hence, are best administered 30min before meals).
- Provide oesophagitis healing rates of ~90% at 8 weeks.
- Complete symptomatic response is approximately 70–80% in erosive disease, but lower in NERD (some studies suggest as low as 45%).
- Side-effects are increased risk of *C. difficile* diarrhoea, increased risk of community-acquired pneumonia and osteoporosis.

H2-receptor antagonists (e.g. ranitidine, cimetidine)

- Block gastric acid secretion by 60–70% (which is much less effective than PPIs).
- Limited effect on meal-stimulated acid secretion, with longest duration of activity when taken at night time.
- Symptomatic relief occurs in 30–80%, with similar figures for mucosal healing in oesophagitis.
- Tachyphylaxis common, so on-demand or infrequent treatment best.

Antacids/alginates

These can be used for short-term symptom relief, but have less of a role in persistent symptoms.

Sucralfate

- Mucosal protectant agent that may block diffusion of noxious elements of refluxate across mucosal barrier.
- Has similar mucosal healing to H2-antagonists is seen, but qds regime is required.

Prokinetics

- Theoretically, can improve strength and competence of LOS, and improve oesophageal acid clearance and gastric emptying.

- Most commonly used agents are dopamine antagonists metoclopramide and domperidone; however, clinical efficacy equivocal and there is no effect on oesophageal or LOS motility.
- May have a role in refractory GORD in patients with delayed gastric emptying.

TLOSR inhibitors

Baclofen has been shown to reduce TLOSRs, but symptomatic benefit is equivocal. It may be useful in some patients with refractory reflux, but its use is limited by its side-effect profile.

Medical treatment failure

Approximately one-third of patients with suspected GORD do not respond to PPI therapy. An empirical approach refractory symptoms (see Box 3.6), or an investigation-directed approach with physiological testing may be taken.

> **Box 3.6 Empirical approach to management of refractory GORD symptoms**
> - Careful history to assess nature of residual symptoms and possibility of alternative diagnosis.
> - Check for treatment compliance.
> - Check for dosing time (15–30min before meals).
> - Double the PPI dose for 2 months.
> - Add-on therapy with alginates/sucralfate.
> - Add-on therapy with H2-antagonists (on demand or infrequent use).

The following mechanisms may be important in PPI failure:
- *Alternative diagnosis:* e.g. functional heartburn, dyspepsia, eosinophilic oesophagitis, or pill-induced oesophagitis.
- *Residual acid reflux:* despite PPI therapy.
- Usually related to insufficient compliance with medication, inappropriate dosing regime (should be taken 30min before meals), or insufficient dose. 24-h reflux monitoring can be helpful to evaluate.
- Education regarding dosing regimen, and increased PPI dose to bd ± pre-bedtime H2-antagonist may be appropriate.
- Very rarely patients have altered PPI metabolism or hypersecretion syndromes to account for residual acid reflux.
- *Weakly acidic reflux and duodenogastro-oesophageal reflux:* some patients remain sensitive to refluxates at pH consistent with PPI treatment (i.e. above 4), either due to pH sensitivity or components such as bile acids. Can be demonstrated on pH-impedance testing 'on' PPI. Alginates or sucralfate may be helpful.

Treatment options for PPI-refractory patients with documented GORD

- Patients with persistent troublesome regurgitation despite adequate heartburn control may benefit from anti-reflux surgery.
- Patients with documented NERD or hypersensitive oesophagus when studied 'off' PPI have satisfactory outcome from fundoplication.
- It is thus-far unknown whether fundoplication helps patients with symptomatic weakly acidic reflux on pH impedance studies.
- Baclofen (initially 10mg tds, increasing to 30mg tds) can be considered in all of these groups, but tolerability can be poor.

Further reading

Bredenoord AJ, Fox M, Kahrilas PJ, et al. Chicago classification criteria of esophageal motility disorders defined in high resolution esophageal pressure topography. *Neurogastroenterol Motil* 2012; **24**(Suppl 1): 57–65.

Dean BB, Gano AD, Knight K, et al. Effectiveness of proton pump inhibitors in nonerosive reflux disease. *Clin Gastroenterol Hepatol* 2004; **2**: 656–64.

Dent, J., El-Serag HB, Wallander MA, et al. Epidemiology of gastro-oesophageal reflux disease: a systematic review. *Gut* 2005; **54**(5): 710–717.

Fass R, Sifrim D. Management of heartburn not responding to proton pump inhibitors. *Gut* 2009; **58**: 295–309.

Lundell LR, Dent J, Bennet JR, et al. Endoscopic assessment of oesophagitis: clinical and functional correlates and further validation of the Los Angeles classification. *Gut* 1999; **45**(2): 172–80.

Mainie I, Tutuian R, Shay S, et al. Acid and non-acid reflux in patients with persistent symptoms despite acid suppressive therapy: a multicentre study using combined ambulatory impedance-pH monitoring. *Gut* 2006; **55**(10): 1398–402.

Pandolfino JE, Sifrim D. Evaluation of esophageal contractile propagation using esophageal pressure topography. *Neurogastroenterol Motil* 2012; **24**(Suppl 1): 20–6.

Pandolfino JE, Kwiatek MA, Nealis T, et al. Achalasia: a new clinically relevant classification by high-resolution manometry. *Gastroenterology* 2011; **135**(5): 1526–33.

Pandolfino JE, Roman S, Carlson D, et al. Distal esophageal spasm in high-resolution esophageal pressure topography: defining clinical phenotypes. *Gastroenterology* 2011; **141**(2): 469–75.

Richter J, Castell D. *The Esophagus*, Wiley-Blackwell, Hoboken, 2012.

Salvador R, Costantini, M, Rizzetto C, et al. (2011), Diffuse esophageal spasm: the surgical approach. *Diseases of the esophagus: official journal of the International Society for Diseases of the Esophagus/ISDE.* Available at: http://scholar.qsensei.com/content/1sl1r9 (accessed 5 June 2013).

Vakil N, van Zanten SV, Kahrilas P, et al. The Montreal definition and classification of gastro-oesophageal reflux disease: a global evidence-based consensus. *Am J Gastroenterol* 2006; **101**(8): 1900–20.

Yazaki, E, Sifrim, D. Anatomy and physiology of the esophageal body. *Dis Esophagus* 2012; **25**(4): 292–8.

Surgical management of gastro-oesophageal reflux disease and hiatus hernia

Hiatus hernia

Aetiology

A widening or weakness in the diaphragmatic crura is instrumental in the development of a hiatus hernia. Increased intra-abdominal pressure forces the abdominal viscera through the path of least resistance, in a similar manner to other abdominal wall hernias. Hiatus hernias can be categorized into four distinct entities (Fig. 4.1).

Sliding (Type I)
- Common (95%).
- Often asymptomatic.
- Contributory to acid reflux due to displacement of LOS mechanism in relation to diaphragm.
- Exposes the LOS to negative intrathoracic pressure.
- Symptoms usually related to reflux, rather than hiatus hernia itself.
- Mass effects from hiatus hernias can lead to dyspnoea and dysphagia.

Rolling/para-oesophageal (Type II)
- GOJ remains fixed in proper location.
- Part of stomach herniates into the chest clinically asymptomatic.
  Or
- Presents with definitive symptoms:
  - Dysphagia.
  - Vomiting/regurgitation.
  - *Chest pain*—different in character to heartburn and difficult to differentiate with a cardiac cause.
  - Pressure symptoms within the chest.
  - Dyspnoea if large.

Mixed sliding/para-oesophageal (Type III)
Both GOJ and part of the stomach herniate into the chest:
- Clinically asymptomatic or presents with symptoms of substernal pain.
- Post-prandial fullness.
- Nausea/vomiting.
- Dyspnoea if large.

Type II or III with visceral herniation (Type IV)
- Some debate about name, some believe this is a variation of a type II or III.
- Clinically asymptomatic.
  Or
- Substernal pain.
- Post-prandial fullness.
- Nausea/vomiting.
- Dyspnoea.

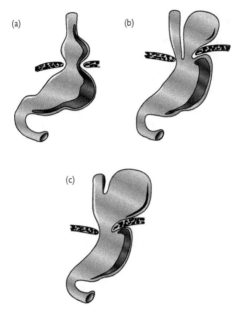

Fig. 4.1 Types of hiatus hernia a) Type I: sliding hernia; b) Type II: rolling/
para-oesophageal hernia; c) Type III: mixed sliding/para-oesophageal hernia.

Anti-reflux surgery

General considerations

Aim of surgery

Improvement in long term quality of life (QoL) as a result of reduction in GORD symptoms and volume reflux:
- No long-term potential systemic effects in comparison with medical treatment.
- Is cost-effective compared with proton pump inhibition.
- When patients demonstrate a particular desire, and when there is clear indication for them to consider surgery, 80% improvement in long-term QoL.
- Effects of successful ARS can decrease over a 5–10-year period.

UK REFLUX trial 2008

This trial compared effectiveness and cost-effectiveness of lap ARS in patients with GORD:
- UK wide. 20 hospitals.
- *Randomized control trials (RCT):* 180 surgery vs. 180 allocated to optimized medical 'recipe' (treatment) (Rx).
- *Parallel cohort:* 261 chose surgery vs. 192 chose to continue with medical Rx. endpoint—QoL.
- Surgical management significantly increases general and reflux specific health-related quality of life (HRQL), at least up to 12 months.
- *Complications rare:* 0.6% open conversion, 2% visceral injury, 0.9% re-operation.
- £20,000 per quality-adjusted life year (QALY). ARS initially more costly as expected benefit from surgery correlates with symptom severity.
- Increased cost of surgery vs. proton-pump inhibitor (PPI) met at 2.5 years if patient remains off PPI.

Long-term results

Booth (2002) 179 patients 2–8 years post-ARS:
- Control of reflux in 85–95%.
- 22% had side-effects, but did not affect overall satisfaction.
- 14% taking PPIs, but not for reflux.
- Results at 1 year predict longer-term outcome.

Indications for anti-reflux surgery

PPIs and lifestyle measures work well for the vast majority of patients reasons to consider surgery:
- Obviates 'dependency' on long-term medication.
- Alternative where side-effects to medication intolerable: such as diarrhoea, headaches, and neurological symptoms.
- Breakthrough symptoms despite full medical treatment.
- Persistent troublesome volume reflux symptoms, such as nocturnal aspiration.
- GORD associated with significant hiatus hernia.
- Extra-oesophageal symptoms of GORD.
- Poor compliance with drug treatment.
- Personal choice and a reluctance to take tablets long-term.

Complicated reflux disease

Constitutes:
- Strictures that require frequent dilatation may do better when reflux is controlled surgically, rather than with proton pump inhibitors.
- Failure of medical therapy in presence of non-healing ulcers or bleeding, especially when Barrett's is present and malignancy has been excluded.

Medical indications

- Learning disabilities, cerebral palsy, recurrent chest infections, and failure to thrive in children.
- Chronic dyspnoea 2° to large para-oesophageal hernias.

Anti-reflux surgery and cancer

Anxiety relating to long-term effects of reflux and malignant potential—there is no data to support the benefit of surgery.
- No clear evidence to show majority of patients well-controlled on PPI receive any true benefit from surgery in comparison with best medical therapy.
- *ARS for cancer risk reduction in Barrett's oesophagus by anti-reflux surgery:* no conclusive supporting evidence.
- *DeMeester:* small study—patients with intact wrap from anti-reflux surgery show less Barrett's progression to dysplasia and cancer than those with a disrupted wrap.

Society of American Gastrointestinal and Endoscopic Surgeons (SAGES) guidelines for anti-reflux surgery

Indications
- Diagnosis objectively confirmed.

Or
- Failed management (inadequate symptom control, severe regurgitation not controlled with acid suppression, or medication side effects).

Or
- Opt for surgery despite successful medical management (quality of life (QoL), lifelong need for PPIs, PPI cost).

Or
- Complications of GORD (e.g. Barrett's oesophagus, peptic stricture).

Or
- Extra-oesophageal sx (asthma, hoarseness, cough, chest pain, aspiration).

Barrett's with GORD considered clear indication for ARS by many, but asymptomatic Barrett's controversial. Evidence: metaplasia may regress, but no change in adenocarcinoma rates.

Medical vs. surgical treatment

- *7 RCTs follow-up 1–10.6-years ARS vs. medical PPI for GORD:* strongly support ARS as effective alternative to PPIs with good symptom control on PPIs or partial relief (level I).
- *pH metry/manometric data:* ARS less acid exposure and significantly increased LOS pressure compared with PPI.
- *ARS:* improved or at least comparable QoL, cf. PPI and high patient satisfaction rates.

- PPI use post-ARS 9–21% up to 8 years post-operatively (level I–III). However, no GORD recurrence on 24-h pH studies for majority (level II).
- *Cost:* RCT Myrvold (2001): ARS vs. PPI over a 5-year period. Total cost lower Denmark, Norway, and Sweden and higher in Finland (level I).
- Cost equivalency point for PPI and ARS 10 years.
- ARS equally effective alternative to PPI and should be offered to appropriately selected patients by appropriately skilled surgeons (Grade A). ARS effectively addresses mechanical issues and results in long-term patient satisfaction (Grade A). For surgery to compete with PPI, it has to be associated with minimal morbidity and cost.

LOTUS trial

- *Attwood 2008:* 5-year randomized, open, parallel-group trial 11 European countries 2001–2009. 554 patients well-established GORD who initially responded to PPIs. 372 patients (esomeprazole, $n = 192$; ARS, $n = 180$) completed 5-year follow-up.
- *266 patients:* esomeprazole, 20–40mg/day vs. 248 ARS standardized Nissen vs. PPI 40 experienced upper gastrointestinal (UGI) surgeons.
  - Opening of phreno-oesophageal ligament in a left to right fashion.
  - Preservation of the hepatic branch of the anterior vagus nerve.
  - Dissection of both crura.
  - Trans-hiatal mobilization to allow approximately 3cm of intra-abdominal oesophagus.
  - Short gastric vessel division to ensure a tension-free wrap.
  - Crural closure posteriorly with non-absorbable sutures.
  - Creation of a 1.5–2-cm wrap with most distal suture incorporating anterior muscular wall of oesophagus.
  - Bougie placement at time of wrap construction.
- *Excellent outcomes cf. PPI:* 2% conversion rate, 3% post-operative complication rate, median post-operative length of stay of 2 days.
- *PPI vs. ARS:* Remission rates: 5 years: 92 vs. 85% in not statistically significant. Symptoms: 16 and 8% for heartburn ($P = 0.14$), 13 and 2% for acid regurgitation ($P < 0.001$), 5 and 11% for dysphagia ($P < 0.001$), 28 and 40% for bloating ($P < 0.001$), and 40 and 57% for flatulence ($P < 0.001$). Serious adverse events were similar in the esomeprazole group (24.1%) and in ARS group (28.6%).

Contra-indications

Patients are unlikely to benefit from surgery if they demonstrate:
- Lack of reflux on pH/bile reflux monitoring.
- A 1° motility disturbance, such as achalasia or nutcracker oesophagus on manometry. These patients will only benefit from anti-reflux surgery if it is combined with a myotomy.
- IBS, gas bloat pre-operatively, fibromyalgia, and arthritis.
- *Impaired oesophageal motility:* presence of weak peristaltic amplitudes or poor oesophageal propagation not a contraindication to ARS.

Patient fitness

- Risk-benefit analysis with patient essential before offering ARS.
- Good cardio-respiratory function, mobility, and an independent lifestyle are desirable in patients being considered for ARS.

- Patients with poorly controlled asthma/chronic obstructive pulmonary disease (COPD) thought to have nocturnal silent aspiration show significant improvement in respiratory function post-operatively therefore an exception.
- *Morbid obesity:* gastric bypass may be a better approach.
- Rheumatic diseases limiting mobility relative contraindication ARS.

Operative considerations for anti-reflux surgery

Aim of ARS

- Improvement in patient symptoms.
- *Restoration of anti-reflux mechanism:* mechanism poorly understood. Increased LOS basal pressure reduced TLOSR, creation of GOJ/ fundal valve.
- *General principles:* mobilize GOJ, reduce any hiatus hernia (HH), repair hiatal defect, fashion fundoplication wrap.

Type of ARS procedure

Posterior wraps

Nissen

- *360°:* originally described as 5-cm wrap, vagal preservation, no Bougie, no short gastric mobilization, no hiatal repair. Hiatal repair consistently incorporated now, 1–2cm wrap, some use 52F Bougie.
- *Floppy Nissen:* Donahu and Bombeck description. Extensive fundal mobilization and short gastric mobilization.
- Currently most common version of 'Nissen fundoplication' short floppy wrap with selective division of short gastrics.
- *Toupet:* partial 270°. Rationale formation of valve at wrap with reduced competence compared with Nissen, degree of competence can be 'tailored' presumed benefit reduction of dysphagia, gas problems. Wrap sutured to left and right walls of oesophagus and right crus.
- *Lind:* 300° as Toupet.

Anterior wraps

- *Watson:* 120° and 180°, posterior hiatal repair, suture of anterior fundal wrap to diaphragm to create neo-angle of His, sutures to right and left oesophagus/crura.
- *Dor:* fundus sutured to left and right oesophagus or crura in modifications.
- *Belsey Mark IV:* left thoracotomy approach, distal oesophagus mobilized, anterior 2/3 wrap sutures to fundus and diaphragm.

General

- ARS predominantly conducted laparoscopically.
- Many modifications or subtle technique changes added by experienced operators.
- Patient fully informed and consented for procedure and possible technical modifications, e.g. conversion to open, and possibility of thoracotomy for large associated HH.
- Thromboprophylaxis should be used according to local guidelines and WHO checklist guidelines adhered to.

Port sites and patient positioning
- Reverse Trendelenburg or French position.
- Patient secured, often by wrapping arms with sheets and tucking under torso.
- 1° operator positioned between patients' legs, with camera holder/ assistant dependent on dominant hand, i.e. left-hand dominant standing on patients left.
- Scrub nurse positioned to patients' right.

Equipment
- Nathanson liver retractor + fast-clamp™ or equivalent.
- Laparoscopic needle holder ×2.
- Laparoscopic knot pusher.
- Harmonic scalpel or equivalent haemostatic dissector.
- Johann tissue forceps (×2 short blade, ×1 long blade).
- Babcock tissue grasper.
- 30° Laparoscope (10mm).

Port sites
See Fig. 4.2.

Positioned to avoid instrument clashing, improve ergonomics, and increased angulation to aid depth of field perception.

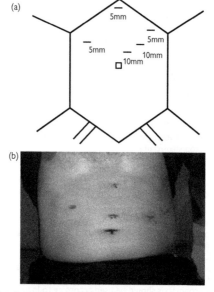

Fig. 4.2 Port site positioning. (a) Suggested port sites for laparoscopic gastric fundoplication. (b) Port site scars after laparoscopic gastric fundoplication.

Camera port (10–12mm)
2/3 from xiphisternum to umbilicus ~40mm left of midline.

Epigastric/xiphisternum (5mm)
Used for liver retraction, such as Nathanson laparoscopic liver retractor.

Right upper quadrant (5mm)
- Approximate angle of 30–45° from midline at xiphisternum.
- Used for left hand instrumentation.

Left upper quadrant (10–12mm)
- Approximate angle of 30–45° from midline at xiphisternum.
- Used for right hand instrumentation and insertion of sutures/needle.

Left flank/costal margin (5mm)
Used for tissue retraction/manipulation by assistant.

Hiatus repair
- For all fundoplication procedures essential to first reduce any HH and repair any hiatal defect (Fig. 4.3).
- Usually straight forward and stomach can be pulled down through diaphragm to its normal anatomical position.
- If condition longstanding and in case of large para-oesophageal herniae dissection up through hiatus and mediastinum required to free adhesions.
- Care taken to avoid pneumothoraces by identifying and carefully dissecting the hernia sac away from pleura.
- Pars flaccida incised to enter lesser sac haemostatic dissection continued up to right pillar of the left crus of the diaphragm.
- Hernia sac dissected from pillar of the crus and this followed posteriorly to where it meets left pillar.
- The oesophagus then mobilized, carefully preserving both Vagus nerves. Essential step to ensure GOJ lies tension free below hiatus.
- Window then made behind oesophagus fully mobilizing it and allowing retraction either with Nylon tape or instrument (Fig. 4.4).
- Hiatus repaired using non-absorbable interrupted sutures to close the defect, e.g. Ethibond.
- Ensure enough space to allow a food bolus to pass equates to passing a 10mm instrument alongside the oesophagus in the hiatus.
- Crural integrity often more robust anteriorly to hold sutures for repair.
- Oesophageal Bougie can be used as a size guide (Fig. 4.5).
- If hiatal defect resistant to 1° suture closure mesh or collagen prosthesis, e.g. surgisys/permacol may be used, risk adhesions, hiatal stenosis, and migration into oesophageal lumen.
- At this stage may be necessary to divide the short gastric arteries to enable adequate mobilization of the gastric fundus (Fig. 4.6).

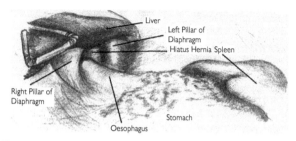

Fig. 4.3 Laparoscopic view of diaphragmatic hiatus anatomy.

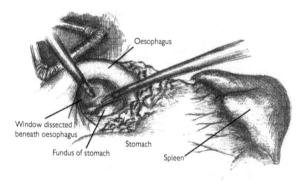

Fig. 4.4 Creation of a posterior window.

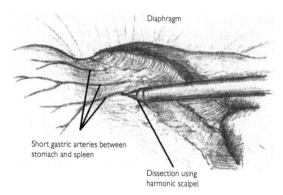

Fig. 4.5 Short gastric vessels.

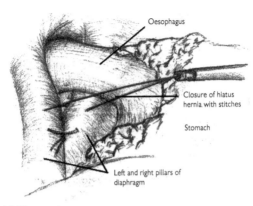

Fig. 4.6 Hiatus repair.

Nissen and Toupet fundoplication

With the fundus adequately mobilized and a window created behind the oesophagus it is now possible to pull the gastric fundus through creating a posterior wrap (Fig. 4.7). The fundus is drawn posteromedially and a 'shoe shine' manoeuvre performed to ensure adequate tension free mobilization.

- *Nissen fundoplication:* full 360° wrap performed and fundus sutured in position with 3–4 interrupted non-absorbable sutures.
- Over a distance of 2–3cm. Wrap fashioned to ensure no posterior redundancy and wrap sits at GOJ (diagram).
- *Variation:* two layers of sutures including either the oesophagus and/or hiatus within one or more stitches (Fig. 4.8).
- 'Floppiness' of wrap should be tested by the ability to elevate the wrap anteriorly from the oesophagus.
- Toupet technique involves a 270° posterior wrap. Sutured using interrupted non-absorbable stitches to both the oesophagus and pillars of the hiatus (Fig. 4.9).

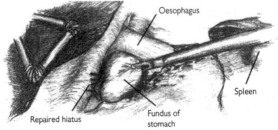

Fig. 4.7 Gastric pull through.

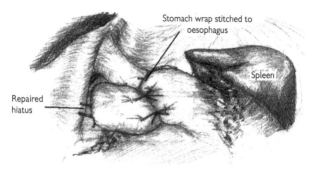

Fig. 4.8 Completed Nissen wrap.

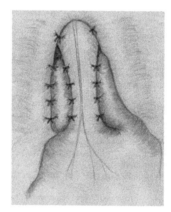

Fig. 4.9 Final view of completed Toupet fundoplication.

Dor fundoplication
- *Dor fundoplication:* often used in conjunction with a cardiomyotomy or a simple Hiatus repair more with paraoesophageal hernias.
- 180° Anterior wrap fundus anchored to diaphragm with non-absorbable interrupted sutures.

Collis gastroplasty
- Oesophageal lengthening procedure largely historic.
- Oesophageal shortening exceedingly rare in post-PPI era.
- Traditionally patients with large HH for many years, often with significant sequelae of long-term reflux difficult to reduce stomach down into the abdominal cavity.

- If undue tension is present, risk of recurrence of hiatus hernia is high.
- *Procedure:* proximal stomach divided in a cranio-caudal manner along the angle of His, essentially elongating oesophagus by including proximal stomach win its length.
- Can be performed laparoscopically using a stapling device, but if gastroplasty is required, surgery may have been converted to open due to difficulty in reducing hernia.
- Extra length available to oesophagus then reduces tension on stomach; wrap can be performed as normal.

Comparisons in outcome according to operative approach: incorporating SAGES guidelines for anti-reflux surgery (2010)

Partial vs. total fundoplication

- 11 RCTs and two meta-analyses have investigated differences between partial and total fundoplications and one randomized controlled trial between two partial fundoplication.
- *1 peri-operative death:* 0.07% oesophageal injury resulting in mediastinitis.
- No differences in peri-operative morbidity across all published studies by two meta-analyses (level I).
- *No differences in the operation time:* average 90min.
- *>Dysphagia, bloating, flatulence, and re-operation rate:* total compared with partial fundoplication (level I).
- No differences in oesophagitis, heartburn, persisting acid reflux.
- Tailoring fundoplication type for oesophageal dysmotility does not change outcome (level I).

Anterior vs. Nissen fundoplication

- *4 RCTs 457 patients:* follow-up 6 months to 10 years.
- Two studies 180° anterior fundoplication and other two a 90°.
- *Anterior fundoplication:* <dysphagia up to 10 years (level I), but < reflux control (based on patient symptoms and objective tests) as more re-operations for reflux control 90 (level I).
- Satisfaction similar between groups in all studies up to 10 years after surgery (level I).
- 90° vs. 180° fundoplication difference unclear, as no comparative studies; however, Engstrom (2007) have suggest 90° is inadequate (level I).

Watson (1999)

- *Prospective double blind randomized trial 107 patients:* Nissen vs. 180° anterior. No outcome difference at 1/12 and 3/12.
- *6/12 & 5-year follow-up:* reduced dysphagia, flatulence, normal belching, overall dissatisfaction.
- Reflux control marginally better in Nissen cohort, but overall satisfaction 94 vs. 86% Nissen vs. anterior.

Watson (2004)

- *112 patients:* multicentre prospective double blind randomized trial Nissen vs. anterior 90° fundoplication. Australia and NZ.
- *Anterior:* reduced dysphagia, flatulence, higher incidence recurrent reflux, greater overall satisfaction, and QoL.

Baigrie (2005)
- *161 patients:* randomized double blind Nissen vs. anterior 180°.
- *Follow-up at 2 years:* reflux control similar, but re-operation for recurrent reflux greater in anterior cohort, ant: reduced dysphagia.

Toupet vs. Nissen fundoplication
- Nine RCTs (including both open and laparoscopic techniques) with follow-up 1–5 years (level I).
- Majority show lower dysphagia for Toupet fundoplication and no difference in heartburn or other symptoms (level I).
- *Lundell (1991):* prospective randomized clinical trial. 137 patients—Nissen vs. Toupet 6/12 similar outcomes.
- *Lundell (1996):* 5-year outcomes—dysphagia, reflux control similar, flatulence worse post Nissen at 2 & 3 years, but same at 5 years. Re-operation for para-oesophageal herniation in Nissen cohort.
- *Hagedorn (2002):* 11.5 year follow-up of Lundell trial—similar reflux control—Nissen 88%/Toupet 92%. Toupet—reduced flatulence and post-prandial fullness.
- *Zornig (2002):* 200 patients reduced short-term dysphagia, partial posterior vs. Nissen.
- *Durability of partial fundoplications:* Jobe (1997), 51% post-Toupet—pathological acid exposure on 24h pH study of which 40% asymptomatic.
- *Mickevicius (2008) lengths of fundoplication (1.5 vs. 3cm):* 3cm Toupet superior reflux control without differences in dysphagia.
- Nissen fundoplication length does not influence reflux control, but a trend for a higher dysphagia rate noted with 3cm wrap at 12-month follow-up (level I).
- Maximal follow-up 5 years for prospective studies retrospective studies suggest inferior long-term reflux control after Toupet (level III).

Anterior vs. Toupet fundoplication
- *Hagedorn (2003):* 120° anterior and 180–200° posterior 95 patients for 5 years (93% follow-up).
- Posterior fundoplication superior to anterior by achieving better reflux control without increased dysphagia.
- Statistically significantly higher PPI intake, more oesophageal acid exposure, higher re-operation rates, and lower patient satisfaction after anterior fundoplication during long-term follow-up and concluded that an anterior repair cannot be recommended for GORD due to insufficient reflux control (level I).

Tailored wraps
- *Rydberg (1999):* retrospective analysis of Lundell trial (1999). Manometrically proven dysmotility does not predispose poor outcomes following Nissen vs. Toupet.
- *Zornig (2002):* 200patients—Nissen vs. partial posterior. 100 abnormal oesophageal motility, 100 normal.
- 4/12 equivalent reflux control 90% overall satisfaction.
- *2 years:* 85% satisfaction. No correlation between dysmotility and outcomes ∴ selective 'tailored' partial fundoplication unwarranted.

- *Patti (2004):* 357 patients. 235 tailored, partial, or Nissen, partial for dysmotility 122 patients not tailored straight to Nissen.
- *Tailored:* 19% heartburn recurrence post-partial, 4% post-Nissen. Dysphagia equivalent.
- *Overall:* little evidence tailoring wraps improves outcomes in context of abnormal oesophageal peristalsis, but confirmed reflux.

Recommendation
- *Partial fundoplication:* less dysphagia, fewer re-operations, and similar patient satisfaction and effectiveness in controlling GORD compared with total fundoplication up to 5 years after surgery (Grade A).
- Tailored approach to oesophageal motility unwarranted (Grade B).
- Paucity of long-term follow-up hard to recommend one type of fundoplication over the other especially in an era where the long-term effectiveness of ARS questioned.
- Anterior partial fundoplication may be less effective in the long term (Grade B) and retrospective data suggests that partial fundoplication may not be as effective as total in the long run (Grade C).
- Surgeons may choose partial fundoplication to reduce dysphagia (Grade A) or a short total fundoplication (1–2cm) over a large Bougie (56 French) (Grade C) and maximize effectiveness of procedure by choosing a total fundoplication (Grade C) or a longer (at least 3cm) posterior fundoplication (Grade C).

Short gastric vessel division
- 5 RCTs: no difference in physiological, symptomatic, and QoL outcomes up to 10 years after surgery 107–111 (level I).
- Division increases operating time (level I–II), increase flatus production and epigastric bloating, and decrease ability to vent air from stomach (level I).
- *Watson (1997):* 102 patients Nissen with/without short gastric division.
- Equivalent outcomes at 6/12, no early post-operative dysphagia.
- *5 years follow-up:* reflux control similar, increased gas bloat, flatulence, and epigastric fullness if short gastrics divided.
- *10 years follow-up:* no significant difference in outcomes. 85–90% success.

Recommendations
- When wrap without significant tension feasible, no division of short gastrics necessary (Grade A).
- Division should be undertaken when a tension-free fundoplication cannot be accomplished (Grade B).

Crural closure: recommendations
- Strongly considered during fundoplication when hiatal opening is large and mesh reinforcement may be beneficial in decreasing incidence of wrap herniation (Grade B).
- Anterior crural closure may be associated with less post-operative dysphagia, but additional evidence is needed to provide a firm recommendation (Grade C).

ARS in the morbidly obese patient
- GORD more prevalent as BMI increases.
- Reduced long-term effectiveness of fundoplication where BMI >30 (level II–III) compared with normal weight patients.

- Laparoscopic Roux-en-Y gastric bypass is the most effective and recommended treatment option. Treats GORD, reduces weight, and improves comorbidities (level II–III).
- Also feasible and efficacious post-ARS surgery, but technically demanding and higher morbidity (level III).
- Gastric banding not procedure of choice.

Use of Bougie
- *Patterson (2000) RCT:* 171 patients 1996–1998.
- *Reduced dysphagia:* 17 vs. 31% at 11/12 follow-up if 56F sizing Bougie placed at the time of surgery. No difference in mortality.
- 1.2% incidence of oesophageal injury due to placement of Bougie.
- Bougie recommended (Grade B).

Predictors of success

Preoperative patient compliance
With anti-reflux medications, significantly reduced HRQL outcome and higher rates of dysphagia in non-compliant.

Age
No significant effect on outcomes, > 65 years excellent outcome after surgery in 90%.

Post-operative diaphragmatic stressors
- *Sudden increases in intra-abdominal pressure:* early post-operative period predispose anatomical failure. Gagging, belching, and vomiting (especially when associated with gagging) are predisposing factors for anatomical failure and the need for revision (level III).
- *Hiatal hernias >3cm:* at predict anatomic failure (level II).

Psychological disease and intervention
Quality of life improvement reduced and severe dysphagia/bloating more common in major depression (level II).

Atypical symptoms
Chest pain, asthma, chronic cough, hoarseness, otitis media, atypical loss of dental enamel, idiopathic pulmonary fibrosis, recurrent pneumonia, and chronic bronchitis predict poor outcome (level II).

Good symptom correlation with reflux
During combined oesophageal impedance and pH monitoring (level II).

Oesophageal function
A normal LOS pressure not associated with increased dysphagia (level II). Non-specific spastic disorders—nutcracker oesophagus, hypertensive LOS syndrome, increased risk for heartburn, regurgitation, and dysphagia after a 360° wrap (level II).

Patterns of reflux
Upright reflux vs. supine
More maladaptive behaviours, reflux, aerophagia, regurgitation, dyspepsia, but Nissen equally effective (level II).

Response to preoperative PPI

Excellent predictor of symptomatic response to fundoplication, but non-response to PPI not a contra-indication to ARS (level II).

Preoperative gastric emptying

Wayman (2007): large prospective non-randomized trial showed no relationship between gastric emptying and outcome following fundoplication (level II).

Revisional surgery for failed anti-reflux procedures

- Same surgical approach for the re-operative patient as for primary procedure recommended (level III).
- *Revisional surgery:* longer operative times, higher conversion rates (level III), higher complication rates (30-day mortality <1%, oesophagogastric perforations in 11–25%, gastric more often than oesophageal perforation, pneumothorax in 7%–18%, splenic injuries in 2% and vagal nerve injuries in 7%, but dysphagia (3–17%) and gas bloat syndrome (5–34%) not higher after re-operation compared with 1° repair.
- Satisfaction after re-operative ARS high (89%). Resolution of heartburn 68–89%, regurgitation in 83–88% at 18/12 13% of patient reflux recurrence at 3/12.
- Should be undertaken only by experienced surgeons using a similar approach to 1° fundoplication (Grade B).

Outcomes

Symptoms

- Heartburn symptoms 87% cure recurrence rates of 10%.
- Regurgitation rates reduced by 87–97% recurrent or new onset regurgitation has been reported in up to 23%: 0–11% common.
- Atypical reflux symptoms to anti-reflux surgery. A typical symptom improvement 67–92%.
- *Cough:* cure rates of 53% short-term improvement rates from 69–100% long-term improvement rates of 71%.
- Hoarseness, sore throat, bronchitis pulmonary symptoms, aspiration asthma laryngitis contradictory reports.

Investigations

- Significant increase in LOS pressure.
- Significant decrease in acid exposure compared with preoperative values are documented in both short- and long-term studies, with pH studies returning to normal in approximately 88–94% of patients.

Post-operative complications

- Conversion rates to open surgery for laparoscopic anti-reflux surgery (LARS) 0–24% high-volume centres <2.4% 32–34, 39 (level I).
- *Specific complications related to LARS:* gastric and oesophageal perforation 0–4% (level I–III) highest after redo ARS pneumothorax during laparoscopic anti-reflux surgery in most series range from 0–1.5% (level I–III).
- *30-day mortality:* rarely reported usually 0% (level I–III). NHS national litigation authority reports multiple cases.
- Wound infections 0.2–3.1% (level II–III).
- Port-site hernias 0.17–9%.

- Herniation of wrap and migration vary related to the technique used and the duration of follow-up 0.8–26% (level I–III).
- Re-operation: 0–15% (level II–III).

Operative time
- 49–210min (level I–III).
- Learning curve 15–20 cases with improved operating times as the number of cases increases (level II–III).
- High-volume centres reporting shorter operating room times (49–120min).

Length of stay post-operative
1–4 days (level I–III).

Quality of life and satisfaction with surgery
62–97% (level II–III) with long-term satisfaction rates (follow-up >5 years) ranging from 80–96% (level II–III). Additionally, 81–95% of patients, in both short- and long-term follow-up, stated that they would undergo surgery again (level II–III). QoL significantly improved after laparoscopic anti-reflux surgery in both early and long-term studies as documented from a variety of QoL surveys including generic and disease-specific QoL (level I–III).

Endoscopic therapies and laparoscopic device insertion

Endoscopic therapies to alter the anatomy of the LOS are an attractive concept. Implant/injection, thermal, and plicating devices developed, but clinical efficacy limited and remain 'evolving'.

Techniques developed
Radiofrequency energy: e.g. Stretta procedure
- Used radiofrequency energy to reduce GOJ luminal diameter.
- Initial results poor: withdrawn.

Injectable polymers: Enteryx
- Used injection of biocompatible non-biodegradeable bulking polymers into oesophagus at level of GOJ to narrow it.
- Poor results and high complication rates: withdrawn.

Suturing techniques: EndoCinch™, or NDO Plicator™
- Use endoscopic sutures to plicate the mucosa of the gastric cardia to reduce reflux.
- Better results than with radiofrequency or polymers, but not as effective as surgical fundoplication.[1,2]

Endoscopic fundoplication (EsophyX™, or Medigus™)
- See Fig. 4.10. Attempt to produce a surgical anterior fundoplication endoscopically.
- Early results are more promising than other endoscopic techniques although comparison of Esophyx™ technique with surgical fundoplication shows long-term results to be inferior.

[1] Schwartz MP, Wellink H, Goozen HG, et al. Endoscopic gastroplication for the treatment of gastro-oesophageal reflux disease: a randomized, sham-controlled trial. *Gut* 2007; **56**: 20–8.

[2] Watson DI, Jamieson GG, Pike GK, et al. A prospective randomized double blind trial between laparoscopic Nissen fundoplication and anterior partial fundoplication. *Br J Surg* 1999; **86**: 123–30.

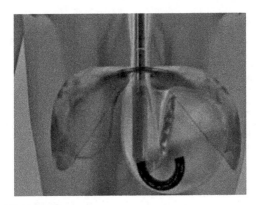

Fig. 4.10 Esophyx™.
Copyright 2013 EndoGastric Solutions®, Inc.

Linx™
See Fig. 4.11.
- Laparoscopic LOS augmentation by magnetic bead band placed around oesophageal sizer.
- Ring of interlinked titanium beads, each with a weak magnetic force that holds beads together to keep distal oesophagus closed. On swallowing, magnetic force overcome, allowing ring to open. After swallowing, beads attract and distal oesophagus closed.
- *Efficacy:* single case series 44 patients up to 4 years follow-up—mean GORD HRQL symptom score improved 25.7–3.8 at 1 year, 2.4 at 2 years (lower scores indicate a higher QoL; $P < 0.0001$ for both) 87% satisfied at 1 year 86% 2 years.
- Decrease in mean time 24h pH< 4, 12%; 3% at 1 year, 2% at 2 years ($P < 0.0001$ for both). 90% cessation PPI at 1 year and 86% 2 years.
- *NICE guidance 2012:* evidence on safety and efficacy limited. Should only be used with special arrangements for clinical governance, consent, and audit or research.

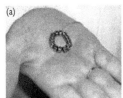
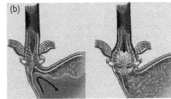

Fig. 4.11 LINX™ reflux management system.
Figure 4.11b with kind permission of Torax Medical Ltd.

Assessment and management of treatment failure and complications

Early complications and failure

Intra-operative complications:

- *Bleeding:* short gastrics, splenic artery, muscular crural branches, liver parenchyma (check liver retractor) inferior phrenic vein, abberant branches of left gastrics, left gastric vessels particularly when encountered high in large paroesophageal herniae. Rare IVC, aorta, cardiac tamponade recognized in litigation data where wrap sutured or tacked to diaphragm underlying pericardium.
- *Damage to local structures:* port puncture of stomach, small bowel, mesenteric vessels, great vessels all recognized, damage to stomach wall, small bowel, colonic splenic flexure. Be aware of delayed thermal injury due to aggressive use of harmonic scalpel and/or diathermy. Omentum can be used as a heat sink. Solid organs—spleen, liver, heart. Also vagus nerves.

Failure of surgery within the first 24h

- Hiatus repair or wrap disruption.
- *Repaired within 12h:* minimal adhesions.
- Consider contrast radiology study to ensure correct position of wrap prior to post-operative feeding.
- Delayed surgical disruption related to retching or attempted vomiting, may be precipitated by bolus obstruction or dysphagia.
- Risk reduced by a modified diet 2–6 weeks post-operative liquid diet, slowly progressing to soft or pureed food, and finally to a normal diet.

Early dysphagia

- Relatively common 2° to new conformation of GOJ/oedema. Can be debilitating.
- If severe usually subsides within 3/12, but occasionally persists.
- *Investigate:* contrast swallow/OGD to ensure correct anatomical position of wrap and exclude recurrence of HH/mediastinal migration of wrap with risk of strangulation. May present as acute emergency post-discharge.
- OGD can also be therapeutic if symptoms necessitate oesophageal balloon dilatation, which can relieve this problem.
- Occasionally, symptoms not relieved by dilatation and further operational intervention required.
- High resolution manometry useful to delineate physiological correlation with symptoms and may detect motility motifs not seen by contrast study or OGD.
- Side effects of surgery occasionally too great for patient to tolerate. Despite extensive counselling before surgery, some patients will still be unhappy with gas bloat or flatulent symptoms, and can request for wrap to be taken down.

Late complications

Recurrent reflux

- Disruption of fundoplication wrap.
- Recurrence of a hiatus hernia.
- *First line therapy:* best medical therapy.
- Exclude a neoplasm in patients with new onset dyspepsia or dysphagia obtain.
- OGD, contrast radiography, pH, and manometry studies of the oesophagus.

Revision surgery

- Consider only if symptoms severe and/or reflux proven on investigation with anatomical disruption of wrap or hiatus.
- Risk of conversion to open surgery due to adhesions, success rate of surgery reduced by half.
- Open surgery frequently required if prosthetic mesh has been employed to close a large hiatal defect as adhesions are often dense and numerous.
- If hiatus hernia has recurred/wrap migration it is also necessary to counsel patient regarding need for a left thoracic approach to hiatus. This carries an increased morbidity, but may be only way to perform surgery safely.

Operative principles

- Divide adhesions between left lobe of liver and wrap.
- Mobilize GOJ and wrap. Concurrent gastroscopy suggested.

Inspect crural repair

- *Tight:* hiatal stenosis—divide adhesions and remove sutures to optimize.
- *Disrupted crural repair with wrap migration:* reduce migrated segment, and repair defect, may require prosthetic mesh. If wrap geometrically adequate retain otherwise refashion.

Inspect wrap

- *If loose:* but geometrically correct, may only require resuturing.
- *If tight:* will require adequate mobilization of stomach/short gastric division and refashioning of wrap.
- *Geometrically incorrect wrap:*
  - *Slipped*—often due to inadequate mobilization of GOJ. Undo wrap, adequate mobilization of distal oesophagus and GOJ, and refashioning of wrap.
  - *Twisted wrap*—mobilize fully and refashion with appropriate repositioning of sutures.
- When refashioning wrap consider conversion to a partial wrap or posterior to anterior depending on configuration encountered.

Persistent dysphagia

Causes

- Redundant fundus forming pouch above or posterior to wrap.
- Hiatal stenosis secondary to tight closure/adhesions.
- Tight wrap.
- General adhesions.
- Missed diagnosis of achalasia.

Management

Exclude a mechanical cause

- Bread contrast, OGD (+ sizing balloons).
- HRM is gold standard investigation.
- 10% have no demonstrable mechanical cause.
- Consider balloon dilatation.
- Laparoscopy and proceed with adhesionolysis, wrap dissection and reconfiguration—partial or anterior.

Fig. 4.12, Fig. 4.13, Fig. 4.14, Fig. 4.15, and Fig. 4.16 demonstrate some of the complications of hiatus hernia repair.

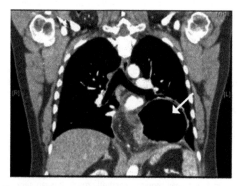

Fig. 4.12 Coronal CT view of hiatus hernia (white arrow).
With kind permission of Torax Medical Ltd.

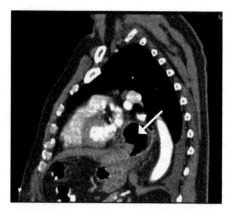

Fig. 4.13 Sagittal CT view of hiatus hernia (white arrow).

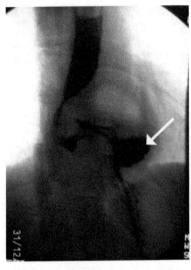

Fig. 4.14 Barium swallow demonstrating pooling of contrast (white arrow) above the left hemidiaphragm, within a mixed hiatus hernia.

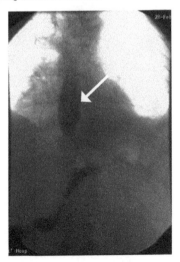

Fig. 4.15 Barium swallow demonstrating pooling of contrast (white arrow) within a sliding hiatus hernia.

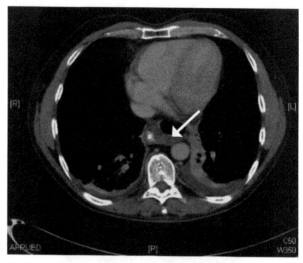

Fig. 4.16 Axial thoracic CT image demonstrating fluid level within hiatus hernia (white arrow).

Further reading

Baigrie RJ, Cullis SN, Ndhluni AJ, et al. Randomized double-blind trial of laparoscopic Nissen fundoplication versus anterior partial fundoplication. Br J Surg 2005; 92(7): 819–23.

Booth MI, Jones L, Stratford J, Dehn TC. Results of laparoscopic Nissen fundoplication at 2–8 years after surgery. Br J Surg 2002; 89(4): 476–81.

Engström C, Lönroth H, Mardani J, Lundell L. An anterior or posterior approach to partial fundoplication? Long-term results of a randomized trial. World J Surg 2007; 31(6): 1221–5.

Hagedorn C, Jönson C, Lönroth H, et al. Efficacy of an anterior as compared with a posterior laparoscopic partial fundoplication: results of a randomized, controlled clinical trial. Ann Surg 2003; 238(2): 189–96.

Hagedorn C, Lönroth H, Rydberg L, et al. Long-term efficacy of total (Nissen-Rossetti) and posterior partial (Toupet) fundoplication: results of a randomized clinical trial. J Gastrointest Surg 2002; 6(4): 540–5.

Jobe BA, Wallace J, Hansen PD, et al. Evaluation of laparoscopic Toupet fundoplication as a primary repair for all patients with medically resistant gastroesophageal reflux. Surg Endosc 1997; 11(11): 1080–3.

Lundell L, Abrahamsson H, Ruth M, et al. Long-term results of a prospective randomized comparison of total fundic wrap (Nissen-Rossetti) or semifundoplication (Toupet) for gastro-oesophageal reflux. Br J Surg 1996; 83(6): 830–5.

Lundell L, Abrahamsson H, Ruth M, et al. Lower esophageal sphincter characteristics and esophageal acid exposure following partial or 360 degrees fundoplication: results of a prospective, randomized, clinical study. World J Surg 1991; 15(1): 115–20.

Mickevicius A, Endzinas Z, Kiudelis M, et al. Influence of wrap length on the effectiveness of Nissen and Toupet fundoplication: a prospective randomized study. Surg Endosc 2008; 22(10): 2269–76. doi: 10.1007/s00464-008-9852-9.

Myrvold HE, Lundell L, Miettinen P, et al. The cost of long term therapy for gastro-oesophageal reflux disease: a randomised trial comparing omeprazole and open antireflux surgery. Gut 2001; 49(4): 488–94.

Patterson EJ, Herron DM, Hansen PD, et al. Effect of an esophageal bougie on the incidence of dysphagia following nissen fundoplication: a prospective, blinded, randomized clinical trial. Arch Surg 2000; 135(9): 1055–62.

Patti MG, Robinson T, Galvani C, et al. Total fundoplication is superior to partial fundoplication even when esophageal peristalsis is weak. J Am Coll Surg 2004; 198(6): 863–70.

Rydberg L, Ruth M, Abrahamsson H, et al. Tailoring antireflux surgery: A randomized clinical trial. World J Surg 1999; 23(6): 612–18.

SAGES guidelines Committee. Guidelines for surgical treatment of gastroesophageal reflux disease. Surg Endosc 2010; 24(11): 2647–69. doi: 10.1007/s00464-010-1267-8.

Watson DI, Jamieson GG, Lally C, et al. Multicenter, prospective, double-blind, randomized trial of laparoscopic nissen vs anterior 90 degrees partial fundoplication. Arch Surg 2004; 139(11): 1160–7.

Watson DI, Jamieson GG, Pike GK, et al. Prospective randomized double-blind trial between laparoscopic Nissen fundoplication and anterior partial fundoplication. Br J Surg 1999; 86(1): 123–30.

Watson DI, Pike GK, Baigrie RJ, et al. Prospective double-blind randomized trial of laparoscopic Nissen fundoplication with division and without division of short gastric vessels. Ann Surg 1997; 226(5): 642–52.

Wayman J, Myers JC, Jamieson GG. Preoperative gastric emptying and patterns of reflux as predictors of outcome after laparoscopic fundoplication. Br J Surg 2007; 94(5): 592–8.

Zornig C, Strate U, Fibbe C, et al. Nissen vs Toupet laparoscopic fundoplication. Surg Endosc 2002; 16(5): 758–66.

Benign gastric and duodenal disease

Gastritis

Gastritis is inflammation of the mucosa of the stomach and is ∴ a pathological, rather than clinical, endoscopic, or radiological diagnosis. There are no characteristic symptoms of gastritis; in fact, the majority of patients are asymptomatic.

Acute gastritis

Classification of acute gastritis
See Table 5.1.

Table 5.1 Classification of acute and chronic gastritis

Gastritis	Synonym
Acute haemorrhagic and erosive gastritis	Acute gastritis
	Acute erosive gastritis
	Acute haemorrhagic gastritis
	Acute stress gastritis
Acute *Helicobacter pylori* gastritis	Type B gastritis (bacterial)
Chemical gastritis	Type C gastritis (reflux, bile, reactive)
Autoimmune gastritis	Type A, diffuse corporal gastritis
Metaplastic gastritis	Atrophic (chronic) atrophic gastritis

Acute (haemorrhagic) gastritis

- *Aetiology:* aspirin, NSAIDs, ethanol, bile acids or from pathological changes 2° to reduced gastric mucosal blood flow in conditions such as trauma, burns (Curling's ulcer), or sepsis.
- *Stress ulcer:* gastritis 2° to severe damage to central nervous system in form of Cushing's ulcer.
- *Presentation:* epigastric pain, haematemesis, or melaena.
- *Prevention:* gastric pH by IV H2 receptor antagonists, proton pump inhibitors, coating mucosa with sucralfate or magnesium trisylicate.
- *Rx:* Endoscopic injection, argon beam laser/ photocoagulation.
- On rare occasions, total gastrectomy may be required if bleeding is life threatening (high mortality).

Helicobacter pylori

Helicobacter pylori plays an important role in upper gastrointestinal disease worldwide, with almost 50% of the world's population being infected with the organism.

- Estimated lifetime risk for peptic ulcer disease and gastric cancer are 20% and 1–2%, respectively.
- In 1983, Warren and Marshall (both awarded the Nobel prize in 2005) successfully cultured *Campylobacter pyloridis*: renamed *Helicobacter pylori* in 1989 when association between organism and gastric inflammation was realized.

Pathophysiology

- *H. pylori*: curved/spiral or S-shaped gram negative rod.
- 4–7 flagellae at one pole.
- Uniquely produces urease.
- *Natural habitat*: human stomach, with highest density in antrum.
- Oral transmission is oro-oral and faeco-oral. Infection in childhood.
- *H. pylori*-related disease depends on bacterial virulence, host genetic susceptibility, and environmental factors.
- ~10% of people with *H. pylori* infestation develop an ulcer in future.
- Proposed mechanism of mucosal injury is either direct assault due to its direct local damage to epithelium, increased gastric acid production, and possible interaction with NSAIDs.

Virulence of the strain

- Virulence factors related to cytotoxin-associated gene (cagA) and vacuolating cytotoxin-associated gene (vacA).
- CagA positive strain causes more intense inflammation and can be associated with ulcer disease and gastric cancer.
- More prevalent in China and Japan; explains higher incidence of gastric cancer in these countries.

Environmental factors

- Diet and smoking.
- 1994 *H. pylori* declared a Group 1 carcinogen by International Agency for Research on Cancer (IARC) as implicated in development of gastric cancer in humans.
- Increases risk of developing gastric mucosa-associated lymphoid tissue (MALT lymphoma).
- Duodenal and gastric ulcers 2° to *H. pylori* infection are usually associated with antral predominant and diffuse gastritis, respectively.
- ~15–20% of patients with the infection are asymptomatic until complications develop.

Diagnosis

There are a variety of tests available for diagnosis. These can be classified into invasive and non-invasive (Table 5.2).

Table 5.2 Sensitivity and specificity rates of tests for *H. pylori*

Test	Sensitivity (%)	Specificity (%)
Biopsy	90	90
CLO test	95	95–100
Serology	85	79
Urea breath	95	95
Faecal antigen	95	95
Culture	85–90	100

- *Invasive:*
  - Endoscopic mucosal biopsy.
  - Histology.
  - Rapid urease test (*Campylobacter*-like organism (CLO) test).
  - Culture.
- *Non-invasive:*
  - Urea breath test.
  - Serology.
- *Biopsy:* two specimens minimum needed for accurate histological diagnosis. Sensitivity and specificity ~90%; however, expensive, labour intensive, and results not available the same day.
- *CLO test:* sensitivity and specificity ~95–100%; considerably cheaper than histology, results available the same day (Fig. 5.1).
- *Culture* of H. pylori: difficult; sensitivity ~80–90%.
- *Significant advantage:* specificity is 100%, but labour intensive, costly, and mainly used for research studies or testing for antibiotic sensitivity in patients resistant to first line medical therapy.
- *(PCR) and confocal endomicroscopy:* both cumbersome and expensive, but can be useful in histologically negative biopsies.
- *Urea breath test:* non-invasive used to check *H. pylori* eradication after treatment.
- Cannot be recommended for pregnant women or children due to radioactive nature of test.
- *Serology:* least expensive, but cannot differentiate between prior exposure and active infection.
- *Faecal antigen test:* a simple test, but inferior to urea breath test; also is cumbersome and may be less compliant.

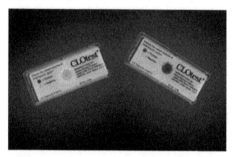

Fig. 5.1 CLO test: a well of indicator gel sealed inside a plastic slide sits flat and can be picked up with theatre gloves on. The gel contains urea, phenol red, buffers and a bacteriostatic agent to prevent the growth of contaminating urease-positive organisms. Urease from *H. pylori* present in the tissue sample changes the gel from yellow to bright magenta.
With kind permission from Trimed Ltd.

Treatment of H. pylori

- *First line:* triple therapy with PPI and two antimicrobial agents:
  - Amoxicillin 1g *or*
  - Clarithromycin 500mg or metronidazole 500mg, all given bd for 7–14 days.
  - Eradicates *H. pylori* ~85% of cases.
- Treatment failure indicates antibacterial resistance or poor compliance.
- Resistance to amoxicillin rare, but to clarithromycin and metronidazole common. Can develop during treatment.
- Consider culture and testing for antibiotic sensitivity.
- *Quadruple therapy:* +bismuth 120mg qds for 7 days recommended.
- *Recent meta-analysis:* efficacy of triple therapy containing levofloxacin 10 days superior to classical quadruple therapy for antimicrobial resistance.
- *Perforated duodenal ulcer: H. pylori* (see Fig. 5.2) is the most important factor for ulcer recurrence and merits eradication along with PPI therapy for about 4-6 weeks. Confirmation of eradication with Urea breath test recommended in patients with resistant ulcer, MALT lymphoma and previous resection of gastric cancer.

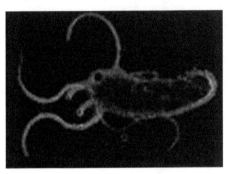

Fig. 5.2 *H. pylori.*

Chronic gastritis

Common forms of chronic gastritis

- Helicobacter gastritis.
- Chemical gastritis:
  - Aspirin and other NSAIDs.
  - Bile reflux.
- Metaplastic atrophic gastritis of which there are two types:
  - Autoimmune.
  - Environmental.
- Chronic gastritis of indeterminate type.

Uncommon forms of chronic gastritis
- Post enterectomy atrophic gastritis.
- Eosinophilic gastritis.
- Infectious gastritis.
- Crohn's disease.
- Sarcoidosis.
- Lymphocytic gastritis.
- Menetrier's disease.
- *Chronic gastritis:* characterized by mucosal infiltration with lymphocytes and plasma cells.
- If persists can progress to atrophic gastritis, which is a precursor of gastric malignancy.

Helicobacter pylori infection can also lead to atrophic gastritis, which can further progress to intestinal metaplasia, dysplasia, and subsequently gastric cancer.
- Association between immune system and chronic gastritis seen in pernicious anaemia (anti-intrinsic factor antibodies).
- 4-fold increase in gastric cancer. Requires regular surveillance OGD.
- Auto-immune gastritis and granulomatous gastritis from Crohn's disease. Can be a manifestation of systemic disease presenting with abdominal pain and weight loss.

Menetrier's disease
- Hyperplastic gastropathy (gastritis).
- Presents with epigastric pain, weight loss, nausea, vomiting, and hypoalbuminaemia.
- Giant gastric folds where albumin leaks into gastric lumen. Weight loss common.
- *Rx:* H2 receptor blockers, PPI therapy, prednisolone, and anti-*H. pylori* therapy all of limited benefit. May require subtotal or total gastrectomy, but this carries a high morbidity and mortality.

Peptic ulcer disease

Surgery for peptic ulcer disease has gone through a significant shift/change in the last 20 years. Modern medical therapy has made the need for elective surgery extremely rare. Operations for peptic ulcer disease, which were once common on an elective surgical list, have virtually disappeared.

Aetiology

The two main factors implicated in the aetiology are NSAIDs and *H. pylori*. Other factors include smoking, chronic liver disease, chronic renal failure, especially during dialysis and transplantation, and hyperparathyroidism.

The role of Helicobacter pylori *in peptic ulcer disease*

- Spiral-shaped Gram negative micro-aerophyllic bacterium. Colonizes gastric epithelium and duodenum.
- More than 50% of world population colonized.
- Humans only reservoir/host for *H. pylori* infection.
- Transmitted orally, probably during childhood.
- *Stomach:* colonizes mainly antral mucosa causing antral gastritis, and increased gastrin production.
- Increased acid production in proximal stomach inhibits colonization of the bacteria.
- ~10% of patients infected develop an ulcer in future.
- Mechanism of mucosal injury is either direct assault due to direct local damage to epithelium, increased gastric acid production, and possible interaction with NSAIDs.
- Antrum-predominant non-atrophic *H. pylori* gastritis basal and stimulated gastric acid output increase, particularly in patients with duodenal ulcer (DU).
- In patients with DU and *H. pylori* infection acid secretion > than infected people without ulcers in response to = gastrin levels.
- Impaired acid response to gastrin in infected people without ulcers, probably caused by intense inflammation of acid-secreting mucosa.
- Patients with duodenal ulcers also have more acid-secreting parietal cells than do people without ulcers, and produce more acid in response to maximum gastrin stimulation.
- Reduction of gastric acid secretion with (PPI) therapy increases intensity of inflammation of acid-secreting mucosa in *H. pylori* patients.
- A high constitutive acid secretory capacity promotes antral-predominant body-sparing gastritis, and duodenal ulceration.
- *H. pylori* infection reduces negative feedback regulation of gastrin release and acid secretion.
- Low antral pH stimulates release of somatostatin from D cells in antral glands, this inhibits gastrin release from G cells.
- *H. pylori* has very high urease activity producing ammonia to protect organism from its acidic gastric environment.
- Alkaline ammonia produced by surface epithelial bacteria and glands of antrum prevents D cells from sensing true acid level, and leads to inappropriate release of somatostatin, an increase in gastrin, and excess acid secretion.

- Hypergastrinaemia induced by *H. pylori* induces hyperplasia of enterochromaffin-like and acid-secreting parietal cells.
- *H. pylori* disrupts neural pathways such as antral-fundic neural connections that down-regulate acid production.
- Impaired inhibitory neural control, in association with hypergastrinaemia, leads to further increase of acid output in patients with duodenal ulceration.
- Resolution of hypergastrinaemia in these patients after *H. pylori* eradication is a common event and occurs much faster than does resolution of acid hypersecretion.
- *H. pylori* induces epithelium-derived cytokines: IL 8 and IL 1β attracting polymorphonuclear leukocytes (PMNs) and macrophages that release lysosomal enzymes, leukotrienes, driving immunopathogeneticulcerogenesis.
- T and B cells release IL 1, 2, 6, 10, TNFα, and antibodies.
- TH1 response promote erosion vs. interleukin-10 mediated protection release confers protection.
- Virulent *H. pylori* in ulcer patients produce greater urease than do those from people without ulcers. Urease catalyses production of ammonia aiding formation of toxic complexes, such as NH_4Cl.53.
- Bacterial phospholipases A and C impair membrane phospholipids eroding gastric epithelial barrier.

NSAIDs
Mechanism of injury
Prostaglandin synthesis disturbance is caused by the inhibition of cyclo-oxygenase enzyme (COX-1). The two independent mechanisms of gastric mucosal injury are, primarily, an irritated topical effect and, secondly, a systemic effect.

Aetiological classification of peptic ulcers
- Positive for *H. pylori* infection.
- Drug, i.e. NSAID, induced.
- *H pylori* and NSAIDs positive.
- *H pylori* and NSAIDs negative.
- Acid hypersecretory state (i.e. Zollinger–Ellison syndrome).
- Anastomotic ulcer after subtotal gastric resection tumours (i.e. cancer, lymphoma).

Rare specific causes
- Crohn's disease of the stomach or duodenum.
- Eosinophilic gastroduodenitis.
- Systemic mastocytosis.
- Radiation damage.
- Viral infections (e.g. cytomegalovirus or herpes simplex infection, in particular, in immunocompromised patients).
- Colonization of stomach with *H. heilmanii*.
- Severe systemic disease.
- Cameron ulcer (gastric ulcer where hiatus hernia passes through diaphragmatic hiatus).
- True idiopathic ulcer.

Diagnosis
Endoscopy
- Mainstay for diagnosis of peptic ulcer disease (PUD).
- Allows biopsy assessment and Rx of bleeding, *H. pylori* assessment by urease testing/histology.
- *Peptic-ulcer diagnosis:* mucosal break of diameter 5mm or larger covered with fibrin; a mucosal break smaller than 5mm is called an erosion; arbitrary, but used in clinical trials.
- Peptic-ulcers, single or multiple, typical location of duodenal ulcer in bulb.
- Site of predilection for gastric ulcers is angulus of lesser curve, but can occur from pylorus to cardia.
- *Difference:* gastritis, duodenitis, marginal ulcers, Mallory–Weiss tear.
- Diagnostic accuracy of endoscopy is almost 95%.
- Gastric ulcers routinely biopsied; malignant risk.
- Repeat endoscopy to confirm healing. Re-biopsy essential for all gastric ulcers.
- Duodenal ulcers do not require biopsy as malignancy exceptional.
- Occasionally, kissing ulcers are seen located face to face on anterior and posterior walls of duodenal bulb. If ulceration is seen in the more distal duodenum, then underlying Crohn's disease, ischaemia, or the rare Zollinger–Ellison syndrome should be considered. On endoscopic diagnosis of peptic ulcer, biopsy samples of the antral and body, or fundus mucosa should be taken for detection of *H. pylori* infection by rapid urease and histological tests.

Barium studies
- May show an ulcer crater in an acute ulcer or scarring of duodenal bulb, indicative of ulcer healing.
- Diagnostic accuracy ~75%.
- Observer-dependent subjective bias in size and active ulceration.
- Reserved for those intolerant of endoscopy or if contraindicated.

Gastric analysis
- Measurement of acid both in fasting state (basal acid output) and in response to pentagastrin stimulation (maximal acid output).
- Cannot diagnose duodenal ulcer, but useful for refractory ulcers or suspected Zollinger–Ellison syndrome.

Treatment
- *Karl Schwarz's dictum:* no acid, no ulcer!
- *Three main principles:*
  - Avoid ulcerogenic agents.
  - Promote mucosal defence with PPIs or H2 antagonists.
  - Eradicate *H. pylori* (e.g. by triple therapy: see 🕮 Treatment of *H. pylori*, p. 99).
- Discontinue NSAID or aspirin use where possible.
- Consider COX-2 selective inhibitors or NSAID with an antacid, in form of proton pump inhibitor, would be the ideal choice.
- *If, despite treatment, ulcer fails to heal:* possible persistent *H. pylori* infection.
- Antibiotic resistance or poor patient compliance.
- *Relapsing resistant ulcer:* consider surreptitious aspirin ingestion, smoking, Zollinger–Ellison syndrome or occult malignancy.

Reinforcement of mucosal barrier

- Useful against NSAIDs and aspirin.
- *Misoprostol:* prostaglandin analogue, abdominal side-effects; diarrhoea and pain; limiting, especially at higher doses.
- *Sucralfate and bismuth salts:* improved mucosal repair, reduced acid secretion, and *H. pylori* infection suppression.
- Bismuth salts with some intrinsic anti-*H. pylori* activity are used in ulcer therapy only in combination with antibiotics.

H. pylori-positive ulcer Rx: Maastricht Consensus Report

First-line options (7–14 days)

- *<15–20% Clarithromycin resistance and >40% metronidazole resistance:* PPI standard dose, clarithromycin 2 × 500mg, and amoxicillin 2 × 1000mg, all bd.
- *<15–20% Clarithromycin resistance and <40% metronidazole resistance:* PPI standard dose, clarithromycin 500mg, and metronidazole 400mg or tinidazole 500mg, all bd.
- *High clarithromycin and metronidazole resistance:* bismuth-containing quadruple therapy.

Second-line option (10–14 days)

- Bismuth-containing quadruple therapy.
- PPI + metronidazole and amoxicillin, if clarithromycin used in first-line Rx (in Latin America and China, furazolidone 2–4 × 100mg is often preferred over metronidazole).

Rescue therapies (10–14 days)

- PPI bd plus amoxicillin 2 × 1000mg with either levofloxacin 2 × 250mg (500mg), or with rifabutin 2 × 150mg.
- Eradication equal duodenal and gastric ulcers.

Duodenal ulcer

- Non-invasive ^{13}C-urea breath test (UBT), stool antigen testing, validated surrogate marker to confirm healing.
- Uncomplicated 7–14 day eradication no further PPIs.

Gastric ulcer

- *OGD and biopsy:* exclude malignancy, ulcer may appear healed.
- PPIs continued beyond eradication phase for 4–8 weeks.
- If complications arise (i.e. bleeding), PPI therapy continued until OGD confirms healing and history confirms eradication; antral and body biopsies, PPI Rx produces false-positive urease test results.
- Eradication depends on drug regimen, resistance, compliance, duration of Rx, and genetic variations in drug-metabolizing enzymes.
- Aim to maintain first-line eradication rates greater than 80%.
- *Duration of eradication Rx:* USA 10 or even 14 days, Europe, 1 week meta-analysis increasing duration 7–10 days eradication increased 4% and 7–14 days, 5%. Minimal clinical significance.
- Quadruple therapies alternative first-line therapies in areas of high resistance.
- Overall failure 10–20%. Bismuth-based quadruple Rx is main option for 2nd line therapy if not used as first-line. Eradication 57–95%.

- If persistent *H. pylori* after two treatments, including clarithromycin and metronidazole, at least single and usually double resistance likely.
- Further Rx based on culture and sensitivity.
- Levofloxacin or rifabutin as a third component besides PPI and amoxicillin can be used for treatment failure. *Eradication rate:* levofloxacin-containing triple salvage therapies 63–94%.
- Rifabutin combined with PPI and amoxicillin > 7 days well tolerated, and highly effective against double-resistant *H. pylori* after failure of standard triple therapy.

Ulceration of gastric or duodenal mucosa in the absence of H. pylori *infection, and NSAID or aspirin*

- Rare.
- Check validity of the test. Never 100% sensitive.
- Eradication is permanent cure of this disease, ∴ repeat test including endoscopic biopsy samples from antrum and body of stomach for histological examination and urease tests.
- Re-examine NSAIDs or aspirin history may be surreptitious.
- Consider rare causes.
- *Zollinger–Ellison syndrome:* gastrin-secreting tumour causes diarrhoea and malabsorption; multiple ulcers extend to duodenojejunal flexure and proximal jejunum. Elevated serum gastrin assess response to IV secretin and gastric secretion tests.

Historic classification and management of peptic ulcer disease

- Modified Johnson classification of benign gastric ulcers (Box 5.1 and Fig. 5.3).
- Five types based on location and importance of acid hypersecretion in pathogenesis. Operative approaches historically used now largely redundant due to PPIs; however, patients may present late in life having had procedures in the past.

Box 5.1 Modified Johnson classification of benign peptic ulcers

- *Type I:* most common: occur along lesser curve, usually at incisura (Billroth I/II) (see Fig. 5.3).
- *Type II:* two ulcers. One ulcer in gastric body, usually around incisura, and another is in duodenum (active or healed) (Billroth I/II + vagotomy).
- *Type III:* prepyloric. Only type II and type III gastric ulcers are associated with acid hypersecretion and require acid-reducing operation (Billroth I/II + vagotomy).
- *Type IV:* high on lesser curve, near gastro-oesophageal junction (subtotal gastrectomy +Roux-en-Y reconstruction).
- *Type V:* anywhere in stomach and caused by medications, such as NSAIDs. Respond to cessation of the offending medication.

Reproduced from 'Gastric Ulcer: Classification, Blood Group Characteristics, Secretion Patterns and Pathogenesis', Johnson, H. Daintree, *Annals of Surgery*, **162** (6), 996–1004, copyright 1965 with permission of Wolters Kluwer Health.

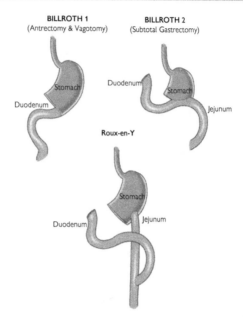

Fig. 5.3 Billroth I (antrectomy and vagotomy), Billroth II (subtotal gastrectomy) and Roux-en-Y gastric bypass procedures.

Historic procedures

Truncal vagotomy and antrectomy

- *Advantages:* least ulcer recurrence, eliminated cancer risk.
- *Disadvantages:* included high operative mortality and development of post-gastrectomy problems in form of dumping, post-vagotomy diarrhoea, and delayed gastric emptying.

Truncal vagotomy and drainage

Has the advantage of being quick and safe biopsy of ulcer performed simultaneously.

Highly selective vagotomy and gastrojejunostomy

- *Advantages:*
  - Low risk procedure treated both ulcer diatheses and obstruction. Preservation of vagal innovation to distal stomach, hence, improved gastric emptying.
  - Gastrojejunostomy potentially reversible.
- *Disadvantages:* increased incidence of marginal ulceration and a slight risk of dumping from bypassing the pylorus.

For gastric outlet obstruction 2° to prepyloric or gastric ulcer, gastric resection is the best option as opposed to a drainage procedure.

- Surgery evolved around concept of acid reduction by denervation of parietal cells by means of vagotomy, resection of parietal cell mass, or resection of antral gastrin-producing cells.
- In the 1970s, truncal vagotomy and pyloroplasty most common operation performed. ∴ truncal vagotomy abandoned in favour of highly selective or proximal gastric vagotomy.
- Significant side effects, ∴ truncal vagotomy abandoned in favour of highly selective or proximal gastric vagotomy.
- *Complications:* delayed gastric emptying, post-vagotomy diarrhoea, dumping syndrome, alkaline reflux gastritis, chronic gastroparesis, and afferent or efferent loop syndrome.
- This surgery has now essentially become a historic footnote no longer part of practical experience of surgeons training today.

Non-variceal upper GI haemorrhage

The most frequent complication of gastroduodenal ulcer disease and accounts for the commonest cause of ulcer related death. Presentation may vary from melaena to occult haemopositive stools, to massive haematemesis and shock.

Causes of upper GI haemorrhage (in UK)

- Peptic ulcers/erosions (45%).
- Idiopathic (25%).
- Oesophagitis (10%).
- Gastro-oesophageal cancer (5%), varices (5%), Mallory–Weiss tear (5%), angiodysplasia, or Dieulafoy ulcer (5%).

Initial resuscitation and management

Initial management of upper GI bleeding involves resuscitation, followed by endoscopy and definitive management as indicated by the overall risk of rebleeding and morbidity.

Resuscitation

- Establish large bore IV access.
- Resuscitation with isotonic crystalloid and blood products.
- Reversal of anticoagulation (if needed).
- Nasogastric tube and aspiration with or without saline lavage.
- If patient is haemodynamically unstable then resuscitate in intensive care unit (ITU), followed by urgent endoscopy or resuscitation in theatre with urgent endoscopy under general anaesthetic.

Risk stratification

See Table 5.3.

- Initial Rockall scoring system appropriate tool for assessment pre-endoscopy—predictive of death and rebleeding in patients with ulcers or varices.
- If initial (pre-endoscopic) score of 0 (age <60 years, no shock, no comorbidity)—extremely low risk of death or rebleeding; consider non-admission or early discharge with appropriate outpatient follow-up.
- *If pre-endoscopic Rockall score >0:* OGD indicated for full assessment of bleeding risk.
- *If full (post-endoscopic) Rockall score <3:* low risk of rebleeding or death consider early discharge and OPD follow-up.

The mainstay of investigation and management is endoscopy.

- Maximum additive score prior to diagnosis = 7.
- Maximum additive score after diagnosis = 11.
- If initial (pre-endoscopic) score above 0, there is a significant mortality (score 1—predicted mortality 2.4%; score 2—predicted mortality 5.6%) Score >8 high risk of death.
- Only those scoring 0 can be safely discharged at this stage.

Table 5.3 Rockall risk score

Variable	0	1	2	3	
Age	<60 years	60–79 years	≥ 80 years		
Shock	'No shock'	SBP* ≥ 100 mmHg, HR < 100bpm	'Tachycardia' SBP ≥ 100mmHg, HR≥ 100bpm	'Hypotension', SBP < 100mmHg	Initial score criteria
Comorbidity	No major comorbidity		CCF, IHD, major comorbid	Renal failure, liver failure, disseminated malignancy	
Diagnosis	Mallory–Weiss tear, no lesion identified and no SRH	All other diagnoses			Additional criteria for full score
Major stigmata of recent haemorrhage (SRH)	None, or dark spot only		Blood in upper GI tract, adherent clot, visible or spurting vessel		

*SBP, systolic blood pressure; *SRH, stigmata of recent haemorrhage.

Reprinted by permission from Macmillan Publishers Ltd: 'Risk assessment after acute upper gastrointestinal haemorrhage', Rockall TA, Logan RF, Devlin HB, et al., *Gut* **38** (3): 316–21, 1996.

The management of non-variceal upper GI bleeding

This is summarized in Box 5.2.

Box 5.2 Management of non-variceal upper GI bleeding (SIGN guidelines: ratified by BSG)

- Initial Rockall scoring system is an appropriate tool for assessment prior to endoscopy, and is predictive of death and rebleeding in patients with ulcers or varices.
- Endoscopic therapy should only be delivered to actively bleeding lesions, non-bleeding visible vessels, and when technically possible, to ulcers with an adherent blood clot.
- Combinations of endoscopic injection of at least 13mL of 1:10,000 adrenaline + either a thermal or mechanical Rx recommended in preference to single modalities.
- Endoscopy and endotherapy should be repeated within 24h when initial endoscopic treatment considered sub-optimal (difficult access, poor visualization technical difficulties) or in patients in whom rebleeding is likely to be life threatening.

(Continued)

Box 5.2 (Cont'd)

- Non-variceal upper GI haemorrhage not controlled by endoscopy should be treated by repeat endoscopic treatment, selective arterial embolization or surgery.
- Patients with peptic ulcer bleeding should be tested for *H. pylori* (with biopsy methods or urea breath test) and a 1-week course of eradication therapy prescribed for those who test positive. A further 3 weeks ulcer healing treatment should be given.
- In non-NSAID users, maintenance antisecretory therapy should not be continued after successful healing of ulcer and *H. pylori* eradication.
- Biopsies for *H. pylori* should be taken at initial endoscopy prior to PPI. Biopsy specimens should be histologically assessed when rapid urease test is negative.
- *H. pylori* eradication should be confirmed by breath test or biopsy to minimize risk of rebleeding from peptic ulcer. Second line treatment should be prescribed in case of eradication failures.
- *H. pylori* testing to confirm eradication should only be taken after proton pump inhibitor and antibiotic therapy has been completed and discontinued: testing within 2 weeks may result in false negative findings.
- Follow-up OGD should be performed to confirm healing of gastric ulcers if suspicion of malignancy.
- High-dose IV proton pump inhibitor therapy (e.g. omeprazole or pantoprazole 80mg bolus followed by 8mg/h infusion for 72h) should be used in patients with major peptic ulcer bleeding (active bleeding or non-bleeding visible vessel) following endoscopic haemostatic therapy.
- Insufficient evidence for use of tranexamic acid in treatment of non-variceal GI bleeding.
- Insufficient evidence for use of somatostatin or synthetic analogues in Rx of non-variceal GI bleeding.
- Patients with healed bleeding ulcers who test negative for *H. pylori* require concomitant PPI Rx at usual daily dose if NSAIDs, aspirin or COX-2 inhibitors indicated.
- If cardiovascular risk is a concern, naproxen with PPI recommended if analgesic therapies fail. COX-2 inhibitors are not recommended in patients with cardiovascular risk.
- Aspirin and NSAIDs should be discontinued when patients present with peptic ulcer bleeding. Once ulcer healing and eradication of *H. pylori* confirmed, aspirin and NSAIDs only prescribed if clear indication.
- Elective SSRIs should be used with caution in patients who have increased risk of GI bleeding, especially in patients taking NSAID or aspirin. A non-SSRI antidepressant may be an appropriate choice in such patients.

Endoscopic management
- Allows visualization of source of bleeding and therapeutic intervention and/or biopsy.

- If haemodynamically stable, OGD on next available list.
- In majority of cases bleeding settles spontaneously.
- If unstable best option OGD under GA in the operating theatre, where airway can be protected to prevent aspiration.
- An appropriate multi-channel gastroscope should be available that allows for insertion of devices such as needles/probes/clips applicators, whilst continue to allow irrigation/aspiration.
- Most patients with bleeding duodenal ulcer can be treated successfully with a combination of endoscopic therapy and PPI.

Adrenalin injection

- Induces vasospasm, local tamponade, and platelet activation: leads to haemostasis.
- 1:10,000 adrenaline injected by an endoscopy injection needle.
- *Volume:* 20, 30, and 40 identical rate of initial haemostasis, perforation significantly higher 40mL adrenaline ($P < 0.05$), rate of recurrent bleeding significantly higher in 20-mL adrenaline group (20.3%) than in 30- (5.3%) and 40-mL groups (2.8%) ($P < 0.01$).
- Arrhythmias, tachycardia, and hypertension, have been known to occur: usually self-limiting.

Bipolar diathermy

- Generates heat to coagulate bleeding vessel.
- Produces local contact heat, which along with pressure of probe stops bleeding.
- Bipolar circumactive probe (BICAP) most commonly used in UK.
- Active spurting blood vessels impede visualization of bleeding point making use of this probe difficult.

Heat probe

- Similar principle to BICAP device.
- Probe coated with a non-stick material, which prevents adherence to coagulated tissue that may dislodge clot.
- Generates temperature as high as 150°C. Should be used with caution.
- BICAP and heat probe associated with perforation and re-bleeding.

Injection sclerotherapy

- Various sclerosants used: alcohol, 1% polidocanol, 3% sodium tetradecyl sulphate (STD) and 5% ethanolamine. For active bleeding ulcer, sclerosant is injected surrounding bleeding point in portions of 0.5mL.
- Technique easily learnt and freely available. Low risk of perforation.

Micro clips (haemoclips/endoclips)

- Preloaded on applicator. Can be used for spurting blood vessel at base or ulcer.
- Now widely available.
- Meta-analysis compared efficacy of endoscopic clipping with injection or thermocoagulation in control of non-variceal GI bleeding ($n = 1156$) 15 RCTs.
- Definitive haemostasis higher with clipping (86.5%) than injection (75.4%; relative risk (RR) 1.14, 95% CI 1.00–1.30).

- Clips significantly reduce rebleeding (9.5%) compared with injection (19.6%; RR 0.49, 95% CI 0.30–0.79) and need for surgery (2.3% vs. 7.4%; RR 0.37, 95% CI 0.15–0.90).
- Clipping and thermocoagulation comparable efficacy (81.5% and 81.3%; RR 1.00).
- No differences in mortality between any interventions.

Laser photocoagulation
- The laser Nd-YAG used exclusively for bleeding peptic ulcer.
- Coagulates bleeding vessel by delivering heat directed without contact with clot.
- Expensive, can be hazardous for staff—need to wear protective goggles. Endoscopy room/theatre needs to be modified and there is risk of perforation.
- Over 90% of bleeding ulcers initially controlled by endoscopic techniques.
- Combination endoscopic Rx superior to single modality therapy, and combination treatment does not increase complications.

The factors that predict failure of endoscopic treatment include those in Box 5.3.

Box 5.3 Predictors of failure of endoscopic treatment
- Haemodynamic instability.
- Significant co-morbidity.
- More than 4–6U blood transfusion in 24h.
- Endoscopic findings of the ulcer:
  - Actively bleeding vessel.
  - Visible vessel.
  - Adherent clot.
  - Ulcer size more than 2cm.

New endoscopic techniques
Fibrin glue has been tried with some success. Simultaneous injection of thrombin and fibrinogen around base of ulcer.

Operative management: general
- Operative intervention is required when bleeding cannot be controlled successfully by endoscopic means or patient is unstable during initial bleeding.
- 10% of patients still require operative treatment to arrest bleeding despite recent advances in medical, endoscopic and interventional radio-embolization.

Indications for surgery
These include:
- Severe haemorrhage not responding to resuscitation.
- Recurrence of bleeding after initial control with endoscopic or medical measures. Interventional radiology failed, inappropriate or unavailable.
- Second admission after treatment of ulcer haemorrhage.

- Prolonged bleeding with loss of 50% or more of blood volume.
- *Blood transfusion:* more than 4–6U in 24h.
- Age 60 or more with shock or anaemia on admission.
- Certain endoscopic features of ulcer, especially ulcer size more than 2cm, visible vessel underneath or on base of ulcer, active oozing or active arterial bleeding from the ulcer.
- Principles of surgery includes an operation that is safest and quickest to arrest bleeding followed by treatment with PPI and *H. pylori* eradication therapy.
- General simple suture control of the bleeding combined with aggressive medical therapy usually proves sufficient.
- Historically, vagotomy and pyloroplasty with suturing of bleeding ulcer was the operation of choice. However, advent of aetiological role of *H. pylori*, role of NSAIDs, and development of PPI therapy has made these operations very rare.

Bleeding duodenal ulcer

Initial resuscitation involves airway, breathing, and circulation (ABC), large bore IV cannula, urinary catheterization, blood transfusions as required, correction of clotting abnormalities, and urgent endoscopy if the patient is unstable.

Operative management: DU

- The surgical technique for peptic ulcer bleeding involves longitudinal duodenotomy distal to the pyloric ring. It is also useful to kocherize duodenum as enables better access to bleeding ulcer.
- Upon opening duodenum, digital pressure over ulcer helps temporize the bleeding and allows resuscitation.
- Adequate control of bleeding requires ligation of gastroduodenal artery proximal and distal to the site of penetration.
- Third stitch often required medially to control transverse pancreatic branch.
- Duodenotomy is closed transversely where possible.
- If pylorus has to be opened then Heineke–Mikulicz pyloroplasty is performed.
- Occasionally, if there is scarring over pylorus or first part of duodenum, whereby transverse closure is difficult, then longitudinal closure with gastro-jejunostomy may be required.
- For giant duodenal ulcers antrectomy is performed, followed by gastroenterostomy, Roux-en-Y. Duodenal stump is then closed primarily or if this becomes difficult then the duodenal stump can be drained either by T tube or Foley catheter. This allows a controlled fistula which usually heals within 4–6 weeks.
- *Small gastric ulcers:* local under-sewing of bleeding point with possible biopsies. Gastrotomy may be indicated.
- Large bleeding distal gastric ulcer a more radical approach, in form of partial gastrectomy, often required to control bleeding.
- *Large lesser curve ulcers:* total gastrectomy or proximal gastrectomy if surgeon experience allows.

Radiological embolization

- Highly useful for patients with recurrent bleeding despite medical or surgical intervention. Local expertise and protocols vary greatly.

- Can also be used in patients who are unfit for surgery, advanced malignant gastric ulcer, occult bleeding not visualized at OGD.
- Bleeding can be controlled by selective infusion of vasopressin into local circulation via left gastric artery or embolization by haemostatic substances, such as metal coils, oxidized cellulose, gel foam, or polyvinyl alcohol.
- *Disadvantage:* angiography will only detect bleeding vessel if bleeding occurs at rate of more than 0.5mL/min. Nevertheless, it is still a useful adjunct in available armamentarium for non-operative management of upper GI bleeding.

Benign gastroduodenal perforation

- *Lifetime risk 10%:* untreated PUD.
- 30–50% of ulcer perforations associated with NSAIDs.
- *80% H. pylori-positive:* ∴ eradication essential. *Pre- H. pylori eradication era:* 80% patients simple omental closure alone develop recurrent ulcers.
- Overall mortality remains between 2 and 8% rising to as high as 30% in the elderly population. Post-operative mortality correlates with pre-op shock, co-morbidity and perforation >48h.
- *Presentation:* (Box 5.4) sudden onset severe epigastric pain, peritonism, rigid abdomen, sepsis. May be non-specific in elderly.
- *Sub-diaphragmatic air:* (Fig. 5.4) may be absent in 20%. CT more sensitive.
- Perforated peptic ulcer is an indication for operation in nearly all cases except when patient is unfit for surgery.
- *Non operative Rx:*
  - Small trials show similar results to operative intervention, 30% for whom non-operative Rx initiated proceed to surgery, particularly if age>70.
  - Advocated in selected patients who do not have generalized peritonitis or continued duodenal leak, and for those in whom there is an absolute contraindication for surgery.
- *Rx:*
  - IV infusion, nasogastric tube (NGT) decompression, broad spectrum antibiotics, analgesia, and IV PPI. Computed tomography (CT)-guided drainage as required.
  - High incidence of intra-abdominal abscesses and sepsis with non-operative management. This has been largely abandoned, even in high risk cases with current advances in anaesthetic approach.

Box 5.4 Key clinical features of gastroduodenal perforation

- *Detailed history:*
  - Epigastric pain.
  - Drugs (NSAIDs, aspirin).
- *Physical examination:*
  - Abdominal guarding, rigidity.
  - Absent bowel sounds.
- *Bloods:* leucocytosis, raised CRP.
- *Abdominal radiograph:* free air under diaphragm.
- *Oral contrast study:* contrast leak in abdomen.
- *CT scan:* free intra-peritoneal air.

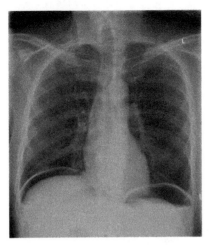

Fig. 5.4 Pneumoperitoneum from GI perforation, as evident on erect chest radiography.
With kind permission from Andrew Stein.

Operative technique
- Simple closure of perforation by suture plication of ulcer, and reinforcement with an omental patch is preferred method of dealing with perforation (Fig. 5.5). Routine drain insertion unproven.
- Formal laparotomy or, in selected patients, laparoscopically.
- Acute ulcers along anterior part of first part of duodenum usually perforate, whereas those on posterior aspect tend to cause bleeding as they erode into gastroduodenal artery.
- With advent of proton pump inhibitors and association with *H. pylori*, definitive ulcer preventing operations, i.e. vagotomy or gastrectomy, have largely been abandoned.
- Laparoscopic repair is a reasonable option in selected patients with a history of less than 24h, no evidence of hypovolaemic shock, and with a perforation <8–10mm.
- Practice depends on expertise and local availability of laparoscopic surgery. Falciform ligament easily mobilized for patch closure.
- *Meta-analysis:* Lau—13 publications; 658 patients—85% success laparoscopic approach. Reduced wound infection, pain, but increase in re-operation.
- Mortality and morbidity is comparable in published series for open vs. laparoscopic approach, there have been no large randomized clinical trials comparing one against the other.
- Mainstay of surgery is thorough normal saline lavage of abdominal cavity to prevent interloop and intra-abdominal abscesses.

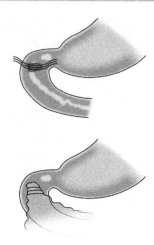

Fig. 5.5 Closure of a perforated duodenal ulcer with an omental (Graham) patch.

Gastric outlet obstruction

- In era of effective treatment of PUD with *H. pylori* and proton pump inhibitors, gastric cancer remains main cause of gastric outlet obstruction as opposed to peptic ulcer disease.
- Surgery for gastric outlet obstruction as a complication of peptic ulcer disease now rare.
- *Symptoms:* post-prandial non-bilious vomiting. Abdominal distension, bloating, vague epigastric discomfort, early satiety, and/or weight loss.
- May present with electrolyte disturbance in form of hypokalaemic metabolic alkalosis.
- Succession splash is present in 25%.
- Most patients malnourished. Consider nasojejunal (NJ) feeding for pre-optimization.

Diagnosis

- Good history.
- Barium swallow/meal.
- Endoscopy.
- CT scan.
- *OGD:* diagnostic and therapeutic. Biopsy is mandatory to exclude malignancy.
- Short strictures amenable to endoscopic balloon dilatation, up to 80% may gain benefit in long run, but in many benefits remain transient.

Operative management
- Surgery is indicated in patients with failed conventional medical treatment, persistent symptoms after 2–3 endoscopic balloon dilatations and finally for perforation (endoscopic or spontaneous), bleeding, or suspicion of cancer.
- Before surgery is contemplated thoroughly exclude previous NSAID or aspirin use. Perform appropriate tests to rule out presence of *H. pylori*.
- Ideal operation relieves the obstruction, controls the ulcer disease, produces very few late complications, and has low morbidity and mortality.
- Currently, there are no published series to suggest a single operation, which meets these criteria.
- Pyloroplasty alone, gastroenterostomy or sub-total gastrectomy most commonly performed.

Other benign gastric disease

Acute gastric dilatation

- Complication of major upper abdominal surgery.
- Commonly seen post-splenectomy.
- Can occur in patients with anorexia and other psychiatric condition when they have been prescribed large doses of psychotropic drugs.
- *DM:* gastric autonomic neuropathy.
- *Presentation:* subtle, persistent left shoulder tip pain, and hiccups are early warning signs, and can be the only presenting symptoms.
- *Treatment:* large bore nasogastric (NG) tube and regular aspiration.
- Correction of biochemical abnormalities, such as potassium, is essential and some cases also require prokinetic drugs to help improve the motility. Unrecognized and untreated cases can have a fatal outcome due to vomiting and aspiration.

Gastric bezoars

Bezoars are persistent concretions of foreign material found in the stomach. The term bezoar was thought to be derived from the Persian word *padzahr*, which means counter-poison or antidote.

Aetiology
See Table 5.4.

Table 5.4 Types and features of GI bezoars

Type	Constituents	Predisposing factors
Phytobezoars	Vegetable matter (cabbage, grapes, celery)	Gastric surgery, especially vagotomy (reduced acid secretion, atony, stenosis
Trichobezoars	Hair	Long hair, gastric stasis (diabetes, hypothyroidism)
Concretions	Foreign material	Ingestion of foreign matter (psychiatric illness)
Pharmacobezoars	Medications (aluminium hydroxide, nifedipine)	GI narrowing, motility disorders
Fungus balls	Yeast	Gastric surgery

Symptoms
- Usually asymptomatic.
- Depending on size can have anorexia, bloating, early satiety, weight loss, epigastric fullness.
- Sometimes presents with complications like ulceration, perforation, intestinal obstruction secondary to migration.
- Peritonitis.

Treatment
See Table 5.5.

Table 5.5 Treatment options for GI bezoars

Medical therapy		
Enzymatic	Proteolytic	Papase tablets (meat tenderizer)
	Cellulitic	Cellulase tablets
	Mucolytic	Acetylcysteine
Mechanical	Removal	Endoscopic snares, baskets and forceps
	Fragmentation	Endoscopic forceps
Others	Motility agents	Metoclopramide and erythromycin
Surgical therapy		
Laparotomy/laparoscopy		Gastrotomy or enterotomy

Gastric volvulus

Gastric volvulus defines abnormal degree of rotation of one part of the stomach around another. It can be mesentero-axial (Fig. 5.6) or organo-axial (Fig. 5.7), and can be partial or complete. It can occur in the newborn and the elderly with peak incidence in the sixth or seventh decade. Predisposing factors include eventration of the diaphragm, hiatus hernia, phrenic nerve injury, trauma or congenital abnormalities of the diaphragm.

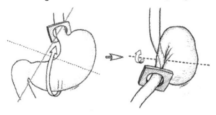

Fig. 5.6 Gastric volvulus: mesenteroaxial rotation.
Reproduced from 'Percutaneous endoscopic gastrostomy tube placement in patients with compound hiatus hernia and intrathoracic stomach: a case series', R Sringeri Manjunath, N C Fisher, *Gut* 2011; **60**: A98–A99, with permission from BMJ Publishing Group Ltd.

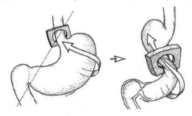

Fig. 5.7 Gastric volvulus: organoaxial rotation.
Reproduced from 'Percutaneous endoscopic gastrostomy tube placement in patients with compound hiatus hernia and intrathoracic stomach: a case series', R Sringeri Manjunath, N C Fisher, *Gut* 2011; **60**: A98–A99, with permission from BMJ Publishing Group Ltd.

Symptoms
- Frequently asymptomatic.
- May be found incidentally on a chest X-ray.
- CT with oral contrast, barium meal (Fig. 5.8) or endoscopy investigation modalities.
- Can create an obstruction, in a similar way to colon.
- Increased likelihood of incarceration and perforation from ischaemia. Carries very high mortality, especially as it tends to affect the elderly, who often have significant co-morbidities.
- Acute gastric volvulus is a surgical emergency.
- Presents with sudden onset left upper quadrant pain and retching.
- *Borchardt's triad:* unproductive retching, acute localized epigastric distension and inability to pass a NGT often diagnostic.

Treatment
- *If asymptomatic:* conservative and expectant.
- *Formal operative management:* elective gastropexy and hiatal repair.
- Can be achieved by open laparoscopically, may entail trans-hiatal approach and/ or thoracotomy.
- If patient high risk and where a non-radical approach favoured: consider percutaneous endoscopic gastrostomy (PEG) insertion.
- *Dual PEG for chronic intermittent volvulus first described by Eckhauser 1985 and single PEG by Tsang 1998:* alpha-loop manouveure used to reduce gastric volvulus single PEG then inserted to prevent recurrent volvulus.
- A combined on-table endoscopic and laparoscopic approach may be necessary to achieve a PEG gastropexy if stomach is infarcted, subtotal or total gastrectomy mandated.
- Mortality is between 30 and 50%.

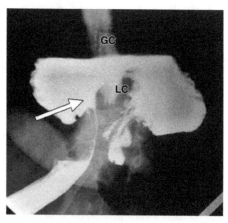

Fig. 5.8 Organoaxial volvulus contrast meal.

Congenital gastric conditions

Hypertrophic pyloric stenosis
- Common in first born male child.
- Results in hypertrophy and hyperplasia of pyloric sphincter in neonatal period.
- Mainly affects circular muscle fibres of pylorus.
- Pylorus becomes elongated and thickened.
- Results in gastric outflow obstruction, vomiting, and dehydration.
- Affects 3 per 1000 live births.
- Male:female 4:1.
- Multifactorial inheritance.
- Strong genetic factor:
  - Risk to son if mother affected = 20%.
  - Risk to daughter if mother affected = 7%.
  - Risk to son if father affected = 5%.
  - Risk to daughter if father affected = 2%.

Aetiology
Unclear due to failure of nitric oxide synthesis.

Symptoms
Typically asymptomatic in the first 3–4 weeks.
- Usually presents between 3 and 6 weeks of age.
- Late presentation up to 6 months can occur.
- Rapidly progressive projectile vomiting without bile.
- Child hungry and often feeds immediately after vomiting.

Diagnosis
Palpable mass in the epigastric and right upper quadrant region particularly while feeding. Dehydration and hypochloraemic alkalosis is a prominent clinical feature:
- Palpable 'tumour' in right upper quadrant best felt from left during test feed.
- Visible peristalsis often seen.

Abdominal ultrasound diagnostic reveals hypertrophic muscle mass.
   Plain X-ray shows large gastric air bubble, but no air beyond stomach and intestine. Barium X-ray shows a long narrow pyloric canal.

Treatment
- Correct the alkalosis with aggressive fluid resuscitation.
- Correct dehydration over a 24–72-h period.
  - NGT often required.
  - Ramstedt's pyloromyotomy—described 1911.
  - Transverse right upper quadrant or circumumbilical incision.
  - Longitudinal incision in pylorus down to mucosa avoiding perforation. Incision extends from D1 to distal antrum (Fig. 5.9).

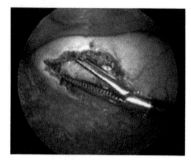

Fig. 5.9 Ramstedt's pyloromyotomy.
Reprinted by permission from Macmillan Publishers Ltd: 'Pediatric Surgery: Laparoscopic surgery safe and effective for infantile pyloric stenosis', Rachel Jones, *Nature Reviews Gastroenterology and Hepatology* **6**, 255, May 2009.

Gastric atresia
The stomach ends blindly in the antrum or pyloric canal.
- *Aetiology:* unclear, but may be familial.
- *Presenting symptoms:* non-bilious copious vomiting and large volume amniotic fluid at birth.
- *Diagnosis:* abdominal X-ray reveals stomach distended with air and typically no air in bowel.
- *Treatment:* surgical, in form of pyloroplasty or gastroenterostomy.

Gastric duplication
Usually occurs with duplications of the digestive tract. Duplication may either be mucosa, submucosa, or three layers of muscle.
- *Symptoms:* abdominal mass or symptoms of gastric outlet obstruction.
- *Treatment:* surgical excision.

Microgastria
This is failure of the stomach to develop from the foregut. The oesophagus dilates and patients present with large volume vomiting of undigested food. Clinical presentation are usually seen at birth and are also associated with cardiac abnormalities. Most patients have a fatal outcome within 3 weeks. If the patient survives, treatment involves reconstruction with a jejunal reservoir.

Gastric teratoma
This is very rare in the stomach and may contain all three 1° embryonic germ cell layers. Presentation is with upper GI bleed, signs of obstruction, or upper abdominal mass. It is found exclusively in male patients, but is present in infancy.
- *Diagnosis:* plain X-ray may show calcification, which may be either teeth or bone within the tumour. Barium studies show a gastric mass.
- *Treatment:* surgical resection.

Further reading

Eckhauser ML et al. The use of dual percutaneous endoscopic gastrostomy (DPEG) in the management of chronic intermittent gastric volvulus. *Gastrointest Endosc* 1985; **31**(5): 340–2.

Tsang TK et al. Use of single percutaneous endoscopic gastrostomy in management of gastric volvulus in three patients. *Dig Dis Sci* 1998; **43**(12): 2659–65.

Chapter 6

Barrett's oesophagus

Aetiology, classification, and historic considerations

Definition

Barrett's oesophagus is a change in the oesophageal epithelium in which any portion of the normal squamous lining has been replaced by metaplastic columnar cells visible macroscopically at endoscopy.

Association with oesophageal adenocarcinoma

- *Barrett's epithelium (BE):* most important precursor lesion for oesophageal adenocarcinoma (OAC).
- 64–86% of all OAC's arise in BE.
- Incidence of OAC for patients with BE increased 30–100-fold above that for the general population.
- OAC develops from BE through a multistep process with progressive dysplasia.

Historic considerations

In 1950 Norman Barrett, a British surgeon, described the columnar lined oesophagus that now bears his name. The disorder had, however, been described 50 years previously by Tileston, a Boston pathologist, who described patients with peptic ulcer of the oesophagus and noted 'the close resemblance of the mucous membrane about the ulcer to that normally found in the stomach'. Later investigators, including Barrett himself, argued that the ulcerated columnar line segment was not oesophagus at all, but a tubular segment of stomach that had been pulled up into the chest due to a congenitally short squamous oesophagus.

It was Bosher and Taylor, in 1951, who first described the intestinal type goblet cells in a columnar-lined oesophagus (CoLO) 'but no parietal cells', which we now refer to as specialized intestinal metaplasia (SIM). Two years later Allison and Johnstone linked the association of GORD and CoLO. Barrett agreed that the columnar lined organ was oesophagus and suggested the condition be called lower oesophagus lined by columnar epithelium. He also recognized the association with hiatal hernia and severe reflux oesophagitis, although maintained, the condition was congenital. By the 1970s it was clear that CoLO, now known as BE, was associated with severe GORD.

Aetiology

Age

- BE is predominantly a disease of middle-aged males.
- Analysis of 5317 BE patients, as part of the UK Barrett's Oesophagus Registry (UKBOR), the M:F ratio of BE patients was 1.7. BE was also found to present at an earlier age in men (62.0 years) than in women (67.5 years).
- Incidence of BE peaked at 60–69 years in males and 70–79 years in females.

Ethnicity
- BE most prevalent in Caucasian males. It is less common in Asian countries, and rare in the Caribbean, Middle East, and much of Africa and South America.
- Cause unclear, but ingestion of a high-fat western diet, and possibly oral and salivary carcinogens that are activated in region of the GOJ, may contribute.

Obesity
- Obesity as measured by BMI strongly associated with both BE and OAC.
- Male pattern of abdominal obesity is a stronger risk factor than total body obesity (as measured by body mass index (BMI)) for both BE and OAC.
- *Mechanisms:* mechanical promotion of GORD in obesity, confounding factors in behaviour of obese individuals that promote GORD and the carcinogenic properties of circulating adipokines.

Reflux
- Association between BE and GORD recognized for many years.
- Presence of both typical GORD symptoms (heartburn or acid regurgitation) and more frequent symptom episodes, are independent predictors of BE.
- Reflux of gastric contents is not the only precursor to BE, duodenal reflux is also thought to contribute—shown through development of BE post-gastrectomy and through detailed analysis of the refluxate reaching the oesophagus.

Helicobacter pylori
- *Helicobacter pylori* promotes development of gastritis role for *H. pylori* in the development of BE and OAC controversial.
- Postulated that individuals with chronic *H. pylori*-associated gastritis have reduced gastric acid production. The acidity of BE generating refluxate is subsequently reduced in turn. A recent meta-analysis supported this inverse association in BE when compared with endoscopically normal controls.

Classification
Prague C&M criteria
- To accurately document the nature of BE the International Working Group for Classification of Oesophagitis (IWGCO) developed the Prague C&M criteria.
- Scoring system is based on circumferential (C value (cm)) and maximal extent (M value (cm)) of BE above the GOJ.
- BE in Fig. 6.1 illustrates a circumferential segment for 2cm above GOJ with a non-circumferential tongue extending to 5cm above GOJ. This would be recorded as C2M5.
- Consensus group in this study decided that 'true islands of squamous and columnar mucosa should not influence the measurement of extent of BE and that only segments of contiguous BE are measured'.

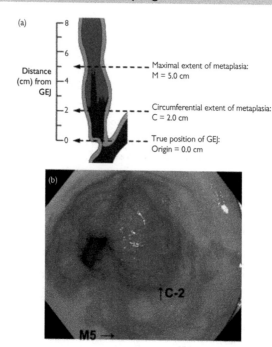

Fig. 6.1 Endoscopic Barrett's oesophagus: (a) diagrammatic representation; and (b) video still.

Reproduced from 'The development and validation of an endoscopic grading system for Barrett's Esophagus: the Prague C & M criteria', Sharma et al., *Gastroenterology* **131**(5): 1392–99, copyright 2006 with permission of Elsevier.

- Proposed scoring system was validated in a study using 29 digital recordings of endoscopies. Internal validation yielded a high reliability coefficient value for agreement on the presence of BE >1cm ($r = 0.72$).

Biomarker predictors of progression to oesophageal adenocarcinoma

Dysplasia

- *Dysplasia:* purely morphological term, defined as 'an unequivocal neoplastic epithelium strictly confined within basement membrane of gland from which it arises'.
- Definition initially proposed for premalignant changes which can develop in inflammatory bowel disease, it has been progressively extended to the entire gastrointestinal tract, including BE.

Classification systems for dysplasia
- 3-tiered system grading dysplasia mild, moderate. or severe.
- *Modified Vienna classification system:* more commonly used— shown in Box 6.1.
- Three-tiered classification, although still in use in some centres, is obsolete because it creates more intra- and inter-observer variability than the Vienna classification.

Box 6.1 **Modified Vienna classification**

- *Category 1:* no neoplasia.
- *Category 2:* indefinite for neoplasia.
- *Category 3:* low-grade adenoma/dysplasia.
- *Category 4:* high-grade neoplasia.
  - *4.1*—high-grade adenoma/dysplasia.
  - *4.2*—non-invasive carcinoma (carcinoma *in situ*).
  - *4.3*—suspicion of invasive carcinoma.
  - *4.4*—intramucosal carcinoma.
- *Category 5:* submucosal invasive carcinoma (carcinoma with invasion of submucosa or deeper).

Reprinted by permission from Macmillan Publishers Ltd: 'The Vienna classification of gastrointestinal epithelial neoplasia', Schlemper RJ, Riddell RH, Kato Y, et al., *Gut* **47**: 251–5, 2000.

Low grade dysplasia
- Characterized by crypts with relative preservation of simple glandular architecture (Fig. 6.2).
- Epithelial cell nuclei are oval or elongated and generally retain polarity. Nuclei are hyperchromatic with mild irregularity of nuclear membrane contour.

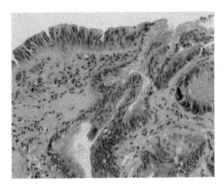

Fig. 6.2 Haemotoxylin and eosin stain of low grade dysplasia—sharp cut off between normal and atypia favours dysplasia. See also Plate 4, colour plate section. Courtesy of Professor Novelli.

The uncertainty of the risk of cancer (Table 6.1) has led to great debate about the advantages and disadvantages of treating low grade dysplasia, particularly with the advent of minimally invasive endoscopic therapies.

- *Argument ablation of LGD is more cost effective than surveillance:* models demonstrate a 65% reduction in progression if complete reversal of dysplasia (CR-D) achieved in 28%.
- A noteworthy feature of LGD not included in these models is phenomenon of regression, demonstrated in recent RCT of radiofrequency ablation (RFA) vs. a sham procedure, when 23% of patients achieved spontaneous regression of LGD in control group. At present time the British Society of Gastroenterology (BSG) recommends that a diagnosis of LGD should warrant close follow-up, with endoscopy every 6 months.

Table 6.1 Risk of developing cancer/high grade dysplasia per patient year with low grade dysplasia

Study	Number patients	Risk of cancer	Risk of HGD	Comments
Reid	43	2.4%		Increased risk with aneuploidy
Weston	54	3%		
Skacel	43	3.7%	12.9%	
Sharma	156	0.6%		
Lim	34	3.4%		
Gatenby	217	2.7%	4.6%	Reduced to 1.4 and 2.2% when prevalent cases excluded
Wani		1.7%		(Meta-analysis)
Curvers (downstaged)	92	0.49%		Unclear how many were prevalent HGD/OAC
Curvers (consensus)	19	13.4%		

HGD, high grade dysplasia.

High grade dysplasia
High grade dysplasia (HGD) is at present the most robust routinely used clinical marker of cancer progression in BE; its presence confers a 56–59% risk of developing cancer within 5 years of the diagnosis of HGD. It is generally accepted that a diagnosis of HGD is an indication for treatment.

In individuals with HGD, particularly with nodular disease, recent UK guidelines recommend that:
- They should all be discussed in a multi-disciplinary team meeting.
- Tissue should be examined with endoscopic mucosal resection (EMR) to confirm diagnosis and depth of infiltration (Fig. 6.3).
- At least two histopathologists report the sample, one of whom should have an interest in GI disease.

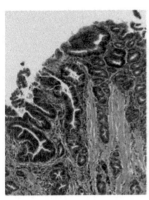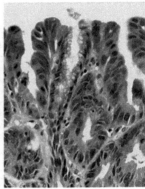

Fig. 6.3 Haemotoxylin and eosin stain of high grade dysplasia - Left ×100, right ×400. See also Plate 5, colour plate section.
Courtesy of Professor Novelli.

Aneuploidy
- Aneuploidy, defined as abnormal DNA content of the nucleus of a cell, is one of the most frequent characteristics of cancer cells that occurs in ~90% of solid tumours.
- In BE, aneuploidy at chromosomes 4 and 8 has been shown to be an early event in carcinogenesis, as have aneuploidy at chromosomes 7 and 17.
- DNA ploidy abnormalities (aneuploidy/tetraploidy) reflect genomic instability and confer an increased risk of cancer progression, when measured by flow cytometry (FC).
- Image cytometry DNA ploidy analysis (ICDA) is a technique with equivalent accuracy to FC and uses formalin fixed tissue, allowing archival analysis.
- DNA ploidy abnormalities have been evaluated in prospective trials of patients with BE, representing phase 4 biomarker development.
- *Patients with both HGD and aneuploidy or tetraploidy:* 5-year cancer risk, 66%, compared with 42% with HGD alone and 28% with DNA ploidy abnormalities alone.
- *Patients with no cytometric abnormality (diploid) and no HGD:* 5-year cancer risk 0%.

Loss of tumour suppressor loci
- *Loss of heterozygosity (LOH):* loss of a chromosome segment after a faulty cell division, and hence the loss of the functioning genes in that lost chromosomal segment.
- LOH of *p53* gene significantly increases risk of progression to cancer in patients with BE with RR of 16 in one study of 325 patients.

Epigenetic changes
- *Epigenetic:* post-transcriptional silencing of specific genes by a variety of mechanisms such as methylation or acetylation. Methylation of DNA cytosine residues in the gene promoter region is common gene-silencing mechanism that has been shown to occur early in tumour genesis, and assessment of promoter methylation at CpG islands provides a novel group of potential biomarkers.
- Promoter methylation of specific genes BNC 2 and CDKN2A has been shown to occur in large areas of contiguous Barrett's epithelium early in progression to adenocarcinoma.
- Methylation induced inactivation of the *p16* tumour-suppressor gene is one of the most common genetic abnormalities in BE and regulates cell cycle progression. In patients with BE, p16 methylation is highly prevalent (34–66%).

Cell cycle markers
- Cell cycle regulator proteins, such as cyclins are potentially useful biomarkers for progression especially because of intimate modulation by p16, a common clonal abnormality in BE.
- Cyclin D1 is an antagonist of p16 and together they regulate cell cycle progression. It has been shown that BE patients positive for cyclin D1 were 6–7 times more likely to develop OAC.

Proliferation markers
- Analyses of markers of DNA proliferation exploited as potential biomarkers for future cancer risk and prognosis.
- In BE Mcm2 and Mcm5 (marker for proliferation) surface positivity correlates with the severity of dysplasia.
- Aberrant surface expression increases along the metaplasia-dysplasia-carcinoma sequence.
- Mcm2 more sensitive than Ki67 for detection of dysplasia.
- *Phase-3 study:* BE biopsies in patients who progressed to OAC had Mcm2 expression in 28.4% of the luminal cells as compared with 3.4% of non-progressors.
- Studies into other potential proliferation markers to predict progression to OAC in BE have shown promising results, but need validation in larger cohorts.

Endoscopic screening and surveillance

Screening

British Society of Gastroenterology guidelines suggest that 'endoscopic screening of patients with chronic heartburn to detect columnar lined oesophagus cannot be recommended, due to a lack of directly applicable studies.'

- American College of Gastroenterology advise gastroscopy for all patients with longstanding GORD for the detection of BE. Remains controversial due to lack of documented impact on mortality from adenocarcinoma.
- A factor to difficulty of applying gastroscopy as a screening tool is lack of an easily identifiable patient group.
- Although GORD is essential to pathogenesis of BE, there is a lack of evidence that symptomatic GORD acutely predicts BE incidence.
- Modiano (2009)[1] 102 patients erosive reflux disease at baseline OGD. Mean follow-up of 25/12.
- 9/102 developed BE, and all nine had severe oesophagitis of Savary–Miller grade 4 (erosive lesion[s] complicated by ulceration or stricture) at their baseline endoscopy. Patients referred for dysphagia (n = 3) or upper GI bleeding (n = 6). None of the patients referred initially for reflux symptoms developed BE.
- Same group evaluated 515 GORD patients (412 with no erosive disease on endoscopy, 103 with oesophagitis) and 169 BE patients. None of 412 GORD patients with non-erosive reflux disease developed BE over a mean follow-up time of 3.4 ± 2.2 years. In group with oesophagitis 5/103 developed subsequent BE. In BE group no patient had a normal endoscopy at baseline.
- Studies present two interesting observations:
  - Presence of severe oesophagitis, in particular grade 4 disease that provokes spontaneous GI bleed, is a significant risk factor for subsequent BE, either because severity of mucosal damage is more likely to heal by metaplastic columnar epithelium or because columnar epithelium is already present, but not visualized.
  - Symptomatic GORD without erosive disease (NERD) is not predictive of future BE incidence, is interesting although follow-up short, and confounding variable. Smoking or PPI usage were not addressed in a multivariate analysis.
- Even if high risk cohort could be identified, cost of OGD-based screening techniques and patient acceptability limit feasibility. Impetus to evaluate new technologies for outpatient screening.

Unsedated transnasal endoscopy
- *Feasible due to introduction of high-quality, small-calibre endoscopes:* outer diameter <6mm.

---

[1] Modiano N and Gerson L Risk factors for the detection of Barrett's esophagus in patients with erosive esophagitis. *Gastrointestinal Endoscopy* 2009; **69**(6), 1014–20.

- Possible as outpatient, sedation unnecessary and acceptable to patients undergoing surveillance.
- *Several types of transnasal endoscope available:* four-directional or two-directional angulation of the tip.
- When biopsies taken, availability of four-way angulation shown to decrease examination time while not significantly altering tolerability.
- Paediatric biopsy forceps necessary due to smaller size of working channel, which limits size of biopsy taken. In a small comparative study of 32 patients, however, there was no significant difference between histological diagnosis of IM or dysplasia between two techniques, despite smaller biopsy size.
- In a feasibility study, unsedated small-calibre gastroscopy and conventional gastroscopy were compared in a randomized cross-over design. Of 121 patients referred for either screening of reflux symptoms or surveillance, 26% had BE using conventional endoscopy vs. 30% using unsedated endoscopy ($P = 0.50$), (71%) preferred unsedated small-calibre endoscopy.
- Despite advantages availability has not increased referral pattern for screening. At present use of this promising screening tool remains in a research setting.

Wireless capsule endoscopy

- Given Imaging were the first company to commercially introduce wireless capsule endoscopy (WCE), a device that has revolutionized imaging of small bowel. Soon after this, a capsule designed for oesophageal use was released, latest model being PillCam ESO 2 (Fig. 6.4).
- The ESO capsules differs from small bowel capsule in having viewing heads at both ends of capsule, which can obtain a total of 18 frames/s, as opposed to 4 frames/s with small bowel capsule.
- To slow oesophageal transit and maximize image capture time, protocol generally involves swallowing capsule recumbent in right lateral position aided by taking sips of water through a straw.
- Studies on utility of WCE as screening tool for BE have followed. In one study 66 screening patients with GORD and 24 surveillance patients with BE were evaluated using WCE with PillCam ESO capsule. This study demonstrated a moderate sensitivity and specificity for the detection of BE, 67 and 84%, respectively.
- Average number of frames in which all four quadrants were visible and presence of bubbles were significant factors in missing diagnosis of BE. In a similar study, a total of 94 patients (41 screening patients with GORD symptoms and 53 known BE under surveillance) had screening with Pillcam ESO.
- The sensitivity and specificity were again moderate, 78 and 75% respectively. A recent meta-analysis that evaluated nine studies, comprising a total of 618 patients, demonstrated a pooled sensitivity and specificity of WCE for the diagnosis of BE were 77 and 86%, respectively. WCE was found to be safe and had a high rate of patient preference.
- One major drawback for use of WCE is rapid transit time through oesophagus, which may lead to inadequate imaging of oesophageal mucosa and GOJ.

- A new approach of string-capsule endoscopy (SCE) using the M2A small bowel capsule has been piloted in feasibility study of 50 patients with BE. Strings were attached to capsule allowing operator-dependent control of probe and acquisition of multiple images around region of interest at squamocolumnar junction. All patients were correctly diagnosed by WCE (mean Barrett's length of 4.47cm), confirmed by subsequent gastroscopy. Procedure was safe and better tolerated by patients than gastroscopy using a simple questionnaire. In addition, probe could be disinfected allowing for multiple uses.
- Same group subsequently conducted a prospective blinded study of 100 consecutive patients with GORD symptoms referred for screening of BE. In the study, 46 patients had endoscopic evidence of BE and 27 were confirmed by presence of specialized intestinal metaplasia (21 with short segment, six with long segment). Sensitivity, specificity, and observed accuracy of SCE for BE when using endoscopic diagnosis as the criterion standard, was again moderate at 78, 83, and 84%, respectively. Of the 16 patients misclassified 10 were false negatives, all of whom had short-segment Barrett's oesophagus (SSBO) at UGI endoscopy.
- Another major disadvantage of using WCE, is inability to collect tissue samples. Although pilot studies have demonstrated feasibility of performing mucosal biopsies using a spring loaded Crosby capsule, no trials have been published to date.
- In summary, WCE has many inherent advantages over endoscopy as a screening tool because it is minimally invasive, safe, well-tolerated by patients, and it can be carried out in a nurse led clinic setting. Despite these advantages, diagnostic accuracy of WCE is not sufficiently high to warrant use as a 1° screening tool, and inability to collect tissue samples make this impractical for Barrett's surveillance.
- Further technological advances in design of WCE that can allow for fluid aspiration, brushings for cytology, multimodal spectroscopic imaging, and immunological cancer recognition may address these limitations.

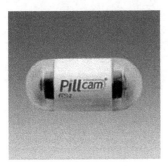

Fig. 6.4 PillCam ESO 2 wireless capsule endoscopy device.
With kind permission of Diagmed Healthcare.

Capsule sponge
- A non-endoscopic capsule sponge device for screening BE has been recently developed in the UK. First tested in Transkei region of South Africa in 1980s for screening of squamous dysplasia.
- Device consists of a polyurethane sponge, contained within a gelatin capsule, which is attached to a string (Fig. 6.5).
- Capsule is swallowed and dissolves within stomach after 3–5min. The sponge can then be retrieved by pulling on string. Cytology specimens retrieved from capsule can then be embedded in paraffin to allow serial sectioning.
- In a pilot study of 92 patients (40 BE, 52 controls) sponge was found to be acceptable and safe.
- Trefoil factor 3 (TFF3) was identified by the group as most promising candidate marker for presence BE with intestinal metaplasia (IM), with a sensitivity of 78% and specificity of 94%. A prospective cohort study further evaluated the capsule sponge in 504 patients in a primary care setting.
- The sponge was swallowed by 99% of patients with no serious adverse events. Prevalence of BE in this cohort (defined as presence of ≥1cm of BE with IM) was 3%. Sensitivity of sponge using TFF3 for detection of BE was 73.3% (95% CI, 44.9–92.2%). For a cut-off of ≥2cm sensitivity increased to 90.0% (95% CI, 55.5–99.7%).
- These promising results are presently being followed up in Barrett's oesophagus screening trial (BEST2). This prospective case controlled study is looking at whether a capsule sponge coupled with a molecular test would offer a suitable alternative to diagnose BE in general population.

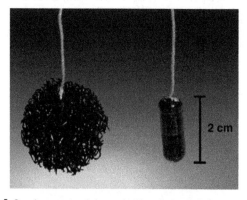

Fig. 6.5 Capsule sponge in gelatin capsule right and expanded left.
Reprinted by permission from Macmillan Publishers Ltd: 'Acceptability and accuracy of a non-endoscopic screening test for Barrett's oesophagus in primary care: cohort study', S.R.Kadri, P.Lao-Sirieix, M.O'Donovan, *BMJ* **341** (2010): c4372.

Surveillance

The rationale of surveillance is the detection of OAC at an early stage when the prognosis is much more favourable, although there is only partial scientific validation to support this view and the value of surveillance is still subject to considerable debate.

- For BE, a four quadrant biopsy protocol (the 'Seattle' protocol) consisting of jumbo forceps biopsies from every 2cm of columnar mucosa, was first proposed for surveillance in 1993.
- National guidelines of many countries recommend this protocol every 2–3 years as standard.
- Observational data to suggest that patients enrolled in surveillance programmes have OAC detected at an earlier stage than non-surveillance detected cancers, with subsequent improved survival.
- Report from the UKBOR cohort on 817 patients, demonstrated a large proportion of dysplastic disease (>90%) was detected on specific surveillance endoscopies, though variation in surveillance practice for BE was observed throughout the UK.
- A 13-fold increase in detection of prevalent dysplasia between patients who underwent four quadrant biopsies every 2cm (median biopsy number; 16) compared with those who had non-systematic biopsies (median biopsy number 4).
- Decision-analysis models have suggested that BE surveillance every two years costs less than £25,000/life-year saved.
- Contradictory evidence in a recent model completed by PenTAG found that surveillance was not cost-effective, with a cost/QALY of approximately £125,000.
- Cost effectiveness analysis of surveillance programmes are dependent on the prevalence of BE, incremental detection rate of dysplasia by endoscopic surveillance and the risk of progression to cancer.
- As the risk of progression and prevalence rates are extracted from observational studies and ∴ represent moderate grade evidence, this in turn makes cost effectiveness models difficult to interpret. This has led to conception of a large UK-based multicentre randomized controlled trial, designed to answer the question of whether surveillance is worthwhile in BE (Barrett's oesophagus surveillance study or BOSS).
- This study has recently completed after randomizing 3400 patients in a 1:1 ratio to either 2-yearly surveillance endoscopy or on-demand endoscopy as symptoms dictate. The results of this trial are eagerly awaited.

Barrett's registries

- A number of Barrett's registries have been set up to answer some key questions into epidemiology and pathogenesis of BE. These include identifying current trends in diagnosis of BE and their relationship to OAC, mapping the natural history of Barrett's metaplasia and identifying associated factors that may influence future cancer risk.
- Currently two main types of registry; institution-based, recruiting patients encoded with a specific diagnosis within institution, and population-based, which usually register patients from histology databases or from links between institutions (Table 6.2).
- Both provide an infrastructure for pathological confirmation of BE, and facilitate co-ordination and recruitment into clinical studies. Follow-up registered patients is allows study of clinically important outcomes.
- Databases recruiting patients from pathological samples have the ability to provide a relevant population denominator for studies, while institutional registries have the ability to draw large numbers of BE patients into studies and access other potentially important clinical information.
- Population databases have a further advantage of facilitating examination of potential geographical and chronological variation in presentation of BE.
- Essential future role of Barrett's registries, however, is to provide data to facilitate accurate cost-benefit analyses for potential future studies in BE population and allow refinement of surveillance strategies, such as targeted surveillance or intervention for only those patients deemed to be at higher risk of progression to OAC.

Table 6.2 Institution and population-based Barrett's registries

Population-based	Institution-based
Northern Ireland Barrett's Registry	Mayo Clinic Barrett's Registry
Danish Barrett's Esophagus Registry	Cleveland Clinic Barrett's Registry
Dutch Nationwide Cohort Registry	Venice Region Barrett's Registry
	UK Barrett's Oesophagus Registry

Management of dysplasia: non-operative

Chemoprevention for Barrett's oesophagus

- *Chemoprevention:* use of pharmacological techniques to reduce cancer risk, is an intense area of research interest in BE. GORD is thought to be essential for BE development, and may have a role in initiating and promoting tumour development.
- Refluxate contains numerous noxious substances, which can cause acute and chronic inflammation, and oxidative stress. An ideal treatment strategy for patients with BE ∴ may be a treatment that prevented reflux and associated inflammatory change with resultant decreased progression to cancer.
- Potential targets that have been identified for chemoprevention include acid suppression with PPI, bile salt manipulation and cyclo-oxygenase (COX) inhibitors.

Proton pump inhibitors

- The hypothesis that PPIs may reduce neoplastic progression in BE by reduction of GORD and inflammation is intuitive, yet evidence from laboratory studies is somewhat conflicting. There is evidence that PPIs have advantageous effects on cellular proliferation, cell cycle control and DNA stability.
- The majority of clinical studies on the use of PPI in BE are retrospective cohort design, with a lack of randomized controlled data and use of surrogate end points for cancer risk. A recent Australian study of 502 cancer-free patients with BE reported that patients not on PPIs at time of diagnosis were 3.4 times more likely to have higher-risk endoscopic features (e.g. ulceration, nodularity, or stricture) or LGD than patients who were on a PPI at time of diagnosis. The same group previously reported that patients who delayed starting PPIs by 2 years or more after diagnosis of BE had a subsequent 5–20-fold increased risk for development of HGD or OAC compared with patients who started shortly after their diagnosis.
- A major concern regarding the long term use of PPIs is the 2° increase in serum gastrin. Increased gastrin expression has been shown to increase risk of dysplasia and cancer in BE in several studies.
- Gastrin is known to increase COX-2 expression and induce proliferation by activation of the cholecystokinin 2 receptor. These experiments are complicated by the variable expression of CCKR in oesophageal tissue and the physiological effects of subtle variations in gastrin concentration. Studies using gastrin antagonists in patients with BE may soon be available for Phase II/III testing.
- Long-term PPI use is also associated with side effects. *Clostridium difficile* infections have been shown to be significantly increased in patients taking long term acid suppression in three separate studies, and incidence seems to be dose related.

- PPI use has also been found to be associated with a small, but significant increased risk of gastroenteritis, pulmonary infections, and hip fractures, which was independent of bone mineral density. Although the effect is moderate, this could amount to a significant morbidity if these drugs were to be used on a large population.
- *BSG guidelines:* routine use of high-dose PPI Rx, beyond need for symptom relief and mucosal healing, is not recommended.

Bile salt manipulation

- One of the major constituents of refluxate, after acid, is bile and it has been shown that a third of patients on PPI therapy will continue to reflux bile salts.
- Bile salts can produce injury over a wide range of pH and chronic injury is dependent on acid dissociation properties of bile salt. Taurine-conjugated bile salts, for example, cause chronic mucosal injury when oesophageal reflux is acidic (pH 4), whereas unconjugated bile salts cause mucosal injury when pH is neutral or alkaline.
- These properties are important as long-term use of PPIs, in addition to increasing pH of lower oesophagus, can cause bacterial colonization of upper gut which deconjugates bile salts.
- Bile salts may play a role in both initiation of tumour development and promotion of growth. Bile salts have been shown to induce DNA damage in a dose-dependent, but non-linear fashion. DNA damage caused by bile salts appears to be mediated by reactive oxygen species, which may lead to potential use of antioxidants for chemoprevention in BE. At present time, no clinical studies of bile salt acid manipulation or antioxidants have been undertaken.

COX-2 inhibitors

- COX-2 is an inducible enzyme that synthesizes prostaglandins from arachidonic acid, and has been found to be increasingly over-expressed along metaplastic pathway to OAC.
- Chemopreventative agents that block COX-2 include aspirin, NSAIDs or more specific selective COX-2 inhibitors.
- Celecoxib, a selective COX-2 inhibitor, has been studied in a phase 2b, multicentre, double-blind randomized placebo-controlled study called the Chemoprevention for Barrett's Esophagus Trial (CBET). In this study 100 patients with LGD or HGD were randomized to either 48 weeks of treatment with 200mg celecoxib or placebo.
- No significant change in the proportion of biopsy samples with dysplasia or cancer was observed between two treatment groups. This outcome was thought to be due to an inadequate dose of celecoxib, however, increased cardiovascular risk for celecoxib is dose dependent and noted at daily doses of 400mg or more, precluding higher dosages being used.
- Non-selective COX-2 inhibition with aspirin or NSAIDs is an alternative strategy for chemoprevention. Protective effect of long term aspirin or NSAID use on risk of progression to OAC has been consistently shown in retrospective cohort and case-control studies.

- A meta-analysis of observational studies evaluating both aspirin and NSAIDs suggests a protective effect for OAC, although aspirin was shown to be more effective.
- Reid study: regular users of aspirin or other NSAIDs had a strong and significant decreased risk of progression to cancer, especially in high-risk individuals with multiple chromosomal instability markers (79 vs. 30% 10-year cumulative cancer incidence).
- Inhibition of COX-2 by these agents may represent a useful chemoprevention strategy that may reduce incidence of OAC in patients at low/medium risk of progression. Safety and efficacy of this treatment strategy needs to be validated in clinical trials and at present time there is insufficient data for chemoprevention with low dose aspirin for BE.
- The Aspirin Esomeprazole Chemoprevention Trial (AspECT trial) hopes to clarify these issues. The trial was formulated in an open, randomized 2x2 factorial design and has recently completed recruitment of 2513 patients. Subject were split into four arms (20mg of esomeprazole alone, 80mg of esomeprazole alone, 20mg of esomeprazole with low dose aspirin and 80mg of esomeprazole with low dose aspirin). Study also hopes to demonstrate whether this treatment strategy can cause 2° cardiac and cancer preventive effects.

Minimally-invasive endoscopic therapy

Endoscopic therapy is now increasingly being considered in the UK as first line therapy for HGD and intramucosal cancer in centres with access to them. Several minimally invasive treatments for BE have been studied and have shown effective eradication of HGD, reducing the risk of progression to cancer.

Photodynamic therapy

- Photodynamic therapy (PDT) is a unique medical technology in which a drug known as a photosensitizer (PS) becomes active when illuminated with light of a specific wavelength. Light triggers a photochemical reaction to convert molecular oxygen into highly cytotoxic reactive oxygen species (ROS). PS can then either kill cell, or fluoresce to highlight it for imaging in a number of ways.
- PDT is attractive as it causes little damage to connective tissue components, such as collagen and elastin, preserving the mechanical integrity of hollow organs such GI tract.
- Furthermore, once a PDT-treated area has healed, it can be treated repeatedly without cumulative toxicity, and it may be safely given to treat areas of recurrent cancer even if they have received maximal radiotherapy, making it ideal as an adjunct to current therapy.
- A multicentre, international randomized controlled trial of 200 patients with high grade dysplasia in Barrett's oesophagus confirmed the effectiveness of Photofrin PDT.

- Complete reversal of HGD (CR-HGD) at 1 year was achieved with Photofrin PDT in 71 vs. 30% in control group ($P < 0.001$). In follow-up evaluation at 5 years CR-HGD was 59% compared with 5% in control arm. Significant decreased incidence of oesophageal adenocarcinoma (13% with Photofrin PDT, 28% with PPI alone) was reported as a 2° end point.
- Two common side effects of PDT using porfimer sodium are photosensitivity reactions and oesophageal strictures. Photosensitivity can occur up to 3 months after treatment and is reported in more than 60% of patients.

Radiofrequency ablation

- Use of HALO RFA (Fig. 6.6 and Fig. 6.7) has recently superseded PDT for the minimally invasive treatment of HGD arising in BE. It has been shown to be successful in both American and European data in eradicated dysplasia in these patients.
- A 16-centre US registry reported initial data on the use of RFA for HGD. Of 142 patients enrolled, 92 patients had at least one follow-up endoscopy and efficacy data was reported at 12 months following initial ablation.
- Among those patients, complete reversal of HGD (CR-HGD) was achieved in 90% (83/92) at a median 1 year follow-up; 80% (74/92) had CR-D and 54% (50/92) had complete reversal of BE with no intestinal metaplasia (CR-IM).
- No serious adverse events were reported and no SSBO was noted. One stricture occurred. Early data from UK HALO registry with over 200 patient has also shown promising results with complete eradication of dysplasia of 95%, which is similar to published data.
- In a randomized controlled trial of 127 patients (63 with HGD and 64 with LGD) randomized in a 2:1 study design, treatment with the HALO360 and HALO90 RFA devices was compared with a sham procedure.
- CR-D was achieved in 81% of those with HGD in the ablation group, as compared with 19% of those in the control group ($P < 0.001$).
- For LGD the CR-D was 91% in the ablation group, as compared with 23% of those in the control group ($P < 0.001$).
- For all patients CR-IM was 77% in ablation group and 2% of patients in sham group at 12-month follow-up ($P < 0.001$).
- Rate of progression from HGD to cancer was significantly lower in those patients treated by RFA than those treated by sham procedure at 12-month follow-up (2% [1/42] and 19% [4/21], respectively; $P = 0.04$).
- No LGD patients progressed to cancer in either group, consistent with known low risk, transient nature and high inter-observer variability of this diagnosis.
- Although length of follow-up in RCT was insufficient to assess recurrence of Barrett's oesophagus after therapy, more recent data emerging has demonstrated that 1-year results seem durable at 3 years.

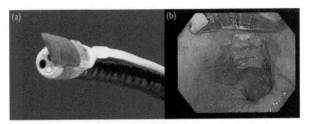

Fig. 6.6 HALO⁹⁰ focal ablation device.

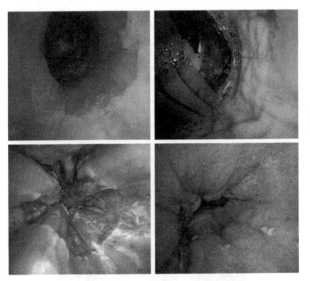

Fig. 6.7 Endoscopic view of Barrett's oesophagus before and after RFA with HALO³⁶⁰ device.

Endoscopic sub-mucosal resection

EMR is an endoscopic technique developed for removal of sessile or flat neoplasms confined to the superficial layers of the GI tract. An example of a combined multi-band ligator device and snare for EMR is shown in Fig. 6.8. EMR is actually a misnomer as the resected specimen can contain tissue down to the submucosa. In contrast to ablative treatments such as PDT and RFA, EMR allows histological assessment of the resected specimen to assess both the pathology and potential infiltration into the lateral basal margins, imitating the surgical situation.

- Several studies have demonstrated that EMR is safe and effective for complete resection of superficial lesions arising in BE (Fig. 6.9).
- *EMR specimens:* much larger than conventional endoscopic biopsies ~10–30mm in size allow assessment of vertical depth of tumour invasion, lateral or deep margin involvement by cancer, which cannot be assessed using standard mucosal biopsy.
- Important as rationale of accurate staging of T1 OAC for potentially curative endoscopic therapy is very low rate of LN metastases limited to mucosa (T1a) of 0–0.03% vs. submucosal cancers (T1b), which have an 18–41% lymph node metastases rate.
- Two recent studies demonstrate less interobserver variability among pathologists for EMR than biopsy specimens for diagnosis of dysplasia.
- Large prospective study 100 patients with low-risk lesions were treated with either cap-assisted or ligation-assisted EMR. Using this approach a 98% CR-D was achieved and overall calculated 5-year survival was 98%.
- Complication rates of EMR are very low from published series. When assessing 12 trials published on EMR alone in 805 patients the overall acute minor bleeding (treated with single modality, no drop Hb>2g/dL or need for transfusion) was in the range 0.6–6%. Strictures occurred in 4% and increased in frequency when greater than 50% of the oesophageal lumen was resected. Perforations are very rare in the oesophagus (0.12% of all patients) when compared with stomach (4.9%).

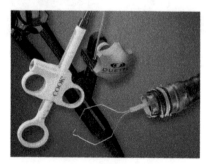

Fig. 6.8 Duette multiband mucosectomy (MBM) kit, Cook, Ireland.
Permission for use granted by Cook Medical Inc., Bloomington, Indiana.

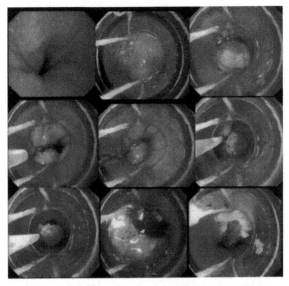

Fig. 6.9 EMR of nodule in Barrett's epithelium. Left to right—(a) Nodular area at 11 o'clock position. (b) EMR cap is seen on tip of endoscope as suction is applied to mucosa. (c) Band placed with some minor haemorrhage. (d) Snare inserted into cap. (e–g) Snare is deployed underneath band and electrosurgical current applied. (h) Polypoid lesion is sucked into cap and removed. (i) Crater formed post-EMR with mucosa visible.

Combination of EMR and field ablation

- Although short-term success rates for complete elimination of all neoplasia are high, ranging from 83 to 98%, complete eradication of all Barrett's mucosa is rarely achieved. Development of new or recurrent lesions during follow-up is seen in a considerable number of patients (0–39%).
- Subsequent studies have addressed the question whether a combination of EMR and field ablative therapy is more effective for long term cure than EMR alone. These are summarized in Table 6.3.
- The overall CR-HGD ranges from 83 to 98% with recurrence rates of 0–33%, although majority of studies have a short mean follow-up of 12 months.
- One study, that evaluated the combination of EMR and ALA PDT in 20 patients with HGD or intramucosal cancer (IMC), reported a significant difference in the success rate that was dependent on the presence of residual HGD after EMR.
- The overall success rate was 15/20 (75%), but when patients were separated into two groups based on the presence or absence of residual HGD in the remaining BE segment, the rate was 55% for residual HGD vs. 100% for no residual dysplasia.

Table 6.3 Clinical results of patients treated with combination of endoscopic mucosal resection and field ablative therapy (EMR, PDT, PS, ALA, RFA, argon plasma coagulation (APC))

Author	Ablation therapy studied	No. patients treated	CR-HGD	Follow-up (months)	No. of treatment sessions	Recurr-ences
(133)	EMR + PS-PDT	24	20 (83%)	12 ± 2	n/a	0
(134)	EMR + PS-PDT	17	16 (94%)	13	2.5	1 (6%)
(123)	EMR + ALA-PDT	9	8 (89%)	34 ± 10	3.8 ± 2.5	3 (33%)
(132)	EMR + ALA PDT	20	15 (75%)	30 (22–31)	2.4	4 (20%)
(118) (subgroup analysis HALO registry)	EMR + HALO RFA	24	21 (88%)	12 ± 4	1 ± 1 RFA, EMR n/a	n/a
(135)	EMR + HALO RFA and/or APC	51	50 (98%)	11.5	4.9	2 (4%)
(136)	EMR + HALO RFA	23	22 (95%)	22	n/a	2 (9%)

- This success rate was calculated at 3 months, however, and 4/15 cases subsequently relapsed to HGD/OAC within 1 year of treatment, and were not amenable to rescue EMR. Therefore, overall CR-HGD was 55%. Criticisms of this paper include study design and dosing of Aminolevulinic acid (ALA, 40mg/kg) which may be considered sub-optimal treatment.
- The only prospective cohort study of combination of HALO, RFA, and EMR published to date was undertaken in 3 European centres on 23 patients, 16 with IMC and 7 with HGD. The worst residual histology results, post-EMR, but pre-RFA were HGD (10 patients), LGD (11 patients), and intestinal metaplasia (3 patients). CR-D and CR-IM after field ablation were 95% and 88% respectively. Two patients required rescue EMR, although none have required additional therapy after a median follow-up of 22 months. Complications included delayed bleeding ($n = 1$) and dysphagia ($n = 1$).
- In a recent US multicentre study (published in abstract form) 51 patients, the majority with HGD or IMC (95%), were treated with RFA (23 patients), APC (13), or both (15). Mean time to achieve CR-IM was 17.4 months (range 2.6–48.1), with length of BE as only significant predictor. Complications included bleeding ($n = 6$), stricture ($n = 3$) and one perforation. After mean follow-up of 11.5 months (range 0–66.1), one patient progressed to cancer, two had recurrent HGD, and one had recurrent IM.
- These studies demonstrate the combination of EMR plus field ablation may be more effective than EMR alone, although recurrence rate of 0–33% is still high and follow-up of these studies is short.

Disadvantages of this approach are number of treatment sessions required to achieve CR-HGD, ranging from 3–5, and need for continued close surveillance during follow-up.

Stepwise radical endoscopic resection

- New approach to endoscopic treatment of BE is complete removal of Barrett's segment by EMR, dubbed 'stepwise endoscopic resection (SER)' in Europe or 'complete Barrett's eradication (CBE)' in US (Typically piecemeal ER of 50% of BO followed by serial ER).
- The efficacy and safety of this approach has been demonstrated in two studies:
  - *Single centre US study*—49 patients (33 HGD, 16 IMC), 32 of whom were analysed. EMR was undertaken using multiband ligator, cap-assisted, and/or 'inject and cut' techniques and mean number of treatment sessions was 2.1. CR-IM was achieved in 31/32 patients after a mean follow-up of 22.9 months. Rate of symptomatic oesophageal stenosis was 37%, and all were successfully managed by endoscopic treatment. No perforations or uncontrollable bleeding occurred.
  - *Multi-centre European study*—169 patients HGD or early cancer Rx, complete EMR of Barrett's segment. After a median of two treatment sessions CR-D was achieved in 95%, and CR-IM 89%, maintained after a median follow-up of 27/12. Recurrence rate for metachronous disease was 1.8%. Most advanced history always at initial EMR session, where most suspicious lesion removed first. Rate of symptomatic oesophageal stenosis 50%. 1/3 graded as severe (>5 dilatation sessions needed).
  - *Serious adverse events:* perforation in 4/169 patients or 2.4% of study population, and bleeding (4/169). These results are largest experience to date with circumferential EMR although retrospective cohort design, enrolment of BE <5cm length and restriction to highly skilled endoscopists at large volume centres limit generalizability of the study.
- *Most effective approach for ablation of Barrett's mucosa unclear:*
  - Preliminary results RCT in Europe to compare SER with combination of EMR + HALO RFA, 47 patients with HGD or IMC and <5cm BE were randomized, 25 to SER and 22 to RFA. CR-IM was achieved in 96 and 95% of subjects in each group, and median number of sessions required to reach this end point was similar. Two in the SER group and three in RFA group.
  - Incidence of stenosis was significantly higher in SER group (86%) vs. RFA group (14%) ($P < 0.001$). Single perforation, from the SER group. Authors recommend a combined approach of focal EMR for visible lesions followed by RFA for complete eradication of remaining BE, although final results of this study with long term follow-up and information on rates of recurrence are awaited.
  - Pouw et al. (2010) showed that SRER of HGD/early cancer arising in patients with BE with a length of <5cm was safe and effective. They demonstrated that complete eradication of all neoplasia and all intestinal metaplasia by the end of the treatment phase was reached in 97.6% and 85.2% of patients. However, >50% symptomatic stricturing that required therapy.

Management of dysplasia: operative

- Historically, it was conventional practice for those with HGD in BE to be referred for operative surgery with oesophagectomy, based on belief that up to 40% of patients may already harbour occult cancer in the Barrett's segment, and that fear that despite comprehensive biopsy protocols, a number of cancers may still be missed.
- In those who receive surgical resection for HGD, survival rates exceed 90%. This is supported by recently published National Oesophago-Gastric Cancer Audit in the UK, which reported hospital mortality for oesophagectomy to be 5.0% (95% CI 3.8–6.4%). Proportion of patients receiving surgery however, had fallen since the last audit. Furthermore, there is strong correlation between surgical mortality and number of operations being performed at an institution and expertise of the surgeon.
- Apart from surgical mortality, up to 50% of patients undergoing surgery suffer significant morbidities such as dumping, regurgitation, anastomotic strictures, and diarrhoea.
- Recently, newer surgical techniques such as minimally-invasive, vagal-sparing oesophagectomy have been to reduce perioperative morbidity, hospital stay and long-term complications, when compared with traditional trans-hiatal or en bloc oesophagectomy in patients with HGD in BE or early cancer.
- At present, studies comparing outcomes between minimally invasive endoscopic and surgical therapy for HGD and early cancer are misleading due to selection bias. Endotherapy was predominantly used in older individuals with smaller segments of BE and earlier tumours.
- The SEER database of the National Cancer Institute (USA) was the first population based study to look at survival in early tumours (Tis and T1 disease without node or metastatic spread) treated endoscopically or with radical surgery. It found equivalent long-term survival in both treatment groups, supporting effectiveness for managing these patients with endoscopic therapy.
- There has recently been a paradigm shift in use of minimally invasive endoscopic therapies for HGD, and question of whether they should be offered to all patients with HGD, as a first line treatment, is subject of great debate.
- The 2011 UK guidelines on management of oesophageal cancer still present surgery as first line treatment option for early oesophageal cancer, recommending further research into minimally invasive endoscopic therapies for HGD and early mucosal cancer despite a growing body of evidence in its favour. In contrast, American College of Gastroenterology guidelines report that 70–80% of HGD can be successfully treated with endoscopic therapy with PDT, RFA, or EMR, and recommend surgery be reserved for disease infiltrating the submucosa (T1b disease) after evaluation by surgical centres that specialize in treatment of foregut cancers and high-grade dysplasia.
- Significance of 'buried glands' with potential for neoplasia, often cited in support of radical surgical Rx, endoscopic ablation can bury metaplastic glands. Even without ablation, buried metaplasia often is found in areas where Barrett's epithelium abuts squamous epithelium.
- Buried metaplasia is reported less frequently after RFA than after PDT: prevalence before ablation: 0–28%. In 22 reports on PDT for 953 patients, buried metaplasia was found in 135 (14.2%); in 18 reports on RFA for 1004 patients, buried metaplasia was found in only nine (0.9%).

Chapter 7

Preoperative assessment and perioperative care

Preoperative assessment of the operative risk profile

Patient selection and risk stratification

Upper GI surgery is major surgery and is associated with a strong systemic inflammatory response both during and after surgery. The patient requires an adequate cardiopulmonary reserve to be able to meet the metabolic demands of surgery. Oesophagectomy, in particular, has one of the highest perioperative mortality rates of all elective procedures (up to 5%), and over 30% of patients suffer a major complication. Therefore, the suitability of a patient for an operative procedure requires careful assessment and optimization of their physiological status.

Preoperative history and examination

Assess for evidence of:

- *Cardiovascular and respiratory system impairment:* pre-existing ischaemic heart disease (IHD), poorly-controlled hypertension, congestive cardiac failure, symptomatic arrhythmias, cerebrovascular disease, and pulmonary dysfunction.
- *Other systemic disorders:* may impinge on cardiorespiratory reserve, in particular renal, hepatic, and endocrine diseases, such as diabetes mellitus and thyroid dysfunction.
- *Smoking:* associated with post-operative pulmonary complications.

Evaluate:

- *Functional capacity:* expressed in metabolic equivalent (MET) levels. Estimated energy expenditure for various activities shown in Table 7.1. Post-operative complications are increased in those unable to meet a 4 MET demand and warrant additional investigation.
- *Impact of age:* not a contraindication to surgery per se, but associated with co-morbidities and increased post-operative complications. May require more intensive perioperative management and a longer hospital stay.

Establish:

- *Medications and their efficacy:* suboptimal Rx IHD, congestive cardiac failure, hypertension, COPD, and asthma contributes significantly to likelihood of avoidable perioperative cardiorespiratory complications. Stop preoperatively: oral hypoglycaemics, insulin, the oral contraceptive pill, anticoagulants, and antiplatelet medications, such as clopidogrel and high dose aspirin. Follow local guidelines.
- *History of allergies:* to drugs, skin preparations, dressings, and latex.
- *Nutritional state:* malnutrition common; increases risk of post-operative complications. Record body weight and BMI.

Table 7.1 The Duke Activity Status Index and AHA Exercise Standards

1 MET	Can you: • Take care of yourself? • Eat, dress, or use the toilet? • Walk indoors around the house? • Walk on level ground at 2–3 mph?
4 METs	Can you: • Do light housework like dusting or washing dishes? • Climb a flight of stairs or walk up a hill? • Walk on level ground at 4 mph? • Run a short distance? • Do heavy work around the house like scrubbing floors • or lifting or moving heavy furniture? • Participate in moderate recreational activities like golf, bowling, dancing?
Greater than 10 METs	Can you: • Participate in strenuous sports like swimming, singles tennis, football, or skiing?

Reproduced from 'A brief self-administered questionnaire to determine functional capacity (The Duke Activity Status Index)', Mark A. Hlatky, MD, Robin E. Boineau, MA, Michael B. Higginbotham et al., *Am. J. Cardiol.* **64**(10): 651–4, copyright 1989 with permission of Elsevier.

Preoperative investigations

- Full blood count (FBC), urea & electrolytes (U&Es), liver function tests (LFTs), coagulation screen, blood cross-match according to hospital guidelines.
- 12-lead electrocardiogram (ECG).
- Pulmonary function tests.

Additional tests that may be required depending on the patient's results and medical history and examination are:

- Arterial blood gases on air.
- Lung diffusion capacity.
- Echocardiography.
- Chest X-ray.
- Exercise testing including cardiopulmonary exercise testing (CPET) controversial with respect to correlation with patient outcomes.
- Pulmonary function tests.
- Requirement for one-lung ventilation (OLV) for oesophageal surgery makes assessment of pulmonary function of particular importance.
- Pulmonary complications are most common cause of morbidity and mortality.
- Patients with significantly impaired preoperative pulmonary function will have difficulties maintaining oxygenation during OLV and in post-operative period.

- Those with shortness of breath at rest, hypoxaemia, and/or hypercarbia will be unlikely to tolerate one-lung anaesthesia.
- Other predictors of post-operative complications are summarized in Box 7.1.
- Risk of developing pulmonary complications cannot be predicted by pulmonary function tests alone and should be considered along with clinical findings and other investigations.

> **Box 7.1 Predictors of post-operative pulmonary complications**
> - Forced vital capacity (FVC) <80%.
> - Forced expiratory volume in 1s (FEV1) <70%.
> - Peak expiratory flow rate (PEFR) <65%.
> - FEV1/FVC ratio <75%.

Cardiopulmonary exercise testing

CPET is a non-invasive assessment of cardiopulmonary function at rest and during stress. Typically, an exercise bicycle or treadmill is used to expose the patient to a gradually increasing work rate until they are unable to continue due to exhaustion, breathlessness, or angina.

- Numerous physiological variables are recorded including breath-by-breath ventilatory parameters, inspiratory and expiratory gases, blood pressure, and ECG.
- Two derived factors, maximum oxygen uptake (VO_{2max}) and anaerobic threshold (AT), have been demonstrated to be predictors of perioperative morbidity and mortality.
- VO_{2max} is the oxygen consumption recorded when oxygen consumption reaches plateau with increasing workload.
- VO_{2max} <15mL/kg/min associated with increased risk of perioperative complications.
- AT is point at which anaerobic metabolism exceeds aerobic metabolism.
- This is generally seen at 47–64% of VO_{2max}.
- It is less effort dependent than VO_{2max}.
- AT of ≤11mL/min/kg has a predictive value in determining increased risk of post-operative complications across a range of surgical procedures.
- An AT ≤8mL/min/kg would suggest such severe systemic disease that surgery would be high risk.
- The interpretation of AT value is open to inter-observer variability.
- Thresholds for different types of surgery may be different, and should be validated for specific types of procedures.
- CPET should be used as one of the tools, along with other clinical findings and investigations, in pre-operative assessment, risk stratification, informed consent, and risk management of a patient presenting for gastric and oesophageal surgery.
- Performance on CPET will be significantly reduced after neoadjuvant chemoradiation. Where results from CPET suggest a higher risk, omitting neoadjuvant chemoradiation and proceeding straight to surgery may be of benefit.

Risk stratification

There are a number of methods by which the perioperative risks of surgery can be quantitatively evaluated. Anaesthetists use the American Society of Anesthesiologists (ASA) classification (Table 7.2). Although it is not a sensitive predictor of morbidity and mortality there is a reasonable correlation with outcome.

A widely used classification is the Physiological and Operative Severity Score for the enumeration of Mortality and Morbidity (POSSUM), and the modified P-POSSUM. It requires the scoring of 12 physiological and six operative parameters to give a percentage risk for morbidity and mortality (Table 7.3). It tends to overestimate risk in low risk groups and becomes increasingly more accurate as risk increases.

Table 7.2 American Society of Anesthesiologists assessment of physical status

Grade	Definition
ASA 1	Normal healthy patient
ASA 2	Mild systemic disease with no functional limitation
ASA 3	Moderate systemic disease with functional limitation
ASA 4	Severe systemic disease that is a constant threat to life
ASA 5	Moribund patient not expected to survive 24h with or without surgery

Excerpted from 'The ASA Relative Value Guide' 2011, of the American Society of Anesthesiologists. A copy of the full text can be obtained from ASA, 520 N. Northwest Highway, Park Ridge, Illinois 60068-2573.

Table 7.3 Physiological and operative parameters in calculating the P-POSSUM score

Physiological parameters	Operative parameters
Age	Operation type
Cardiac status	Number of procedures
Respiratory status	Operative blood loss
ECG	Peritoneal contamination
Systolic blood pressure	Malignancy status
Pulse rate	Urgency of surgery
Haemoglobin	
White blood cells (WBC)	
Urea	
Sodium	
Potassium	
Glasgow Coma Score (GCS)	

Anaesthetic considerations

- *History of previous GA complications:* difficulties with tracheal intubation, a family history of malignant hyperthermia and pseudocholinesterase deficiency (or 'sux apnoea') should be alerted to anaesthetist well ahead of surgery.
- Tumour involvement with major airways can obstruct positioning of tracheal or double lumen endobronchial tube, or cause serious or life-threatening airway trauma. If suggested by CT scans, airway anatomy may require further investigation with bronchoscopy.
- *Gastro-oesophageal reflux common in this group of patients:* risk of aspiration under GA and leading to aspiration pneumonitis within hours. Potentially life-threatening condition caused by inflammatory reaction of lung parenchyma to acid gastric contents.
  - *Prophylaxis*—antacids or H2 receptor antagonists should be continued up to the day of surgery.
  - If significant risk of reflux rapid sequence induction (RSI) performed to intubate trachea in shortest possible time.
- *Deep vein thrombosis (DVT) prophylaxis:* anti-embolism stockings[FM] and low molecular weight heparin (LMWH). If post-operative epidural analgesia planned, last dose should be given at least 12h before epidural catheter is sited (or removed post-operatively) and must not be restarted within 4h of epidural catheter being sited (or removed post-operatively). Dynamic Flowtron boots used intraoperatively.
- If on Rx doses of LMWH for thromboembolic disease require it to be discontinued for 24h before epidural insertion.
- The case for low-dose aspirin (75mg) is less clear and the decision to stop it pre-operatively is a matter of personal preference. Evidence that it is safe to insert an epidural catheter in presence of aspirin.
- Stop clopidogrel 7 days prior to surgery. If drug-eluting coronary stent inserted recently, seek cardiology advice.
- Excessive preoperative fasting for food and fluids should be avoided. Fasting time for food/milk is 6h and clear, non-carbonated fluids should be continued up to 2h preoperatively. In fact, small amounts of water (150mL) given preoperatively reduce volume and acidity of gastric contents.
- In absence of disorders of gastric emptying or diabetes preoperative administration of carbohydrate rich beverages 2–3h before induction of anaesthesia may attenuate preoperative thirst, anxiety, and post-operative nausea and vomiting. It also substantially reduces post-operative insulin resistance, thereby improving efficacy of post-operative nutritional support.
- Preoperative overnight IV fluids unnecessary when patients are able to take oral fluids.

Perioperative optimization

Beta blockade

- Patients with coronary artery disease should be receiving beta-blockers unless contraindicated.
- Patients already on beta-blockers should be maintained on their medication throughout perioperative period. Stopping beta-blockers perioperatively associated with significant increase in cardiac complications.
- In practice, for most oesophagogastric surgery, this would require local protocols for IV beta-blocker.
- Adjusting dose of beta-blocker to maintain tight heart rate control throughout perioperative period should be considered, with careful titration of dose to effect.
- Patients not taking beta-blockers, but in whom indicated should commence them at least 1 week pre-operatively.
  - Acute perioperative beta-blockade for at risk patients may significantly reduce myocardial infarction (MI), need for coronary revascularization and incidence of AF, but associated with significant increase mortality, cerebrovascular accident (CVA) clinically significant hypotension and bradycardia, and ∴ cannot be recommended for majority of patients.

Statins

- Patients already on statins should be maintained on their medication throughout perioperative period.
- In these patients, statins should be resumed as soon as possible post-operatively and preferably within 4 days.
  - Some evidence supports use of statins perioperatively to reduce cardiac complications, particularly new or recurrent atrial fibrillation (AF) in vascular and cardiac surgery. For oesophagogastric surgery benefit is less clear.

Nutritional status

- All patients should have their weight and BMI (in kg/m^2) measured.
- History of weight loss over preceding 6 months should be sought.
- Malnutrition is associated with increased risk of post-operative infectious complications.
- Hypalbuminaemia as a marker of malnutrition is a predictor of adverse surgical outcome.
- Role of preoperative nutrition in form of total parenteral nutrition (TPN) and total enteral nutrition (TEN) is unclear. Some evidence that it can reduce complications. Disadvantages of preoperative TPN include complications and increased cost of treatment.
- Feeding jejunostomy inserted during a staging laparoscopy procedure prior to surgical resection can be of benefit in severely malnourished.
- Oral nutritional supplements are cheaper and easier to administer than parenteral or enteral nutrition, and have few disadvantages. Evidence to support their use post-operatively, but there is less evidence to support their use preoperatively.

Goal-directed haemodynamic pre-optimization

- Haemodynamic optimization is concerned with adequate perioperative perfusion of organs.
- Achieving it requires adequate perfusion pressure, oxygenation of blood, and systemic blood flow (cardiac output).
- Perfusion pressure can be easily measured by non-invasive and invasive blood pressure monitoring. Oxygenation can be measured by pulse oximetry and intermittent measurement of arterial oxygen partial pressures and haemoglobin levels.
- Other clinical parameters, such as heart rate, central venous pressure (CVP) and urine output give some information about the adequacy of the intravascular volume and end organ perfusion, but lack sensitivity and specificity in identifying volume deficit.
- Pulmonary artery catheter (PAC) can measure cardiac output. Although still regarded as gold standard, it is cumbersome, invasive, has major risks, and in practice cannot be used intraoperatively.
- Measuring cardiac output has been made easier by development of new flow-based technology. Now there are several non-invasive devices available that can measure cardiac output and, in some cases, patient's ability to respond to fluid challenges (Table 7.4) Advantages and limitations to each of these monitors.
- Goal-directed therapy (GDT) pertains to the protocolized use of fluid and inotropic therapy to achieve pre-determined goals for cardiac output and systemic oxygen delivery.
- GDT initiated before surgery. Has been shown to improve post-operative surgical outcomes, but requires preoperative admission to intensive care unit (ICU). The problems with utilizing this scarce resource have focused development of intra- and post-operative GDT.
- Of all available monitors, oesophageal Doppler has most outcome benefit data of reducing both rates of post-operative complications and mortality, as well as significantly reducing both length of hospital stay and overall number of ICU and high dependency unit (HDU) bed days used. Unfortunately, use in oesophagectomy is limited.
- There is outcome benefit data on lithium dilution monitor, arterial pulse contour and transpulmonary thermodilution monitor when used intra- and or post-operatively in a GDT protocol.
- Advantage of these monitors is that they are easier for awake patient to tolerate post-operatively than oesophageal Doppler monitor.

Table 7.4 Examples of some commercially available cardiac output monitoring devices.

Minimally invasive cardiac output monitoring devices	Examples	Comments
Oesophageal Doppler	Cardio-Q ODM (Deltex Medical, Chichester, UK)	Requires oesophageal probe
Thoracic electrical bioimpedance	Bioz DX (Cardiodynamics Intl, San Diego, CA)	Poor reliability. No outcome data
Lithium dilution	LiDCO plus (LiDCO, London, UK)	Requires arterial cannulation
Arterial Pulse Contour	LiDCO Rapid (LiDCO, London, UK) FloTrac (Edwards Life Sciences LLP, Irvine, CA)	Requires arterial cannulation
Transpulmonary thermodilution	PiCCO (Pulsion Medical Systems, Munich, Germany)	Requires cannulation of large artery and central vein

Operative anaesthetic management

Lung isolation techniques in oesophageal surgery

Surgical access to the oesophagus is facilitated by the intra-operative collapse of one lung. There are two techniques by which this can be achieved—by the use of an endobronchial tube or by an endobronchial blocker. The choice of technique is one of individual preference.

Endobronchial tubes
- Mainly double lumen endobronchial tube (DLT), of which there are many types (Fig. 7.1).
- Has cuffed endobronchial and cuffed tracheal portion. Endobronchial portion may be left- or right-sided.
- Connected to ventilator via double catheter mount.
- Ventilation to one lung can be maintained through corresponding lumen of tube.
- Collapse of other lung achieved by occluding gas flow through corresponding lumen and opening lumen to atmosphere.
- Two-stage oesophagectomy will require deflation of right lung.
- Thoraco-abdominal approach will require deflation of left lung.
- Regardless of surgical approach most anaesthetists will insert left-sided DLT.
- Right-sided DLT more difficult to position as right upper lobe bronchus is in close proximity to carina and can be occluded by endobronchial cuff.

- Correct positioning of tube can be confirmed clinically by auscultation, confirming that each lung can be isolated and ventilated independently of the other.
- Correct positioning should be further confirmed by fibre optic endoscopy through tracheal lumen. Carina should be visualized, endobronchial lumen should be seen inserted into intended bronchus and endobronchial cuff herniation that may obstruct trachea can be excluded.

The complications of endobronchial intubation include:
- Trauma to lips, teeth, oropharynx, laryngeal nerves, larynx, or trachea.
- Misplacement in to oesophagus or incorrect bronchus.
- Incorrect positioning or movement during re-positioning of patient can cause inadequate ventilation and impaired gas exchange.
- Damage to mucosal of bronchus due to prolonged or excessive endobronchial cuff inflation can lead to bronchial rupture or ulceration causing stenosis as late complication.

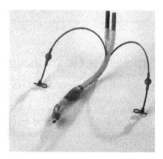

Fig. 7.1 Left-sided Robertshaw double-lumen endobronchial tube.
With kind permission of P3 Medical Ltd.

Endobronchial blockers
- Used in conjunction with traditional endotracheal tube.
- Passed into bronchus and cuff inflated, thereby blocking ventilation to lung, while allowing lung to deflate through lumen of endobronchial blocker that is open to atmosphere (Fig. 7.2).
- There are a number of different designs. Modern examples often require insertion under direct vision with a fibre optic endoscope.
- Surgical exposure is equal to that of DLT tube.
- Can be easier to position in some patients, such as those of short stature or with difficult airways, than double-lumen endobronchial tube (see Table 7.5).

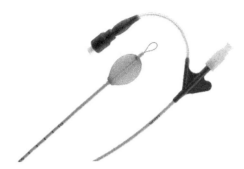

Fig. 7.2 Arndt Endobronchial blocker.
Permission for use granted by Cook Medical Inc., Bloomington, Indiana.

Table 7.5 Advantages and disadvantages of the endobronchial blocker and the double lumen tube

Device	Advantages	Disadvantages
DLT	Quicker to position Faster lung collapse Larger lumen to allow suction of secretions	Appropriate size needs to be selected Positioning may be difficult in some patients Bulky Potential for tracheo-bronchial injury Problems in difficult airways Need for tube exchange if ventilation required post-operatively
Endobronchial blocker	One size only Suitable for difficult airways Rapid sequence induction Critically ill intubated patients who require OLV Tracheostomized patients who require OLV Does not require tube exchange if ventilation is required post-operatively	Longer time to lung collapse or assisted suction to expediate lung collapse Potential for obstruction from secretions Poor collapse of right upper lobe due to obstruction of right upper lobe bronchus by cuff. Greater potential for dislodgement Potential bronchial injury from cuff over-inflation

One-lung anaesthesia during oesophageal surgery

- The management of one-lung anaesthesia requires good communication between the anaesthetist and surgeon to prevent and/or manage hypoxia (i.e. arterial oxygenation <90%).
- OLV is commenced in thoracotomy stage of oesophagectomy.
- Dependent left lung is ventilated and non-dependent right lung allowed to collapse.
- All ventilation is with dependent lung.
- Dependent lung is preferentially perfused due to gravity (60% of blood flow).
- Collapse and surgical manipulation of non-dependent lung causes mechanical obstruction and further diverts blood towards dependent ventilated lung.
- Hypoxic pulmonary vasoconstriction is reflex vasoconstriction of pulmonary arterioles in response to low PO_2 in alveoli. This reduces flow of blood to poorly ventilated areas of lung. In one-lung anaesthesia, this results in up to a further 50% reduction in flow of blood to non-dependent lung and reduces ventilation/perfusion mismatch (V/Q mismatch). These mechanisms allow patient to tolerate such a large reduction in area available for respiratory exchange.
- Blood flow to non-dependent lung is reduced to 20%. Blood is no longer oxygenated and will mix with oxygenated blood leaving dependent lung in heart causing venous admixture and fall in PaO_2. This is a form of V/Q mismatch referred to as shunt. The greater the venous admixture, the larger the shunt and fall in PaO_2.
- In lateral position, weight of mediastinal contents, elevated position of paralysed diaphragm, and abdominal contents pushing up on dependent diaphragm, all reduce compliance and functional residual capacity of dependent lung, which can result in areas of patchy atelectasis, which will also cause a degree of shunt and hypoxia.
- Hypoxia can often be greater in normal lungs. In diseased lungs blood flow will have already adapted somewhat pre-operatively leading to smaller drop in PaO_2.
- There are other causes of hypoxia during one-lung anaesthesia other than shunt from non-dependent lung (Box 7.2), and these need to be ruled out or treated.
- Low cardiac output states will worsen hypoxia because of decrease in mixed venous saturation of blood passing through shunt.
- Once other causes of hypoxia have been excluded, suggested sequence of manoeuvres to manage hypoxia from one-lung anaesthesia is outlined in Box 7.3.
- CO_2 elimination increases through dependent lung and will be maintained provided minute ventilation is unchanged.
- If airway pressures are high (<25–30cmH$_2$O), tidal volume should be reduced and respiratory rate increased to maintain minute ventilation.
- If airway pressures remain high despite altering tidal volumes and respiratory rate, permissive hypercapnia to spare barotrauma should be allowed.
- At end of surgery, bronchus of collapsed lung is suctioned and lung re-inflated by manual ventilation under direct vision.
- Post-operative chest X-ray should be performed to exclude pneumothorax, haemothorax, collapse, and misplaced chest drain.

Box 7.2 Aetiology of hypoxia during one-lung anaesthesia

Ventilatory causes of hypoxia
- Problem with breathing circuit, connections, or anaesthetic machine.
- Occlusion of double lumen tube.
- Displaced double lumen tube or endobronchial blocker.
- Pre-existing disease in dependent ventilated lung.
- Intraoperative deterioration in dependent ventilated lung, i.e. retained secretions, bronchospasm, pulmonary oedema.

Circulatory causes of hypoxia
- Hypovolaemia.
- Surgical manipulation of mediastinum.
- Compression of inferior vena cava or right atrium.
- Arrhythmias, i.e. excessive peritoneal traction, surgical manipulation of heart.

Box 7.3 Sequence of manoeuvres to correct hypoxia during OLV

- Increase inspired oxygen concentration to 100%.
- Insufflate oxygen to non-dependent lung.
- Apply continuous positive airway pressure (CPAP) of 5–10cmH$_2$O to non-dependent lung. This will slightly distend lung, but should not interfere with surgical access.
- Consider application of 5–10cmH$_2$O of positive end expiratory pressure (PEEP) to the dependent lung. This may improve oxygenation by increasing functional residual capacity and compliance of dependent lung. However, may worsen hypoxia by increasing pulmonary vascular resistance and diverting blood to non-dependent lung, thereby increasing shunt from non-dependent lung.
- Consider removing PEEP if previously applied.
- *Intermittent inflation of collapsed lung*: should be done after communication with surgeon.
- Proceed with two-lung ventilation and retraction of non-dependent lung.
- Consider temporary occlusion of pulmonary artery supplying non-dependent lung.

Fluid therapy and blood transfusion
- Use of flow-based technology to measure intra-operative cardiac output and stroke volume should be considered.
- When flow-based measurement not available, fluid therapy will be guided by pulse, peripheral perfusion, capillary refill, CVP, measured blood loss, acid-base, lactate, and haemoglobin measurements.

- Due to stress response of surgery, patients are prone to salt and water retention. There is natural anti-diuresis due to vasopressin, catecholamines, and renin-angiotensin-aldosterone system activation. Low urine output can be misleading and needs to be interpreted in context of patient's cardiovascular parameters.
- Where flow-based measurements are available 200–250mL fluid challenges with suitable colloid or crystalloid solution should be given to achieve and maintain maximal stroke volume.
- Most fluid is required at beginning of surgery, when anaesthesia and epidural analgesia is established.
- Vasopressors, either intermittently or as an infusion, should be given where hypotension is not fluid responsive.
- 0.9% Saline carries risk of inducing hyperchloraemic acidosis when used routinely for fluid replacement or resuscitation. In these circumstances:
  - Balanced salt solutions, e.g. Ringer's lactate, Hartmann's solution, or balanced colloid solutions should be used.
  - Adequate haemoglobin concentration must be maintained. Adequate tissue oxygenation can be maintained at a haematocrit of 30%, coexisting cardiopulmonary disease may raise threshold for transfusion.
- Serious complications of blood transfusion are outlined in Box 7.4.
- Transfusion-related immune suppression is manifest as increased risk of post-operative infections and increased tumour recurrence after surgical resection.

Box 7.4 Serious complications of blood transfusion

Early
- Haemolytic reactions:
  - Immediate haemolysis (e.g. ABO incompatibility).
  - Delayed haemolysis (e.g. minor groups).
- Allergic reactions to proteins, immunoglobulin A (IgA).
- Transfusion related acute lung injury.
- Circulatory overload.
- Thrombophlebitis.
- Metabolic (e.g. hyperkalaemia, hypocalcaemia, alkalosis).
- Hypothermia.
- Impaired coagulation (after massive transfusion).

Late
- Infective.
  - Viral (e.g. hepatitis, human immunodeficiency virus (HIV), cytomegalovirus (CMV)).
  - Bacterial (e.g. Gram negative).
  - New variant Creutzfeldt-Jacob disease (vCJD).
- Graft vs. host disease.
- Immune sensitization (Rhesus D antigen).
- Iron overload (chronic transfusions).

Post-operative care

Timing of extubation

Post-operative ventilation may be associated with an increased risk of barotrauma, acute respiratory distress syndrome (ARDS) and ventilator-associated pneumonia. With improvements in patient selection, operative technique and anaesthetic management most patients can now be safely extubated immediately post-operatively provided the following criteria are met:

- A stable cardiovascular system.
- Normal acid-base balance, with near normal base deficit.
- Absence of hypoxia and/or hypercarbia on arterial blood gas measurements.
- Active cough and gag reflex.
- Ability to respond to commands.
- Normothermia.
- Adequate analgesia.
- Absence of confusion.
- Other operative and preoperative factors, which may lead to reventilation or lead to a decision for elective post-operative ventilation are:
  - Massive blood transfusion intra-operatively.
  - Prolonged duration of surgery, particularly of one-lung anaesthesia.
  - Low preoperative FEV1.
  - Low preoperative FEV1/FVC ratio.
  - Extenuating comorbidities.

Post-operative analgesia

- Post-operative pain associated with pulmonary complications.
- Adequate post-operative analgesia is associated with lower cardiopulmonary complications.
- Epidural is commonest and generally considered to be most effective analgesic technique for oesophagectomy. Attenuates stress response and may reduce post-operative morbidity and mortality.
- Epidural analgesia can avoid some systemic side effects of systemic opioids, such as nausea and vomiting, sedation, respiratory depression, hallucinations, confusion, urticaria and GI ileus.
- Epidural analgesia involves the infusion of local anaesthetic agent, often in combination with an opiate in to the extradural space. The dose of opiates in an epidural is low therefore the likelihood systemic effects are also lower.
- Contraindications to epidural analgesia are shown in Box 7.5.

Box 7.5 Contraindications to epidural analgesia
- Patient refusal.
- Infection (localized or generalized).
- Abnormal coagulation.
- Epidural catheter should not be inserted/removed within:
  - 12h prophylactic LMWH.
  - 24h treatment doses of LMWH.
  - 4h subcutaneous prophylactic unfractionated heparin.
  - 7 days of stopping clopidogrel.
- For patients on warfarin the INR must be <1.4.
- Individual risk and benefit should be considered.
- The next dose of heparin (LMWH or unfractionated heparin) can be given 2h after catheter removal.
- Platelet count should ideally be >80 × 10⁹/L.
- True safe value is unknown.
- Individual risk and benefit should be considered.

- Potential complications and side effects are shown in Box 7.6. Epidurals require active management in the post-operative period to maintain optimal analgesia. They must be cared for by appropriately trained staff, who are familiar with the side effects and potential complications.
- Paravertebral nerve blocks and incisional wound catheters in combination with morphine can be useful adjuncts in those in whom an epidural has failed or is contraindicated.
- Paravertebral nerve block blocks nerves as they pass through intervertebral foramina into paravertebral space. Catheter can be placed to allow continued infusion of local anaesthetic (LA).
- Paravertebral nerve block in thoracic region can be of benefit for thoracotomy wound following oesophagectomy and can be placed by surgeon under direct vision. In these circumstances additional analgesia for abdomen will be required.
- Complications of paravertebral block include extradural, subarachnoid and IV injection, but it is associated with fewer haemodynamic effects.
- Incisional wound catheters provide a continuous infusion of LA directly in to the surgical site. It may have an opiate sparing effect.
- Opiates delivered initially by IV loading and continued with patient-controlled analgesia (PCA) device can be effective where an epidural cannot be given. This should be part of a multimodal analgesic approach combined with NSAIDs and/or paracetamol.
- Continuous infusion of LA catheters also highly effective and easily placed. Useful as an alternative to an epidural.

Box 7.6 Complications of epidural analgesia

Related to insertion of needle/catheter
- Neurological damage (rare).
- Bloody tap (needle/catheter inserted into extradural blood vessel).
- Extradural haematoma.
- Dural tap (subarachnoid needle/catheter).
- Post-dural puncture headache.
- Failure to locate extradural space.

Related to injection/infusion of drug
- IV injection of local anaesthetic.
- Inadvertent spinal blockade.
- Extensive high block (following prolonged infusion or top-ups).
- Failure or incomplete blockade.
- Hypotension (sympathetic block below level of block).
- Anterior spinal artery syndrome (probably related to severe hypotension).
- Abscess/meningitis (rare).
- Shivering.
- Leg weakness (more likely in lower thoracic or lumbar placement).
- Pruritus (due to opiate component of infusion).
- Respiratory depression (due to opiate component of infusion).
- Hallucinations and/or confusion (due to opiate component of infusion).

Post-operative management

- Approximately 30–50% will experience some post-operative complication (see Box 7.7).
- HDU facilities for post-operative care must be available prior to commencing surgery. This facility can offer basic respiratory support (i.e. non-invasive ventilation, $FiO_2 \leq 50\%$) and/or cardiovascular support (i.e. invasive arterial and central venous pressure monitoring, IV vasoactive drug therapy to support arterial pressure, anti-arrhythmic drug therapy).
- In some cases, where a period of post-operative ventilation is anticipated, an ICU will be required.
- Approximately 25% of patients can suffer pulmonary complications following oesophagectomy, and it is leading cause of mortality.
- Post-operative hypoxia is common after upper GI surgery and its causes are multifactorial (see Box 7.7).
- Measures to minimize hypoxia include adequate analgesia, semi-erect posture, regular physiotherapy, early mobilization, and humidified oxygen.
- Avoiding hypo- and hypervolaemia of utmost importance in these patients.
- Hypovolaemia will exaggerate any hypotension 2° to epidural or opiate analgesia.
- Hypervolaemia will lead to third space fluid shifts in pulmonary and GI tissue. Following oesophagectomy there is increase in pulmonary vascular permeability, making lung increasingly susceptible to fluid overload.
- Use of flow-based technology to measure cardiac output and stroke volume should be considered.

Box 7.7 Complications

Medical
- *Pulmonary:*
  - Pneumonia.
  - Acute lung injury (ALI)—syndrome of acute respiratory failure from acute pulmonary oedema and inflammation.
  - ARDS—a more severe form of ALI.
  - Air leak.
  - Aspiration.
  - Pulmonary embolus.
- *Cardiovascular:*
  - Arrhythmias—AF; supraventricular tachycardia.
  - Myocardial ischaemia/infarction.
  - Congestive cardiac failure.
  - Cerebrovascular event.
- *Other:*
  - Renal failure.
  - Hepatic failure.

Surgical
- Anastomotic leakage.
- Anastomotic stricture.
- Gastric outlet obstruction.
- GI ileus.
- Intra-abdominal sepsis.
- Haemorrhage.
- Chylothorax.
- GI ischaemia/infarction.
- Recurrent laryngeal nerve palsy (in cervical oesophagogastric anastomosis).

Enhanced recovery

- Originally developed by Professor Henrik Kehlet (Copenhagen).
- Used in UK since 1999; initially established in colorectal surgery, but now a cornerstone for improving outcomes.
- Founded on four working principles (see Box 7.8).
- Standardized perioperative clinical pathways improve outcomes in patients with oesophageal cancer.
- Multidisciplinary role essential. All members should feel empowered to promote, design, and influence patient pathways.
- While surgeons only part of the process, surgical leadership is a key requirement to institute and initiate change and quality improvement.
- Attention to dietary and nutritional needs with clear targets shared with patients.
- Engage patient and family in discussions and planning.
- *Seattle pathway (Don Low) 2007:* 340 consecutive oesophagectomy patients 1991–2006 managed according to an evolving perioperative clinical pathway. Prospective data capture.
- Mean age 64 (33–90), Barrett's oesophagus (17), or invasive cancer stages I-87, II-133, III-94, IV-9. 139 (41%) neoadjuvant therapy. 63% ASA class III or IV, 5 different operative approaches used.
- Patients managed intraoperatively with a 'fluid restriction' protocol. Mean intraoperative blood loss, 230mL. 99.5% extubated immediately, mean ITU and hospital stays, 2.25 (1–30) and 11.5 (6–49) days. Post-operative analgesia, patient-controlled epidural analgesia in 98.5, and 86% mobilized on day 1.
- Complications in 153 patients (45%), AF (13%), delirium (11%). Anastomotic leaks (3.8%). Mortality (0.3%). No significant differences were seen in length of stay, operative time, blood loss, or complications in patients receiving neoadjuvant therapy. For stages I, II, and III, patients between 1998–2004 Kaplan–Meier 5-year cumulative survival was 92.4, 57.1, and 34.5%.
- Standardized perioperative clinical pathways can provide the infrastructure for treatment ensuring low mortality (aim for <2%: approaches 0% in best high volume centres) should include increased efforts to minimize blood loss and transfusions, improve post-operative pain control and extubation rates, and facilitate early mobilization and discharge.
- *Perioperative fluid management by anaesthetist:* data driven, based on algorithms developed when nephrotoxic anaesthetics were more commonly used. Excessive fluid compromises cardiovascular, pulmonary, thromboembolic, and renal function.
- *Relative intraoperative oliguria not of clinical significance:* 'fluid restriction' reduces complication rates, length of hospital stay, and cost. 'Fluid overload' may be associated with poor outcome and increase.
- Standard fluid replacement algorithms not at all evidence-based.
- *Early extubation:* requires immediate pain control and pulmonary toilet, but provides faster recovery, fewer complications, and earlier mobilization.

- Regional anaesthesia and analgesia techniques, specifically patient-controlled systemic or epidural analgesia, improve pain control and lead to earlier extubation and decreased pulmonary complications facilitates aggressive chest physiotherapy, early mobilization (walking day 1 post-operatively) and early discharge.
- ITU step-down dependent on demonstrating early mobilization achieved in 95%.
- Minimally invasive oesophagectomy (MIO) and approaches such as transhiatal oesophagectomy (THO) designed specifically to avoid painful incisions (particularly thoracotomy) and so minimize post-operative discomfort.
- Success in improving morbidity and mortality rates with improved perioperative management pathways will allow the emphasis to shift to HRQL and cancer survival rates.

Box 7.8 Enhanced recovery principles
- *All patients should be on a pathway to enhance recovery:* enables patients to recover from surgery, treatment, illness leave hospital sooner by minimizing physical, and psychological stress responses.
- *Patient preparation ensures patient is in the best possible condition:* identifies risk and commences rehabilitation prior to admission or as soon as possible.
- *Pro-active patient management components of enhanced recovery are embedded across the entire pathway:* pre-, during, and post-operation/ treatment.
- Patients have an active role and take responsibility for enhancing their recovery.

Enhanced recovery: anaesthetics

Minimizing the risk of post-operative nausea and vomiting
- Avoid use of nitrous oxide.
- Consider intraoperative anti-emetics/prescribe first-line and rescue anti-emetics routinely.

Anaesthetics a key role in enabling early mobilization
- Effective analgesia to allow early mobilization.
- Regional anaesthesia/nerve blocks used, long acting opiates avoided.
- Regular paracetamol and NSAID reduce opiate requirements.
- Where regional analgesia not used, PCA morphine.
- *Spinal analgesia:* low complication and insertion failure rate, improved mobility.
- *Thoracic epidurals:* excellent analgesia, but hinder mobilization. Transversus abdominis plane (TAP)/paravertebral block, with or without in-dwelling catheter useful.

Maintain normothermia pre- and post-operation
- Reduces risk of bleeding and wound infection.
- Hypothermia prevention: monitoring, air-warming system, IV infusion warmers, as per NICE guidance.

Enhanced recovery fluid management
- Maintain good pre-operative hydration.
- Give carbohydrate drinks pre-operatively.
- Use intraoperative fluid management technologies to deliver individualized goal-directed fluid therapy.
- Avoid crystalloid excess (salt and water overload).
- Avoid post-operative IV fluids.
- Encourage early post-operative drinking and eating.

Aims of enhanced recovery fluid management (by the end of surgery)
- Patient is warm and well perfused with no evidence of hypovolaemia.
- and/or tissue hypoperfusion/hypoxia.
- Hb >7g/dL. No clinically significant coagulopathy.
- 'Zero balance' (i.e. less than 1L positive fluid balance).
- Minimize use of vasopressors.

Predictors of poor outcome
- Greater age.
- Higher ASA status.
- High blood loss.
- Protracted surgery.
- Hypovolaemia and/or hypoperfusion (e.g. metabolic acidosis, blood lactate > 2mmol/L, central venous O_2 <70%).
- Greater vasopressors.
- High volumes of IV fluids (>3.5L total), positive fluid balance (>2L positive on day of surgery).
- Failure to achieve aims suggests quality of care should be reviewed, and/or the need for ongoing care in a higher care environment (e.g. extended recovery, HDU or ITU).

Intra-operative fluid management
- *Indicators of central hypovolaemia:*
  - Blood and/or fluid loss, tachycardia, hypotension cool peripheries low CVP low cardiac output.
  - Reduced stroke volume pulse pressure variation (during intermittent positive pressure ventilation (IPPV)). Pre-load responsiveness. Low central venous O_2 saturation.
  - Central hypovolaemia responds to volume infusion.
- Use of intraoperative fluid management technologies is recommended from outset by NICE guidelines in high risk surgery and in high risk patients undergoing intermediate risk surgery. Includes:
  - Major surgery with a mortality rate of >1%.
  - *Major surgery:* anticipated blood loss of greater than 500mL.
  - Major intra-abdominal surgery.
  - Intermediate surgery high risk patients (patients aged >80 years).
  - Unexpected blood loss and/or fluid loss requiring >2L fluid replacement.
  - Patients with ongoing evidence of hypovolaemia and/or tissue hypoperfusion (e.g. persistent lactic acidosis).
  - Perceived lack of resources not a viable excuse in the NHS.
- *NICE conclude:* cannot afford *not* to have cardiac output measuring technologies available.

British Consensus Guidelines on Intravenous Fluid Therapy for Adult Surgical Patients guidelines

Intraoperative IV infusion to achieve optimal stroke volume should be used, where possible, as this may reduce post-operative complication rates and duration of hospital stay (see Box 7.9).

Box 7.9 2010 enhanced recovery implementation guide: delivering enhanced recovery

'Individualized goal-directed fluid therapy...When intravenous fluid is given, the benefits of maintaining circulatory filling and organ perfusion must be weighed against the risk of excess fluid accumulation in the lungs causing hypoxia, and, in the gut, causing nausea and delayed return of gut motility (ileus).'

Reproduced from 'Delivering enhanced recovery: Helping patients to get better after surgery', Department of Health, March 2010. ©Crown copyright 2010.

Oesophageal cancer

Epidemiology, presentation, and clinical evaluation

Epidemiology
- Variable incidence depending on worldwide location.
- Highest rates in Ethiopia, China, Japan, Iran.
- In UK, 12.6 men/5.9 women per 100 000 population.
- Increasing incidence in Western world—particularly adenocarcinomas near oesophagogastric junction.
- *Parallel increases in adenocarcinoma of gastric cardia:* now 50% of all gastric cancer: similar epidemiological profile suggesting a similar aetiology.
- 9th most common cancer in UK (comprises 3% all UK cancers).
- 7000 new diagnoses/6700 deaths per year (UK).
- 5-year survival rates 8% overall (UK).
- 1-year survival rate 30% men/27% women (UK).
- Mean age 65–70 years/very rare under 40 years. Peak age UK 50–60.
- 2/3 of those diagnosed >65 years age.
- Male > female. Between 2:1 and 12:1.

Aetiology
- GORD leading to Barrett's metaplasia and dysplasia.
- *Obesity:* 3–6-fold risk, independent of reflux.
- *Hiatus hernia and reflux:* mechanical risk.
- 67% >risk (BMI) >25, and increases >BMI.
- Women (BMI >30) men overweight (BMI 25–29.9) and obese (BMI >30).
- *Male pattern obesity associated with metabolic syndrome and malignant transformation:* growth factor/cell cycle dysregulation.
- Metabolic syndrome 10–20% population.
- 46% of Barrett's patients and 36% GORD.
- *Million women study:* 50% oesophageal adenocarcinoma in postmenopausal women due to obesity.
- *H. pylori:* hypochlorhydria and ammonia from urea by bacteria may protect lower oesophagus by changing content of refluxing gastric fluid.
- Decreasing *H. pylori* in countries associated with > GOJ cancer.
- Community *H. pylori* eradication may increase GOJ cancer.
- Other data suggests cardiac inflammation and metaplasia associated with *H. pylori* infection despite reflux.
- *H. pylori* seropositivity and gastric atrophy associated with non-cardia gastric cancer.
- *Cardia cancer two distinct groups:*
  - *H. pylori* serology negative—no evidence of gastric atrophy.
  - *H. pylori*—positive evidence of atrophy.
- *Type 1:* behave like non-cardia cancer more diffuse type.
- *Type 2:* behave like oesophageal adenocarcinoma and more intestinal type.
- Possibly different carcinogenic process at the two sites.

Presentation

Elderly male with short history of dysphagia is commonest:

- *Progressive dysphagia*: solids initially, then liquids.
- Site identified by patient as area of blockage, usually above actual site.
- 25% of all presenting with true dysphagia will have oesophageal cancer.

Other history

- Past medical history/ongoing history of symptomatic reflux.
- Regurgitation of food and saliva.
- Weight loss, anorexia, and emaciation—usually rapid onset.

Occasional symptoms

- Odynophagia (painful swallowing).
- Hoarse voice/bovine cough—laryngeal irritation and invasion of recurrent laryngeal nerve.
- *Chest pain:* bolus food impaction and local infiltration.
- *Respiratory symptoms:* overspill symptoms or rarely.
- Tracheo-oesophageal fistula.
- *Halitosis:* residual food or bronchial involvement.

Clinical evaluation

Often absent clinical signs:

- Weight loss/cachexia.
- Anaemia.
- Cervical lymphadenopathy.
- *Jaundice/hepatomegaly:* metastatic disease.
- *Chest signs:* overspill/fistula/metastatic disease.

Referral guidelines for suspected upper gastrointestinal cancer

- Dysphagia.
- Dyspepsia combined with weight loss, anaemia, recurrent vomiting, GI blood loss, or anorexia.
- Dyspepsia in a patient aged over 55 years with onset of dyspepsia less than a year ago, or continuous symptoms since onset.
- Dyspepsia combined with at least 1 of the following risk factors— Family history of upper GI cancer in more than 1 first-degree relative, Barrett's metaplasia, pernicious anaemia, peptic ulcer surgery over 20 years ago, known dysplasia, atrophic gastritis, intestinal metaplasia.
- Jaundice.
- Upper abdominal mass.

Current UK national guidelines dictate all patients referred should be seen within 2 weeks by a team specializing in the management of upper GI cancer.

- Patients diagnosed with oesophageal cancer should be offered written information with a named contact on the multi-disciplinary team.
- All results should be confirmed by a second pathologist in cases where radical intervention is contemplated based upon histology.

Barrett's oesophagus

See Chapter 6.
- Pre-malignant condition referring to glandular epithelium cephalad to the GOJ.
- Can lead to dysplasia and malignant change to adenocarcinoma.
- Usually 2° to GORD (oesophageal epithelium undergoes metaplasia from squamous to columnar epithelium following chronic reflux), but can be due to ectopic mucosa.
- Usually acquired, but possible genetic import—family clusters.
- 10% with GORD will develop Barrett's—bile reflux appears to be of greatest significance.
- 1% per year will progress to carcinoma (30× increased risk).

Presentation

Typical patient
- Obese.
- Male.
- >45 years.
- *Poor lifestyle:* heavy smoker/poor diet.
- *Symptomatic reflux for over 10 years:* heartburn, indigestion, nausea, and vomiting.
- Family history of oesophageal/gastric cancer.
- *Barrett's per se is usually asymptomatic:* may have dysphagia or odynophagia.
- Usually nil to find on clinical examination.

Diagnosis

By upper GI endoscopy
- Irregular edge of pink mucosa (metaplastic gastric mucosa) seen extending more than 3cm above GOJ.
- *Long segments (8–10cm):* increased risk carcinoma.
- Significance of short segments (<3cm) unknown and often missed on endoscopy anyway.
- *Ultra-short segments (intestinal metaplasia at the cardia only detectable histologically):* much lower malignant risk—probably related to *H. pylori*, rather than GORD.
- *Structured biopsy protocol:* multiple biopsies from all four quadrants, at 2-cm intervals throughout the length of the oesophagus (± cytological brushings) and biopsy any visible lesion or ulcer (can develop in Barrett's).
- *If dysplasia:* more biopsies can be taken for accurate assessment.

Histology
- Three types of glandular epithelium can be seen:
  - Gastric fundal type epithelium with mucous secreting cells.
  - Gastric junctional type epithelium with mucous secreting cells.
  - Specialized columnar epithelium with mucous secreting goblet cells, amounting to intestinal metaplasia.
- 10–20% with Barrett's develop dysplasia (low to high grade, as per revised Vienna classification).
- Dysplasia most commonly occurs in intestinal type mucosa.
- 40% with dysplasia have carcinoma focus within dysplastic area.
- Low-grade dysplasia can convert to high grade and then cancer, but can undergo spontaneous regression.
- Those more likely to progress to malignancy are:
  - Male.
  - >60 years.
  - *Endoscopy signs:* ulceration and severe oesophagitis, nodularity, stricture, or dysplasia.

Treatment
- *High-grade dysplasia (Tis) is indication for resection:* re-evaluation demonstrates malignant change in up to 40%.
- If malignancy ruled out, those with high-grade dysplasia should undergo endoscopic treatment (endoscopic mucosal resection/ablation). See ▭ Management of dysplasia: non-operative, p. 139.
- Oesophagectomy for dysplasia has excellent prognosis (80% 5-year survival) and is necessary in longer segments.
- *Also:*
  - *Lifestyle changes*—lose weight, stop smoking, drink less alcohol, small regular meals, avoid foods aggravating symptoms, raise head of bed to help reflux.
  - *Life-long acid suppression*—PPI/H2 receptor blocker (little evidence this leads to regression of metaplasia).
  - *Also*—photodynamic therapy, cold coagulation, argon plasma coagulation, radiofrequency ablation, multipolar electrocoagulation endoscopic plication.
  - Reduction of risk of progression to adenocarcinoma is not an indication for anti-reflux surgery.

Follow-up
- *3-month to 3-year endoscopies:* to detect dysplasia before progression to carcinoma (interval depends on degree of dysplasia and hospital protocol).
- ∴, oesophageal cancers diagnosed in Barrett's patients tend to be early and have a good prognosis.
- However, studies have reported a large number of endoscopies with little overall effect upon diagnosis and survival.

Adenocarcinoma

- Comprise ~50% of all oesophageal carcinomas.
- Increasing in incidence.
- More common in Western Europe/USA, and now more prevalent than SCC.

Risk factors
See Table 8.1.

Table 8.1 Risk factors for adenocarcinoma

Proven strong association	Barrett's oesophagus Male gender (M:F, 5–10:1) Symptomatic GORD leads to: • Barrett's metaplasia • Obesity and high BMI • Previous mediastinal radiotherapy, e.g. breast cancer (2× risk) • Hodgkin's
Proven weak association	• Heavy smoking and alcohol (weaker association than SCC). • *Poor diet:* low in fruit and veg • *Achalasia, scleroderma, caustic or chemical injury to oesophagus:* associated with metaplasia, anticholinergics, β - agonists, aminophyllines—relax lower oesophageal sphincter and increase reflux
Possible association	• Trichloroethylene (dry-cleaning) • Silica dust

Protective factors
- *Regular NSAIDs/aspirin use:* weaker association than SCC.
- *H. pylori:* may protect against reflux effects.

Diagnosis
- History and clinical examination.
- *Rapid access endoscopy and biopsy:* principal method of diagnosis—can take biopsies and evaluate small lesions more accurately than radiological techniques.
  - *Site*—predominantly lower 1/3 of oesophagus or GOJ.
  - *Appearance*—papilliferous mass, annular stricture, ulcer.
  - *Biopsy*—multiple biopsies to confirm histology and grade.

Treatment
Treatment should be arranged and planned by MDT.
- Surgery ± neo-adjuvant chemotherapy.
- Chemoradiotherapy (if not fit for or refused surgery), although adenocarcinoma tends to be resistant to radiotherapy.
- Palliative procedures in metastatic or advanced disease.

Oesophagogastric junction tumours

- Evidence shows they should be classified as a separate entity.
- Siewert's classification (Box 8.1) considers GOJ adenocarcinomas to be centred within 5cm from the GOJ (identifiable by proximal margin of gastric folds).
- True GOJ tumours behave more aggressively than oesophageal tumours.
- It is also argued that these tumours should undergo different surgical approaches to ensure clear surgical margins.

Box 8.1 Siewert's Classification of gastro-oesophageal junction adenocarcinomas

- *Type I—distal oesophageal:* centre of tumour lies 1–5cm above anatomical cardia.
- *Type II—cardia of stomach:* centre of tumour from 1cm above to 2cm below anatomical cardia.
- *Type III—proximal stomach:* centre of tumour from 2–5cm below anatomical cardia.

Reproduced from 'Classification of adenocarcinoma of the oesophagogastric junction', Siewert JR, Stein HJ, *Br J Surg* **85**: 1457–9, copyright 1998 with permission of John Wiley and Sons.

Squamous cell carcinoma

- Comprise roughly 50% of oesophageal malignancies. Likely to decrease as adenocarcinoma incidence increases.
- More common in China, Japan, parts of Africa, Iran. Very high incidence.
- No strong gender link (unlike adenocarcinoma).

Risk factors

- *Heavy alcohol intake:* acts synergistically with tobacco.
- *Tobacco:* chewing or smoking increases risk 9-fold (much stronger association than adenocarcinoma).
- *Diet:* low in fruit and vegetables, high in pickled, smoked, and salted foods, high in nitrosamines, trace element and vitamin deficiencies, mycotoxins, and aflatoxins.
- *Previous mediastinal radiotherapy:* e.g. breast cancer (2× risk), Hodgkin's.
- *Achalasia:* cardiac sphincter malfunction (16× increased risk).
- *Coeliac disease:* gluten sensitivity, malabsorption.
- *Tylosis:* autosomal dominant condition with palmoplantar keratosis.
- *Paterson–Brown–Kelly (or Plummer–Vinson) syndrome:* Fe-deficiency anaemia, glossitis, and oesophageal web.
- *Human papillomavirus (types 16 + 18):* 15% malignancies analysed +ve for human papillomavirus (HPV) DNA.

Protective factors

- Aspirin.

Diagnosis

- History and clinical examination.
- *Barium/Gastrografin® swallow:* irregular filling defect identified, but will miss a proportion of early cancers and can lead to confusion with other conditions that may mimic cancer.
- *Rapid access endoscopy and biopsy:* principal method of diagnosis. Can take biopsies and evaluate small lesions more accurately than radiological techniques.
  - *Site*—predominantly middle 1/3 or upper 1/3 of oesophagus.
  - *Appearance*—papilliferous mass, annular stricture, ulcer.
  - *Biopsy*—multiple biopsies to confirm histology and grade.

Treatment

Treatment should be arranged and planned by a multi-disciplinary team.

- Surgery ± neo-adjuvant chemotherapy.
- Chemoradiotherapy alone (if not fit for or refused surgery).
- Palliative procedures in metastatic disease.

Other oesophageal tumours

Other tumours of the oesophagus are rare (Box 8.2).

Box 8.2 Other tumours
- *Benign:*
  - Leiomyoma—commonest benign tumour, usually asymptomatic + discovered incidentally.
  - Gastrointestinal stromal tumour (GIST).
  - *Malignant*—leiomyosarcoma.
- *GIST:*
  - *Secondary*—direct invasion from stomach/lung.

Staging classification

Staging needs to be accurate and thorough so that therapeutic strategies can be planned appropriately and potentially curative therapy can be targeted to those likely to benefit.

Modes of spread

- Both squamous cell and adenocarcinomas spread in a similar fashion.
- Longitudinal submucosal spread is feature of all types of oesophageal cancer and accounts for high rate of resection margin positivity.
- *Direct*—circumferentially/longitudinally within mucosa (intra-epithelial), submucosa, and muscle layer (intramucosal).
- *Local*—to adjacent structures, e.g. trachea, bronchi, pleura, aorta, pericardium, thoracic duct, recurrent laryngeal nerves.
- *Lymphatic*—intramural lymphatic permeation and embolization to para-oesophageal, tracheo-bronchial, supraclavicular, and sub-diaphragmatic nodes.
- *Blood*—to liver, lung, and bone.

Staging

American Joint Committee on Cancer (AJCC) designated staging by the tumour, node, and metastasis (TNM) classification 6 differs from TNM 7 (2010; Box 8.3 and Box 8.4). Any tumour within 5cm from GOJ considered Oesophageal (not gastric).

Regional nodes: TNM 6

- Dependent on site of 1° tumour along length of oesophagus.
- *Coeliac nodes classified as M1a*: not considered as unresectable disease. Should undergo resection of 1° tumour and lymphadenectomy, where appropriate.
- *Distant metastases or lymph nodes in three compartments (neck, thorax, and abdomen)*: not candidates for curative therapy.

Regional nodes: TNM 7

- Any nodes within the drainage field of the oesophagus independent of the site of the 1° tumour.
- *Includes*: coeliac, para-oesophageal, and paratracheal in neck, but *not* supraclavicular.
- Decision to offer surgery should be pragmatic considering in hospital mortality, docetaxel, cisplatin, and fluorouracil combination chemotherapy regimen, and HRQL.
- 50% stage IV patients have distant haematogenous spread—amenable to palliation only.

Reasons for poor survival

- *Present late*: once symptoms present, tumour has usually invaded muscularis propria, or beyond.
- Often elderly with multiple co-morbidities.

Box 8.3 TNM classification system for oesophageal cancer

T: primary tumour
- *TX*: primary tumour cannot be assessed.
- *T0*: no evidence of primary tumour.
- *Tis*: carcinoma in situ/HGD.
- *T1*: tumour invading lamina propria, muscularis mucosa, or submucosa.
  - *T1a*—tumour invading lamina propria, muscularis mucosa.
  - *T1b*—tumour invading submucosa.
- *T2*: tumour invading muscularis propria.
- *T3*: tumour invading adventitia.
- *T4*: tumour invading adjacent structures.
  - *T4a*—pleura, pericardium, diaphragm (potentially resectable).
  - *T4b*—*other structures*: aorta, vertebrae, trachea.

N: Regional lymph nodes
- *Nx*: nodes cannot be assessed.
- *N0*: no regional lymph node metastasis.
- *N1*: 1–2 regional lymph node metastases (1–6 TNM 6).
- *N2*: 3–6 regional lymph node metastases (7–15 TNM 6).
- *N3*: >7 regional lymph node metastases (>15 TNM 6).

M: distant metastasis
- *M0*: no distant metastasis.
- *M1*: distant metastases.
- *TNM 6 Presence of distant metastases*: depends on site of 1° tumour.
- *Upper oesophagus*:
  - *M1a*—mets in cervical nodes.
  - *M1b*—other distant metastases.
- *Middle oesophagus*:
  - *M1a* —not used (same prognosis as distant nodes).
  - *M1b*—non-regional nodes ± other distant mets.
- *Lower oesophagus*:
  - *M1a*—mets in coeliac lymph nodes.
  - *M1b*—other distant metastases.

Reproduced from Edge SB, Byrd DR, Compton CC, eds. *AJCC Cancer Staging Manual*. 7th ed. New York, NY: Springer, 2010.

Box 8.4 AJCC Anatomical stage groupings (major changes from TNM6)

- *Stage 0*: Tis/N0/M0.
- *Stage Ia*: T1/N0/M0.
- *Stage 1b*: T2/N0/M0.
- *Stage IIa*: T3/N0/M0.
- *Stage IIb*: T1 or 2/N1/M0.
- *Stage IIIa*: T4a/N0/M0, T3/N1/M0 or T1/2 N2 M0.
- *Stage IIIb*: T3N2M0.
- *Stage IIIc*: T4aN1/2M0, T4b any N/M0, Any T/N3/M0.
- *Stage IV*: any T/Any N/M1.

Staging and preoperative preparation

Patients who should undergo staging
- Patients diagnosed with malignancy.
- Patients diagnosed with high-grade dysplasia (to exclude co-existing malignancy or focus of malignancy).
- Patients that have undergone neo-adjuvant therapy should always be re-staged.

Diagnosis by oesophagogastroduodenoscopy and biopsy
- Site, size, proximal, and distal extent of tumour.
- Pre-operative dilatation or stenting if appropriate to improve nutrition (may consider biodegradable stent).
- Biopsy for histological grade.
- Assess suitability of oesophageal replacement (stomach, colon, jejunum).
- Minimum eight biopsies should be taken to diagnose malignancy.
- Routine use of chromo-endoscopy is not advised, but may be of use in those patients at high risk of oesophageal cancer.
- *EMR:* submucosa present in up to 88% samples cf. 1% of biopsies interobserver diagnosis of neoplasia greater for EMR than biopsy.
- Assess penetration, differentiation, vascular, and lymphatic involvement.
- EMR superior to endoscopic ultrasonography (EUS) in staging early T1 cancers.
- *Barium swallow:* irregular filling defect, miss a proportion of smaller tumours. Now largely defunct in this context.
- OGD may be repeated by surgeons at time of laparoscopy to plan operative approach.

Staging: mandatory
History and clinical examination
CT thorax/abdomen/pelvis
- Assess local spread, exclude distant, unresectable disease.
- Spiral, IV contrast-enhanced scans, thin (2.5–5mm) collimation, and gastric distension with water or oral contrast 1l (200mL pre-scan). Gas forming granules useful.
- Scan obtained in prone position.
- Liver imaged in the portal venous phase.
- Poor delineation of layers of oesophageal wall, cannot differentiate T1 and T2 tumours (volumetric analysis may improve this) or microscopic invasion in T3 tumours.
- Predicts mediastinal invasion > 80% cases and involvement of aorta, tracheobronchial tree, and crura are easily identified.
- Multi-planar reformats delineate T3/4.

Endoscopic USS
- All candidates for curative resection should be considered for EUS ± FNA if indicated. Preferably in unit with >100 cases/year, radial + linear acquisition as supported by the current BSG guidelines. EUS (alone or in combination with CT) sensitivity 91% for detecting local nodal disease.
- Assess tumour size, depth of invasion, and local LN.
- *Distinguishes layers of oesophageal wall:* superior to CT for local tumour staging, assessment of lymphadenopathy, volume and characteristics of LN.
- Nodal metastases suggested by 4 echo pattern characteristics of size >10mm, well-defined boundary, homogeneously low echogenicity, and rounded shape.
- All four present in ~25% of cases significantly reducing sensitivity.
- Establish local resectability by EMR/ESD at specialist centres.

Laparoscopy
- Primarily to assess peritoneal spread. Consider in all oesophageal tumours with a gastric component, additional information 17% GOJ tumours and 28% gastric.
- *Assess:* peritoneal deposits; may require biopsies; falciform ligament and pelvis not to be missed, liver, tumour extension from GOJ, serosal disease, lesser curve, and coeliac nodal extension and fixity of conduit.
- *Also exclude colonic disease:* may be required as conduit.
- *Peritoneal washout cytology:* debated, oesophageal, and junctional cancers with positive peritoneal cytology have a poor prognosis, median survival of 13 (range 3.1–22.9) months.
- Jejunostomy may be placed at this stage.

PET-CT
- Combination of metabolic assessment with 2-[^{18}F]fluoro-2-deoxy-D-glucose (^{18}F-FDG) PET and CT provides integrated functional and anatomical data.
- Exclude distant metastases such as bone and delineate significance of equivocal lesions, such as pulmonary radio-opacities.
- For regional and distant nodal disease, PET-CT has been shown to have a similar or better accuracy than conventional.
- EUS-CT (sensitivity and specificity 46 and 98% vs. 43 and 90%, sensitivity and specificity 77 and 90% vs. 46 and 69%).
- Addition of PET significantly improves unsuspected metastatic disease detection rates (sensitivity 69 vs.78%, specificity 82 vs.88%), present in up to 30% of patients at presentation.
- *Limitations:* American College of Surgical Oncology Group trial of PET 3.7% false positive and 5% false-negative rates.
- *Reduced sensitivity:* early stages (T1 and T2) and poorly cellular mucinous tumours. Peritoneal metastases.
- *Reduced specificity:* smooth muscle activity and GORD, false positives.
- *Gastric cancer:* tumour size, site, and history affect avidity. Distal tumours, T1 and T2 tumours, and diffuse low sensitivity.
- Tumour standard uptake value does not predict outcome.

Staging: adjuncts

- *Abdominal triple phase CT, USS, or MRI:* assess equivocal hepatic lesions.
- *MRI thorax:* reserve for those who cannot undergo CT or use for additional investigation following CT/EUS. No convincing evidence of benefit over CT/PET/EUS although high resolution triple MRI/PET/CT scanners may change this.
- *Bronchoscopy ± USS:* if imaging evidence of tracheobronchial invasion.
- *Thoracoscopy:* if there is evidence of suspicious nodes that are not amenable to biopsy or assessment by CT or other image-guided techniques.
- *Neck imaging:* EUS or CT in patients with cervical tumours.

Preoperative assessments

- Preferably achieved at a multidisciplinary clinic with surgeons, anaesthetists, dieticians, and physiotherapists.
- Formal assessment of performance status, but largely subjective at present absence of accepted evidence-based data, and an agreed protocol.

Exercise testing

- Poor exercise tolerance correlates with perioperative risk independent of age and other factors.
- Exercise capacity is surrogate for functional cardiorespiratory reserve.
- Tolerance of climbing flights of stairs, hill walking, running, cycling, swimming, or performing heavy physical activity may predict tolerance of UGI surgery.
- *Inability to climb two flights of stairs correlates:* >ASA, 90% risk post-operative cardiorespiratory morbidity.
- Subjective clinical assessment/exercise testing does not exclude latent cardiorespiratory disease in the absence of cardiopulmonary monitoring.
- Desaturation climbing 3 flights of stairs suggests poor metabolic reserve and predicts post-operative complications in lung reduction surgery.
- Exercise-induced hypotension suggestive of ventricular impairment secondary to coronary artery disease is ominous mandating investigation.

CPEX testing

- Dynamic non-invasive objective test of the cardiorespiratory system to adapt to sudden increase in oxygen demand.
- *Ramped exercise test with cycle ergometer, monitoring:* expired CO_2, ECG monitoring and O_2 consumption.
- O_2 consumption related to delivery and linear function of CO when exercising.
- 24% incidence of 'silent' IHD.
- Lactate rises when O_2 consumption exceeds delivery O_2 consumption at this point is AT.
- Greater mortality AT <11mL/kg/min in major abdominal surgery particularly with IHD.
- Perioperative risk stratification by CPET debated.

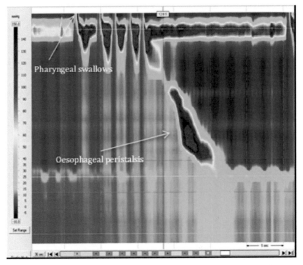

Plate 1 High resolution oesophageal manometry study demonstrating deglutative inhibition. Five pharyngeal swallows are seen, but only final swallow results in peristalsis. See also Fig. 3.1.

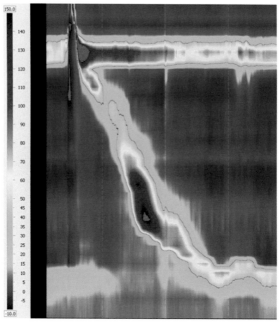

Plate 2 A normal swallow on HRM. See also Fig. 3.3.

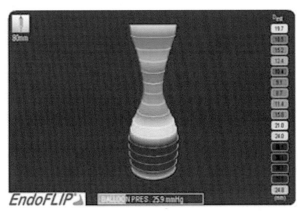

Plate 3 EndoFLIP® device performing intraoperative pressure and volume measurements. See also Fig. 3.4.

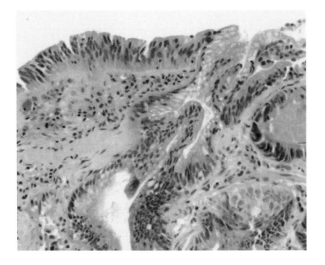

Plate 4 Haemotoxylin and eosin stain of low grade dysplasia—sharp cut off between normal and atypia favours dysplasia. See also Plate 4, colour plate section. See also Fig. 6.2.
Courtesy of Professor Novelli.

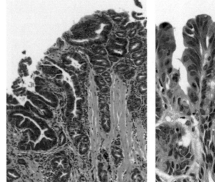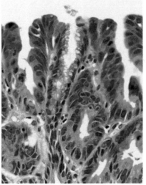

Plate 5 Haemotoxylin and eosin stain of high grade dysplasia - Left ×100, right ×400. See also Fig. 6.3.

Courtesy of Professor Novelli.

- *Japanese study:* Nagamatsu (2001), 91 patients transthoracic oesophagectomy, maximum O_2 uptake during exercise correlated with post-operative cardiopulmonary complications, transthoracic oesophagectomy safe if max O_2 uptake >800mL/min/m².
- UK study Forshaw (2008), 78 consecutive patients CPET testing prior to oesophagectomy. Limited predictive value of post-operative cardiopulmonary morbidity.
- Limitations of CPET testing can occur in patients with reduced lower limb function related to osteoarthritis or limb dysfunction.
- Malnutrition also reduces exercise tolerance.

Shuttle walk testing

- Incremental and progressive shuttle walk testing (SWT) endurance correlates with CPET O_2 utilization.
- Preoperative SWT can be a sensitive indicator of 30-day operative mortality.
- Patients who walk >350m on have reduced risk of death.
- Exercise tolerance of <350m may be associated with inadequate O_2 delivery correlating with impaired wound healing and increased anastomotic failure.
- Patients with musculoskeletal disease and morbid obesity may be unable to complete any form of dynamic exercise testing.
- Upper limb ergometry, pharmacologically-induced myocardial stress testing monitored by thallium imaging or ECHO cardiography may be an alternative.
- *Bloods:* FBC/U&E/LFT/clot/G&S.
- *Arterial blood gas and Lung function tests*—assess lung function in terms of tumour effects and comorbid disease.
- *ECG ± exercise test:* assessment of cardiac status.
- *Anaesthetic review:* suitability for single-lung anaesthesia and thoracic epidural. Only patients with an ASA score of 3 or less should be considered for surgery.

Preoperative preparation

- *Nutrition assessment ± hyperalimentation:* using a validated nutritional risk tool. At risk patients are offered advice and considered for pre-operative nutrition. Those with BMI <18.5 or >20% weight loss—increased risk of post-surgical complications (obesity also increased risk of complications, but rare in these patients).
- *Nutritional pre-loading:*
  - Malnourished patients (inadequate intake >5/7) considered for pre-operative nutritional support for 10–14 days.
  - *Post-operative supplementation:* reduces hospital stay.
  - *Liquid nutritional support with immunonutrients:* arginine, omega-3 fatty acids and nucleotides.
  - *RCTs:* reduction in post-operative infections in both malnourished and normally nourished patients when used for 5–7 days preoperatively.
- Prolonged jejunal feeding routine in some centres. Specific evidence lacking and mounting evidence of complications.

- *Psychological preparation:* counsel patients about treatment options and supply detailed description of peri-operative period. Psychological counselling should be available if needed.
- Smoking cessation.
- Dental treatment.
- *Thrombo-embolic prophylaxis:* anti-thromboembolic stockings, low molecular weight heparin, and pre-operative pneumatic calf compression.
- *IV broad-spectrum antibiotics:* immediately pre-operatively or at induction (cefuroxime, co-amoxiclav).
- *X-match 4 Units blood:* avoid use if possible due to risks associated with transfusion.
- HDU or ITU bed available.
- *Colon prepared:* if required as conduit (Picolax®, Fleet Phospho-soda®, Klean-Prep®).
- *Epidural placement:* for post-operative analgesia.

Management algorithms

See Box 8.5, Table 8.2, Table 8.3.

Box 8.5 Palliative support
- *Pain:* deep X-ray therapy (DXT) and/or analgesics.
- *Obstruction:* dilation, stenting, argon beam laser, photodynamic therapy.
- *Bleeding:* endoscopic Rx, DXT.
- *Nutrition:* oral support, gastrostomy, jejunostomy.

Table 8.2 Resectabilty criteria

Resectable	• Patient fit • >5cm from cricopharyngeus • T1a endoscopic mucosal resection • T1–T3 ± N1 • T4 if diaphragm, pleura, or pericardium involved only • *Lower oesophageal Stage IVa:* any T, any N/M1a coeliac nodes <1.5cm and no major arterial or other organ involvement • Salvage oesophagectomy following 1° chemoradiation if conditions above met and no distant metastases
Unresectable	• Patient unfit • Systemic metastases or non-regional nodes • Stage IVa involving major arteries or other organs or coeliac nodes >1.5cm • T4 heart, great vessels, or contiguous organs invaded

---

Table 8.3 Metastatic disease

Metastatic disease	*Good performance status:* ECOG < 2, Karnofsky >60	*Chemotherapy:* • FU-based • oxaliplatin-based • cisplatin-based • irinotecan-based • taxane-based • Up to second line then palliative support
	Poor performance status	Palliative support

Neo-adjuvant chemoradiotherapy for oesophageal cancer

- Pre-operative treatment currently recommended for all, but the earliest resectable carcinomas of the oesophagus, both squamous cell cancer and adenocarcinoma.
- Chemotherapy is administered concurrently with radiotherapy and acts as a radio-sensitizer.
- Neo-adjuvant chemoradiotherapy is the standard treatment in the USA as recommended in the current National Comprehensive Cancer Networkguidelines (2010).
- Evidence of benefit over neo-adjuvant chemotherapy alone limited.
- *Gebski meta-analysis (2007)* of 10 RCTs comparing neo-adjuvant chemoradiotherapy to surgery alone.
- *Significant survival benefit at 2 years:* HR 0.81, corresponding to a 13% absolute difference in survival.

Two further trials

Dutch trial
- Paclitaxel and carboplatin + surgery vs. surgery alone.
- 74% Distal oesophageal 12% GOJ.
- *Mean survival:* 49/12 vs. 26 months for the surgery alone arm.
- Benefit more pronounced in SCC (HR 0.34; 95% CI 0.17–0.65) adenocarcinoma (HR 0.82; 95% CI 0.58–1.16).

FFCD 9901 trial
Fluorouracil (FU)/cisplatin + DXT + surgery vs. surgery.
- 195 patients with localized stage I and II oesophageal SCC (70%) and adenocarcinoma (29%).
- *Aborted:* no advantage to chemoradiation and significantly increased operative mortality (7.3%).
- Neo-adjuvant chemoradiotherapy as an option is also included in British and European guidelines, although trials are ongoing to determine optimum radiation dose and most effective chemotherapeutic agents.
- Neo-adjuvant chemoradiotherapy should be considered for tumours above T2 or N1 (excluding T1 N0 tumours), in patients who are medically fit for both resection and chemoradiotherapy.
- Measures of fitness include WHO PS 0 or 1, adequate renal function (GFR >50), cardiac reserve and pulmonary function. The tumour is localized using all available data from CT and PET-CT scans, EUS, and endoscopy and the radiotherapy is planned using CT scans performed in the treatment position and conformal radiotherapy techniques used to minimize the dose to normal tissues.
- Target volume includes 1° tumour and involved nodes.
- Dose to normal tissues should be kept within internationally accepted dose limits, particularly the spinal cord and lung. Typical DXT doses are between 40 and 50Gy in 20–30 daily fractions (lower than doses for definitive chemoradiotherapy as 1° Rx).

- Standard chemotherapy agents are cisplatin and FU. Newer agents that have shown promise in trials include paclitaxel, carboplatin, and capecitabine.
- *Acute side effects:* neutropenia and anaemia, nausea, and progressive dysphagia.
- Nutritional support via jejunostomy often required.
- Surgery should not take place for at least 4 weeks after radiotherapy is complete to allow inflammation to settle and maximum response to occur.
- Earlier trials suggested an increase in post-operative morbidity, but more recent studies have shown no increase in post-operative complications or in-hospital mortality.
- Individual randomized trials of neo-adjuvant chemoradiotherapy against surgery alone have not all been positive, but meta-analyses have suggested there is an improvement in median survival and overall survival at 3 and 5 years.
- *CROSS study:*
  - Paclitaxel and carboplatin with radiotherapy.
  - Median survival 49/12 in chemoradiotherapy arm vs. 26/12 in surgery alone arm and the 3-year survival rate was increased from 48–59%.
  - *R0 resection:* 90 vs. 65%.
  - *Complete pathological response:* 25% of cases and associated with a significantly better prognosis, 5-year survival rates of up to 60%.
  - Quality of life deteriorates during the treatment, but recovers to pre-treatment levels by 1 year.
  - Principal criticism adenocarcinoma and SCC combined and control arm surgery alone, rather than chemotherapy as standard of care.

Neo-adjuvant radiotherapy

- Cochrane meta-analysis (2005) of preoperative radiotherapy for patients with resectable oesophageal carcinoma (any histological subtype).
- 3–4% absolute improvement in OS (HR 0.89; 95% CI 0.78–1.01; $P < 0.062$).
- Preoperative radiotherapy not recommended for potentially resectable oesophageal SCC or adenocarcinoma.

Neo-adjuvant chemotherapy for oesophageal cancer

The Medical Research Council (MRC) OE02 study of 802 patients with carcinoma of the oesophagus was published in 2002 and set the standard for neo-adjuvant therapy for oesophageal cancer in the UK.

- Two cycles of cisplatin and FU (CF) chemotherapy prior to definitive surgery.
- The OE02 trial randomized 802 patients:
  - 31% SCC, 66% adenocarcinomas, 3% undifferentiated.
  - 75% male.
  - 64% lower third, 10% cardia, 25% middle third, and 1% upper third.
  - 97% WHO performance score 0 or 1.
- *R0 resections:* from 54–60%, although fewer patients in the chemotherapy arm proceeded to surgery (92 vs. 97%), with some pre-operative deaths observed in the chemotherapy group (3 vs. <1%).
- *Dysphagia:* improved prior to surgery in 37% of patients.
- *Median survival:* improved from 13.3–16.8 months.
- *2 year survival:* from 34–43%.
- See Box 8.6 for the standard (OE02) chemotherapy regime.
- Toxicities include nausea, neutropenia, anaemia, fatigue, neuropathy, diarrhoea, and mucositis. Surgery should be planned within 6 weeks of completion of chemotherapy.
- MRC Medical Research Council Adjuvant Gastric Infusional Chemotherapy (MAGIC) (2006) trial of peri-operative chemotherapy (three cycles of epirubicin, cisplatin and infusional FU (ECF) before and after surgery) produced impressive results in GOJ oesophageal and stomach adenocarcinoma, and this regime is currently recommended for lower third and junctional adenocarcinomas in Europe and USA.
- Median survival improved from 13.3–16.8 months, and 2-year survival from 34–43%. There was no increase in post-operative mortality (10% in both arms).
- Majority of western oesophageal cancers are distal oesophageal or junctional leading to use of adaptations of gastric regimes.
- Current trials are aiming to optimize chemotherapy regime, by adding third drug, giving four cycles of chemotherapy and incorporating oral capecitabine, instead of infusional FU, thus avoiding need for central line.
- MRC OE05 trial (ongoing).
- Adenocarcinoma only.
- Cis/FU vs. epirubicin, cisplatin, capecitabine (ECX; four cycles).

Box 8.6 OE02 chemotherapy regime
- Two cycles of cisplatin (80mg/m^2 day 1 with hydration).
- FU (1g/m^2 by continuous infusion days 1–4), given at three weekly intervals. Patients should be fit, WHO performance score 0 or 1, with adequate renal function (glomerular filtration rate (GFR) > 50) and have no significant active IHD.

US intergroup-0113 study

- 467 patients: surgery alone or three cycles of cisplatin/FU/surgery and post-operative cisplatin/FU in responders.
- No significant difference in median OS.
- Failure may relate to excessive toxicity of chemotherapy regimen and delay to surgery for non-responders.

Gebski meta-analysis of preoperative chemotherapy

- HR for all-cause mortality for neo-adjuvant chemotherapy 0.90 (95% CI 0.81–1.00; $P < 0.05$) 2-year absolute survival benefit of 7%.
- *Subtype analysis:* significant survival benefit in adenocarcinoma (HR 0.78; $P < 0.014$), but not SCC (HR 0.88; $P > 0.12$).
- No phase III trial comparison of chemoradiation + surgery vs. chemotherapy + surgery exists to date.

HRQL

- Few of the trials to date have considered HRQL outcomes in detail.
- Preoperative chemo may not delay post-operative recovery of HRQL, but persistent reflux, diarrhoea, and dyspnoea may continue for at least 3 years after surgery.

Definitive chemoradiotherapy for oesophageal cancer

- Radical chemoradiotherapy is a curative option in oesophageal cancer and is recommended treatment for localized upper third squamous cell cancers <5cm from cricopharyngeus.
- *Alternative to resection:* patient choice or unfit for cardio-oesophagectomy.
- *Randomized trials:* combination chemo-DXT superior to DXT alone.
- *Published case series:* survival rates for chemoradiotherapy can be similar to surgery alone. Many studies include patients whose tumours were deemed too advanced for curative surgery.
- Trials aiming to demonstrate that radical chemoradiotherapy is an effective alternative to resection slow to recruit, but few that have completed seem to confirm non-inferiority for overall survival.

Standard treatment

Herskovic regime
Cisplatin and FU/ DXT 50Gy in 25 fractions over 5 weeks, with chemo weeks 1 and 5.

RTOG 85-01 trial (1992)
- *SCC:* DXT 64Gy vs. four cycles Cis/FU + concurrent DXT 50Gy at 2Gy/day.
- 2-year survival 36% and 5-year survival (26 vs. 20% and 0 at corresponding time points in the radiotherapy alone arm). Both adenocarcinomas and SCC included.
- Median survival 14/12 vs. 9/12. 8 year survival 22% vs. 0% in the DXT alone arm.

RTOG 94-05 (2002)
- Regime modified to give induction cisplatin and FU chemotherapy prior to chemoradiotherapy.
- No advantage in increasing radiation dose from 50Gy to 60.4Gy.

INT 0123 trial
- 85% SCC, 15% adenocarcinoma 50.4 and 64.8Gy DXT otherwise same regime as RTOG 85-01.
- Higher dose radiation gives no significant improvement in survival or local/regional control recurrence.

French study (FFCD 9102, Bedenne, 2007)
- Assessed definitive chemoradiotherapy for responders to induction CT-XRT as an alternative to resection.
- Equivalent OS, but higher local recurrence in the non-surgical arm.
- Infiltration of the trachea-bronchial tree is a contraindication to use of CT-XRT, because of risk of fistula formation, and pretreatment bronchoscopy is recommended for middle third tumours.
- Similar results obtained in later studies, 5-year survival up to 25%. Where results quoted separately for SCC or adenocarcinomas, survival seems better for SCC.

Planning

- DXT target volume determined endoscopy, CT, PET-CT, and EUS.
- Radiation field planned using CT scans taken in treatment position encompassing 1° tumour with craniocaudal margin of 5cm, and radial margins of 1.5–2cm. Local enlarged nodes are included within target volume. Normal tissue tolerances are considered and volume of lung receiving above 20Gy calculated and radiation technique adjusted if necessary.

Toxicities

Infection, mucositis, progressive dysphagia, fistula formation, cardiac toxicity, and pneumonitis. Late effects include radiation induced oesophageal stricture, which may be amenable to endoscopic dilatation.

Treatment mortality

Standard dose chemoradiotherapy: less than 5% and figures of less than 2% are quoted in more recent single centre series.

Loco-regional relapse

- Most common site of treatment failure after chemoradiotherapy.
- More frequent than after surgical resection.
- Local persistence or progression 15–30% with local relapse as first event in about 30% of cases.
- *Salvage surgery* for residual disease after chemoradiotherapy may be considered in fit patients.
- *Limitations:* difficult plane between oesophagus and aorta, increased in-hospital mortality up to 17%. Survival benefit limited. Informing patients of potential high risks and poor outcomes is critical part of decision-making process.
- *New trials* are looking at addition of biological and targeted therapies to cytotoxic chemotherapy, and at novel radiotherapy fractionation regimes. Infusional FU is commonly replaced with oral capecitabine and use of docetaxel, paclitaxel, irinotecan, or oxaliplatin has been studied.
- The question of whether increasing radiation dose improves response is being reconsidered given availability of modern radiation techniques. These include image-guided (IGRT) and intensity modulated radiotherapy (IMRT) both of which could allow use of smaller radiation fields and ∴ reduced normal tissue toxicity.

Operative considerations

Operative settings
- All patients should be discussed in multi-disciplinary setting and surgery only undertaken if it is general consensus of team—surgical decisions should be taken based upon predicted prognosis and effect of intervention upon quality of life.
- Surgery should only take place in high volume centres with sufficient surgical and anaesthetic experience. Individual surgeon experience should be > 20 cases/year.
- Laparoscopic and thoracoscopic techniques should only take place in specialist centres, by experienced surgeons, with full informed consent and local clinical governance committee support.

Operative indications
- *Malignancy:* fit patients with early lesions should undergo resection with curative intent (T1–3/N0/M0).
- High grade dysplasia in a long Barrett's segment (consider endoscopic treatments in short segments).
- Surgery has no place when haematogenous spread has occurred.
- Where radical surgery is based upon histology alone, results should be confirmed by second pathologist.

Operative rationale
Radical surgery and lymphadenectomy should aim for R0 resection—proximal, distal, and circumferential margin clearance.
- Achieve optimal staging.
- Control local disease.
- Improve cure rates.

Operative results
Surgery is the only treatment modality that has consistently been shown to prolong survival, albeit only in ~20% cases.
- Excellent results for early squamous and adenotumours—5-year survival >80% when tumour confined to mucosa and 50% when submucosa involved.
- Overall surgical treatment gives 5-year survival of 5–20%.
- In-hospital mortality should be <10%.
- Clinical anastomotic leak rates should be <5%.
- Curative resection rates (R0) should exceed 30%.

Choice of operative procedure
Type of surgical procedure is determined by:
- Site and type of tumour.
- Extent of lymphadenectomy needed.
- *Surgeons expertise*—type of reconstruction and use of pyloric drainage procedures should depend on surgical preference.

Upper 1/3 tumours
This requires a cervical incision—transhiatal or 3-stage oesophagectomy.

Carcinoma above diaphragm

Requires thoracotomy for formal lymph node dissection—Ivor–Lewis procedure. Third cervical stage can be added to improve clearance and anastomosis performed in neck or left thoraco-abdominal approach for distal. Transhiatal approach for Type I/II tumours in which tumour is mobilized under direct vision is an alternative.

Tumours below diaphragm

- Require radical excision of lower thoracic oesophagus and gastric cardia, entire stomach—left thoraco-laparotomy.
- *In 2-stage:* 2-incision procedures—possible with careful positioning to have 2 teams working simultaneously.

Transhiatal versus transthoracic approaches

- *Dutch randomized trial:* Hulscher, Sandick et al.
- Extended trans-thoracic vs. trans-hiatal resection.
- Siewert type I and II GOJ tumours. 220 patients.
- Median FU 4.7years.
- Operative morbidity significantly lower in the transhiatal group, but in-hospital mortality rates similar.
- Transthoracic trend towards survival benefit, not statistically significant (p0.06) at 5 years.
- *Subgroup analysis:* slight advantage for transthoracic resection for type I GOJ and node positive.
- *HRQL:* activity levels and pain better in transhiatal group in early post-operative months patients undergoing transhiatal surgery.
- By 12 months scores similar in both groups.
- *Proximal 1/3 and SCC in general:* lymphadenectomy likely to be compromised by trans-hiatal approach.

Studies claiming benefits for a particular approach usually hide multiple confounders, of which the potential for stage migration as a result of inadequate lymphadectomy is usually important.

Resection margins

- Extensive studies show resection margins should be 10cm proximal to macroscopic tumour and 5cm distal (when oesophagus is in natural state).
- Adenocarcinoma of lower oesophagus commonly invades gastric cardia, fundus, and lesser curve—some degree of gastric excision essential for adequate resection and lymphadenectomy in the abdomen.
- Adequate radial margins also need to be considered and contiguous excision of the crura and diaphragm needs to be considered particularly for junctional tumours.

Resection specimen

As a minimum, the pathology report should include:

- Type of tumour.
- Grade of tumour.
- Depth of invasion.

- Involvement of resection margins.
- Vascular invasion.
- Presence of Barrett's metaplasia.
- Number of nodes resected and the number containing metastatic tumour.

Lymphadenectomy

Aims of lymphadenectomy

- *Improve staging*: minimum 15 LN excised.
- Reduce loco-regional recurrence.
- Increase the number of patients undergoing R0 resection—improve 5-year survival rate.

The majority undergoing surgery have lymph node metastases at presentation and the extent to which lymphadenectomy reduces local recurrence is unknown. The existing evidence that thorough lymphadenectomy improves survival simply represents more adequate staging.

In squamous cells, the number of lymph nodes involved are of prognostic significance, as is the ratio of invaded to resected lymph nodes.

- Most SCC patients have extensive proximal para-oesophageal LN extending proximally.
- Extent of mediastinal lymphadenectomy.
- In upper half of the mediastinum, remains unclear.
- *Munich study*: type II GOJ tumours that the pattern of lymph node involvement—mediastinal (2.1%), para-oesophageal (15.6%) and intra-abdominal (56–72%) suggesting a three-field dissection is unlikely to be of prognostic benefit.

Abdominal single field dissection

Dissection of right and left cardiac nodes, nodes along lesser curve, left gastric, hepatic, and splenic artery territories.

Two-field dissection

This involves thoracic lymph nodes, including para-aortic nodes (with thoracic duct), para-oesophageal nodes, right and left pulmonary hilar nodes, and tracheal bifurcation nodes. In Japan, it is extended superiorly to include para-tracheal nodes, including those along left recurrent laryngeal nerve.

Three-field dissection

This is advocated in Japan and extends lymphadenectomy to the neck, including brachiocephalic, deep lateral and external cervical nodes, and deep anterior cervical nodes adjacent to recurrent laryngeal nerve chains in neck. Three-field operation is advocated in Japan for squamous cell tumours, but its benefits may simply reflect decreases in staging error as nearly ¼ of all Japanese patients will have cervical lymph nodes. No robust evidence that three-field lymphadenectomy improves outcome for adenocarcinoma and it is associated with a higher incidence of poor outcome. Single operator studies advocating three-field dissection for adenocarcinoma in the USA include Altorki at Cornell and DeMeester.

Guidelines
- Studies show that two-field dissection is associated with no increase in operative mortality or morbidity.
- In UK, two-field lymphadenectomy should not be extended into superior mediastinum or neck.

Other treatment options
- Superficial cancer limited to the mucosa should be treated by EMR—endoscope injects fluid below tumour to make it more prominent and tumour is then removed with an endoscopic snare. Can be combined with other therapies, e.g. post-procedure photodynamic therapy. Commonest side-effects are bleeding and stricture.
- Mucosal ablative techniques such as photodynamic therapy, argon plasma coagulation or laser, should be reserved for the management of residual disease following EMR, and not for initial management in patients with invasive cancer that are fit for surgery.

Surgical anatomy of the oesophagus

The course of the oesophagus
- The oesophagus is a hollow muscular tube, 25cm in length.
- Extends from cricopharyngeal sphincter (C6) to cardia of stomach (Table 8.4).
- Passes through lower part of neck, passing slightly to left and then returns to midline at T5.
- Then passes down and forwards through superior and posterior mediastinum, before piercing diaphragm through an elliptical opening in the right crus (oesophageal hiatus) at T10.
- Last 4cm lies below diaphragm and is retroperitoneal with peritoneum covering anterior and lateral borders only.
- Terminates at GOJ to left of midline at T11—junction marked by abrupt change from oesophageal (bluish) to gastric columnar (florid pink) mucosa—the 'Z-line'.
- 3 anatomical narrowings—strictures (benign or malignant) commonest at these sites (measured from incisors):
  - 15cm—cricopharyngeal sphincter.
  - 25cm—aortic arch and bronchial bifurcation.
  - 40cm—diaphragmatic hiatus.

Table 8.4 Anatomical divisions of the oesophagus

Cervical oesophagus	Lower border of cricoid cartilage to jugular notch
Upper oesophagus	Jugular notch to tracheal bifurcation
Middle oesophagus	Tracheal bifurcation to midpoint of carina and GOJ
Lower/abdominal oesophagus	Midpoint of carina and GOJ downwards, includes lower thoracic and abdominal oesophagus

Layers of the oesophageal wall
- *Mucosa:* non-keratinizing stratified squamous epithelium. May have gastric-type columnar epithelium in lower 3–4cm (non-acid secreting cells). If columnar epithelium higher up Barrett's metaplasia has taken place. Mucosa is thick and thrown into multiple folds in collapsed state.
- *Submucosal:* contains sparse mucous glands (mainly upper + lower 1/3).
- *Musculature:* striated in upper 1/3 + smooth muscle in lower 2/3 internal circular layer + external longitudinal layer.
- *Areolar tissue:* thin external covering.
- *Serosa:* no serosa except for short abdominal segment (last 4cm).

Relations
- *Anterior:* trachea in neck—trachea, left bronchus, and left atrium in thorax.
- *Posterior:* cervical vertebrae in neck, aorta in thorax—starts on left and then moves posteriorly.

• *Right and left:* in neck, carotid artery and thyroid, subclavian artery, and thoracic duct also on left at root of neck in thorax—pleura and lung. Vagus nerves closely associated on right and left, crossed only by azygos vein and right vagus on the right. Least hazardous surgical approach.

Arterial supply

Requires varied sources of vascular supply and drainage due to its length.

• *Upper 1/3:* inferior thyroid artery.
• *Middle 1/3:* oesophageal branches of thoracic aorta and bronchial arteries.
• *Lower 1/3:* oesophageal branches from left gastric (from coeliac axis) and also from left inferior phrenic artery.

Venous drainage

• *Upper 1/3:* inferior thyroid and brachiocephalic veins.
• *Middle 1/3:* azygos system.
• *Lower 1/3:* azygos system (systemic) and left gastric vein (portal)—provides a site of porto-systemic anastomosis.

Lymphatic drainage

• *Lymph channels exist within the oesophageal walls:* allow lymph to pass for long distances before draining out to nodes—drainage from one area does not necessarily follow particular pattern.
• *Cervical/upper oesophagus:* peri-oesophageal lymph plexus drains to deep cervical nodes, then thoracic nodes, tracheobronchial, and finally posterior mediastinal nodes.
• *Lower/abdominal oesophagus:* peri-oesophageal lymph plexus drains to nodes around left gastric and then to coeliac nodes.

Nerve supply

• *Parasympathetic:* vagus nerves form intrinsic and extrinsic nerve plex.
• *Uses on the oesophageal surface:* anterior and posterior vagal trunks contribute to plexus—anterior trunk mainly left vagal fibres and posterior trunk mainly right vagal fibres (but both are mixed).
• *Sympathetic:* upper part from middle cervical ganglia running with inferior thyroid arteries, middle and lower parts from thoracic sympathetic trunks, and greater splanchnic nerves.

Operative technique

Left thoraco-abdominal oesophagectomy

General
- Used for bulky tumours of GOJ, lower and middle third oesophagus.
- *Contra-indicated for malignancy above aortic arch:* due to poor access.
- Excellent access to lower thoracic oesophagus and upper stomach.
- Relatively poor access to infracolic abdomen and thoracic duct.
- Historically high levels of R1/R2 resections reported.
- *Japan Clinical Oncology Group Trial (largely SCC):* increased complications, no survival benefit. May be appropriate for cardiac tumours only.
- *Maynard 2010:* 211 patients in hospital mortality 5.7%, 52% single complication, 7% anastomotic leak, 71% R0, 1- and 5-year survival 70 and 21%. respectively.

Preparation
- Patient on right side, left leg extended, right leg flexed at knee and hip, arms flexed with forearms before face (Fig. 8.1).
- Fix hips with encircling band and support left shoulder with padded post.
- Double lumen ET tube allows exclusion of one lung.
- Prophylactic antibiotics.
- DVT prophylaxis.

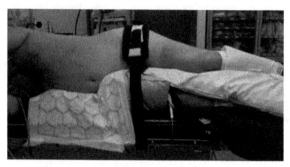

Fig. 8.1 Left thoraco-abdominal oesophagectomy: patient position.

Incision
- Incise midway between xiphisternum and umbilicus and continue obliquely up and left (Fig. 8.2).
- At this stage perform laparotomy to assess fixity and nodal involvement (ensure no unresectable disease).
- *If resection possible:* extend incision across costal margin to continue along line of 6th/7th intercostal space to the tip of left scapula.
- *In elderly or those with fixed ribs:* sometimes necessary to excise few cm of bone near rib neck to allow access to chest. Rare for this approach.
- Deepen incision by dividing thoracic wall muscles with diathermy and open pleura at upper border of rib (Fig. 8.3).

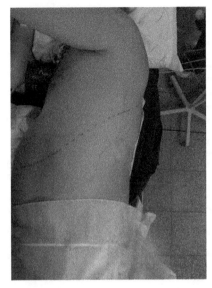

Fig. 8.2 Left thoracoabdominal oesophagectomy: incision.

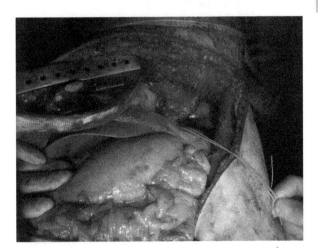

Fig. 8.3 Left thoracoabdominal oesophagectomy exposure: above/below: left lung, oesophagus, heart, cut edge of costal margin and diaphragm, left lobe: liver, stomach.

- Divide costal margin and incise diaphragm radially 10–25cm towards oesophageal hiatus or peripherally parallel to chest wall (phrenic nerve sparing).
- Insert self-retaining rib retractor.
- Use double lumen tube to collapse lung and anchor incised edge of diaphragm to skin to prevent lung prolapsing into operative field.
- Divide peritoneum from rectus sheath to costal margin.

Abdominal phase
- *Assess tumour:* if stomach largely involved, plan for total gastrectomy.
- Open lesser sac, dissect greater omentum from transverse colon and divide avascular portion of lesser omentum.
- Divide gastro-hepatic, gastro-splenic, and gastro-colic ligaments (preserve right gastric and right gastroepiploic vessels).
- Divide short gastric vessels and extend mobilization to fundus and the left crus, phreno-oesophageal ligament and join the line of mobilization at the lesser curve/right crus.
- Ligate and divide left gastric artery and vein separately performing a formal lymphadenectomy at the left gastric origin, splenic artery, and common hepatic, isolating this with a sling if necessary.
- Dissect and carefully divide all peri-aortic tissue proximal to the coeliac in a cranial direction to end at the inferior angle of the crura.
- Gently mobilize oesophagus at hiatus, taking a cuff if needed.
- Perform pyloroplasty and kocherize duodenum (for length) if desired.

Thoracic phase
- Divide pulmonary ligament to free inferior lobe of left lung (take care not to injure pulmonary vein).
- Incise mediastinal pleura anterior to lower thoracic aorta and dissect to expose oesophageal vessels.
- Ligate and divide aortic oesophageal vessels.
- Elevate and pull forward lower lobe of left lung to expose posterior mediastinum and incise mediastinal pleura posterior to pericardium.
- Oesophagus can now be gently mobilized by blunt dissection, (take care not to injure inferior pulmonary vein, thoracic duct or azygos vein on right side).
- Mobilize oesophagus from hiatus upwards to aortic arch.
- Take care to preserve left recurrent laryngeal nerve while mobilizing at level of aortic arch.
- Transect oesophagus and perform intra-thoracic oesophagogastric anastomosis placing a purse string, insertion of an anvil and fashion a circular stapled anastomosis, curved end-to-end anastomosis size 25–29 is common. Fashion the gastric conduit using a linear stapler sequentially around the greater curve from the apex of the fundus to the mid-point of the vascular anastomosis between the right and left gastric arteries at the lesser curve. Residual conduit can be divided using a linear or TA stapler.

Closure
- Close diaphragm and costal margin with continuous, strong, absorbable suture.
- Insert apical and basal underwater seal chest drains to left chest and right if pleura breached.
- Re-expand collapsed lung.
- Re-approximate ribs with interrupted, strong, absorbable suture, e.g. 0 vicryl.
- Close muscle in layers with 1 PDS and clips to skin.
- Insert feeding jejunostomy via Witzel tunnel.
- Close abdomen with routine mass closure.

Ivor–Lewis oesophagectomy

General
- The most widely practiced approach—initial laparotomy, then right postero-lateral thoracotomy to excise tumour and form anastomosis at apex of mediastinum.
- Classic procedure for mid-oesophageal tumours, but can also be used for lower third tumours.
- Also known as *Lewis-Tanner* or *abdominal and right thoracic subtotal oesophagectomy*.

Preparation
- Patient's supine for abdominal phase and in left lateral position for thoracic phase.
- Prophylactic antibiotics.
- DVT prophylaxis.
- Double lumen ET tube for one lung exclusion.

Abdominal phase
- Upper midline incision to xiphisternum or rooftop.
- Peritoneum opened to left of falciform ligament.
- Assess fixity and nodal involvement (assess suitability for resection).
- If resection possible—ligate and divide ligamentum teres and falciform ligament.
- Assistant elevates liver with flat-bladed retractor and draws down stomach to enable oesophagus to be palpated through oesophageal hiatus.
- Can divide left triangular ligament and remove xiphoid process to improve exposure if necessary.
- Mobilize stomach, but preserve right gastric and gastroepiploic vessels as for left thoraco-abdominal approach, see 📖 Abdominal phase, p. 202.
- Transversely incise peritoneum and fascia over abdominal oesophagus to expose lower thoracic oesophagus.
- Incise diaphragmatic crus to enlarge the hiatus and mobilize lower oesophagus up into thorax by blunt and finger dissection.
- Insert feeding jejunostomy via Witzel tunnel.
- Close abdomen with mass closure as routine.

Thoracic phase

- Right thoracotomy at level of 5th or 6th rib.
- Divide intercostal muscles and muscles of thoracic wall with diathermy and excise neck of lower rib for better exposure.
- Control intercostal vessels and diathermize intercostal nerve (better post-operative pain control).
- Collapse right lung.
- Pull lung down and forward to expose and incise mediastinal pleura.
- Mobilize, divide, and doubly ligate azygos vein, as it arches over lung root (2/0 vicryl).
- Divide right pulmonary ligament until inferior pulmonary vein can be seen.
- Excision thoracic duct and para-aortic lymph nodes *en bloc*.
- Incise mediastinal pleura over anterior border of aorta and ligate oesophageal aortic branches.
- Oesophagus is now exposed and can be mobilized by blunt dissection from lung hilum and pericardium, taking all lymph nodes *en bloc*: a tape can be passed around oesophagus to aid retraction and dissection.
- Excise carinal, bronchial, para-aortic and para-tracheal lymph nodes *en bloc*: take care not to damage fragile posterior membranous aspect of the trachea.
- Ligate and divide thoracic duct just above diaphragm (prevents chylothorax) at around T10.
- Continue thoracic oesophageal mobilization until it meets abdominal mobilization.
- Divide all pleural attachments to allow stomach to pass into thorax.
- Withdraw NGT, place proximal oesophageal stay sutures and transect oesophagus at level of apex of thorax.
- Divide stomach along lesser curve with linear stapler and remove specimen with lymph nodes en bloc.
- Perform gastro-oesophageal anastomosis within thorax.

Closure

- Insert basal, apical, and left pleural underwater seal chest drains as deemed appropriate.
- Re-approximate ribs with strong, absorbable, interrupted sutures, e.g. 0 vicryl.
- Re-expand lung.
- Close muscles in layers with 1 polydioxanone suture (PDS) and clips to skin.

Transhiatal oesophagectomy

General

- Advocated for intraepithelial SCC and HGD in Barrett's very low incidence nodal disease and surgeon preference.
- Fewer pulmonary complications than transthoracic routes, but often achieve sub-optimal lymphadenectomy. Some report higher rates of local recurrence.

- Similar mortality figures to other approaches, although in-hospital mortality as low as 0.9% reported.
- Oesophagus resected by blunt dissection with anastomosis of conduit (stomach/jejunum/colon) via neck incision.
- Modern retractors allow resection and anastomosis to be performed under direct vision in neck. Technique often used for benign disease.
- *Can have major blood loss due to surrounding structures:* low threshold for thoracotomy in this eventuality.

Preparation

- Supine with neck extended and head turned to opposite side.
- Prophylactic antibiotics.
- DVT prophylaxis.

Abdominal phase

- Upper midline incision to xiphisternum or rooftop.
- Assess fixity of stomach and lymphadenopathy (exclude distant or unresectable disease).
- *Routine gastric mobilization:* to facilitate tension-free passage to neck care taken to divide all posterior adhesions to stomach and close to right gastroepiploic origin.
- *Perform pyloroplasty and kocherize duodenum:* if favoured.
- Free the GOJ taking a cuff of crura if needed.
- Ligate inferior phrenic vein, and dissect plane between diaphragm and pericardium. Transect diaphragm anteriorly to widen hiatus. Place a deep St Mark's lipped retractor in hiatus.

Mediastinal phase

- Mobilize lower 1/3 to1/2 of oesophagus by combination of blunt and finger dissection, and sweep oesophagus to left and right to identify strands that require division with the harmonic scalpel.
- Divide anterior connections to tracheobronchial tree, posterior connection to aorta and lateral connections to pleura and lung.

Cervical phase

- 5–8-cm incision along anterior border of sternocleidomastoid—centred at level of cricoid cartilage.
- Incise through platysma, cervical fascia, and omohyoid muscle.
- Ligate and divide middle thyroid vein.
- Enter space between oesophagus, larynx, trachea, and thyroid medially and sternocleidomastoid and carotid sheath laterally, by retracting medial and lateral structures.
- Inferior thyroid artery crosses this space and can be divided if necessary (leave intact if possible).
- Identify recurrent laryngeal nerve in tracheo-oesophageal groove—even small retractors cause damage. Nerve on opposite side cannot be seen and is at risk.
- Rotating medial structures (oesophagus, trachea, larynx, thyroid) to opposite side exposes posterior surface of oesophagus and tracheo-oesophageal groove.

- Separate oesophagus from trachea with blunt forceps (e.g. Lahey's).
- Pass a tape around oesophagus and into jaws of forceps to form a sling.
- The sling can now be used for retraction and oesophageal blunt dissection continued down cervical and thoracic oesophagus to level of carina.
- Divide proximal oesophagus in neck.
- Insert a vein stripper from cervical oesophagus to lesser curve of stomach. Attach a long suture to this. Placing a hand in mediastinum, stripper is gently drawn caudally as oesophagus inverts. Take care around carina. The specimen is delivered and a gastric conduit fashioned. A chest drain is sutured to tip of conduit and long suture extending from neck. This is now drawn into neck.
- Hand-sewn anastomosis with interrupted sutures fashioned (Fig. 8.4).
- A transhiatal chest drain is placed in the mediastinum and/or right and left thoracic cavities if the pleura is breached.
- Jejunostomy fashioned if needed.

Closure
- Leave corrugated drain close to anastomosis and bring out near cervical wound.
- Re-approximate platysma (2-0 vicryl) and close skin with clips.
- Insert feeding jejunostomy via Witzel tunnel.
- Close abdomen with routine mass closure.

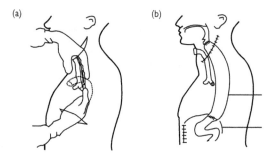

Fig. 8.4 Transhiatal mobilization of oesophagus.
Reproduced from *The Oxford Specialist Handbook of Operative Surgery*, eds. McLatchie & Leaper, copyright 2006 with permission of Oxford University Press.

Further approaches

3-stage oesophagectomy

- Also known as McKeown oesophagectomy.
- Same abdominal and thoracic phases as Ivor–Lewis technique, although thoracic phase precedes abdominal and cervical.
- Oesophageal mobilization extended with incision of superior mediastinal pleura along right vagus nerve.
- Right brachiocephalic vein and SVC are protected as is the right recurrent laryngeal nerve.
- Addition of cervical phase (as per transhiatal technique) for neck anastomosis.
- Used for proximal tumours where slightly more dissection and resection required to achieve safe proximal margin.
- Some prefer to anastomose oesophagus in neck routinely.

Radical curative surgery (Akiyama technique)

- Performed in Japan.
- Initial Ivor–Lewis abdominal and thoracic phases, and then bilateral cervical incision with extensive lymphadenectomy in neck, mediastinum, and abdomen.
- Not used in west—less incidence of lymphadenopathy (higher incidence of Squamous in Japan, whereas higher incidence of adenocarcinoma in west) and additional morbidity, such as recurrent laryngeal nerve injury.
- Need reliable pre-operative assessment by conventional methods.
- Operative survival is similar to western figures and 5-year survival over 50% in those undergoing curative resection.

Pharyngo-laryngo-oesophagectomy

- For carcinoma of the upper cervical oesophagus or hypopharynx.
- Usually performed by head and neck surgeons.
- Usually use free jejunal graft as interposition.

Minimally invasive oesophagectomy

Multiple approaches

Poor nomenclature at present with multiple hybrid approaches and poorly comparable approaches in literature.

See Box 8.7 for AUGIS recommendations.

- MIO technique considered an adjunct to open surgery provided by individual surgeons: open unlikely to be replaced in near future.
- Patients considered for MIO should be fit for open surgery as well.
- *Evidence that MIO reduces peri-operative insult:* less pain, less wound-related complications and faster return to normal activities, no good evidence that MIO reduces hospital stay, overall complication rates or peri-operative mortality.
- *Some complications more frequent:* conduit necrosis, airway injury.
- Comprehensive prospective outcomes submission advocated.
- Surgeons should be fully trained in laparoscopic surgery at hiatus, intra-corporeal suturing and lap stapling.
- *'Learning curve' long:* 20–50 cases.

- Only performed in recognized cancer centres with open operative proficiency.
- Surgeons should enter their patients into high quality.
- RCTs of MIO vs. open oesophagectomy.
- Fitness criteria used same as for open resection.
- Patient suitability for MIO should be discussed in the specialist upper GI MDT.
- BMI >30, T4 tumours, perceived risk of invasion into an adjacent structure, proximal tumours or patients with large LN burden on EUS/CT should be avoided until proficiency established.
- Ideal patient characteristics for MIO therefore include:
  - Low BMI.
  - Non-arthritic shoulders and spine.
  - Small early tumours of the mid- and distal third of the oesophagus.
- Usually slower and not suitable for all tumours, but often less painful and shorter in-hospital stay.
- May require open conversion.
- *NICE guidelines:* effective enough to be available on NHS, but only if surgeon has sufficient experience and training.
- Needs full informed consent and local clinical governance committee support.
- Convincing data in terms of long-term outcome and comparisons with other techniques needed.

Box 8.7 AUGIS recommendations

- MIO + cervical anastomosis: laparoscopic and thoracoscopic approach.
- MIO + intrathoracic anastomosis: lap and thoracoscopic approach.
- Laparoscopically-assisted oesophagectomy (LAO) + standard thoracotomy and intra-thoracic anastomosis.
- LAO + mini-thoracotomy and intra-thoracic anastomosis.
- LAO + thoracotomy and cervical anastomosis.
- Thoracoscopically-assisted oesophagectomy (TAO) + laparotomy and cervical anastomosis.

Reproduced from *A Consensus View and Recommendations on the Development and Practice of Minimally Invasive Oesophagectomy*, Hardwick RH, September 2008, with permission of The Association of Upper Gastrointestinal Surgeons (AUGIS) and The Association of Laparoscopic Surgeons of Great Britain & Ireland (ALS).

Anastomosis

Aims
- Tension-free.
- Good vascular supply (note colour and temperature)—blood supply tenuous when oesophagus is mobilized so care must be taken to maintain as much as possible.
- Close apposition of epithelial margins.

General advice
- Can be hand-sewn or stapled.
- Can be sited in neck or thorax. No evidence for one being preferable in outcome or functionality.

- Ensure two ends to be anastomosed are not twisted.
- Avoid trauma from non-crushing clamps.
- Advance NGT through anastomosis at end of procedure.
- Ensure drain (24 Fr Robinson) placed close to anastomosis, prior to closure.

Stapled

- Circular stapling devices usually quicker and can be used in difficult positions, e.g. under aortic arch/high in abdomen or thorax.
- Can use with any type of conduit, in neck or thorax, and can perform end–end or end–side anastomoses.
- If stapler fails, it is usually difficult to hand-sew and often requires higher transection of conduit, as well as causing crushing effect on tissues.
- Withdraw NGT from proximal oesophageal remnant while aspirating.
- Hold oesophageal lumen open with sponge forceps to pass a test head or measuring device. Choose largest that fits.
- Hold oesophageal lumen open with stay sutures and place purse-string suture to proximal oesophageal remnant at 5mm intervals and 5mm depth (2/0 prolene on small round-bodied needle) (Fig. 8.5).
- Insert correct size head of stapling gun into proximal oesophagus and tighten purse-string around its neck—insert second purse-string if oesophagus not drawn tight to neck (Fig. 8.6).
- Open stapling device (Fig. 8.7) so that gun spike passes through distal conduit (stomach, colon, jejunum) and secure around neck of gun with a purse-string suture.
- Reattach head to body of stapling device.
- Ensure there is nothing interposed between the 2 ends, release the safety catch and fire the gun.
- Inspect completeness of toroidal oesophageal and viscous remnants (doughnuts)—ensure they contain all layers of the wall.
  - Separate jaws of instrument and carefully rotate it to withdraw it.
  - Some over-sew with 2/0 PDS.

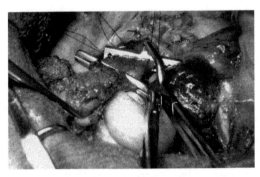

Fig. 8.5 Purse string clamp across the oesophagus 5–6cm proximal to tumour.
Reproduced from *The Oxford Specialist Handbook of Operative Surgery*, eds. McLatchie & Leaper, copyright 2006 with permission of Oxford University Press.

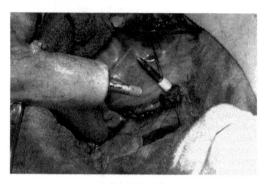

Fig. 8.6 Staple gun in the gastric conduit with the staple head in the proximal cut end at the oesophagus.
Reproduced from *The Oxford Specialist Handbook of Operative Surgery*, eds. McLatchie & Leaper, copyright 2006 with permission of Oxford University Press.

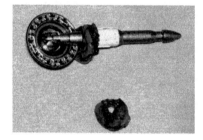

Fig. 8.7 Gastric and oesophageal donuts with the staple head.
Reproduced from *The Oxford Specialist Handbook of Operative Surgery*, eds. McLatchie & Leaper, copyright 2006 with permission of Oxford University Press.

Sutured
See Fig. 8.8.
- Often preferable in neck as often insufficient distal conduit to place gun through.
- Many different techniques—key to success is care with which they are applied.
- Oesophageal wall largely composed of longitudinal muscle. Longitudinal sutures can cut out, particularly as longitudinal muscle leads to shortening of oesophagus after anastomosis. This must be allowed—oesophagus has large lumen when relaxed and action of circular muscle makes lumen appear smaller. Unless lumen is dilated, closely-spaced sutures will be widely spaced when muscle relaxes, leading to leaks.

- Withdraw NGT, while aspirating.
- Lie two ends together, ensure hole in distal conduit matches size of oesophageal lumen after dilatation.
- Insert traction sutures through all coats of both conduits, and slightly posteriorly to the lateral angles.
- Draw traction sutures apart to oppose posterior walls, while leaving anterior walls slack.
- Place traction suture in middle of anterior walls and draw them apart so that posterior walls can still be seen.
- Carefully place sutures at 2–3-mm intervals and with 2–3-mm bites. Include all layers of the wall, and take mucosa on both sides. Sutures cut easily through longitudinal muscle so suture strength depends largely on submucosa and partly mucosa.
- Use fine 4/0 or 5/0 sutures on a small, round-bodied needle, in a continuous or interrupted fashion. Use absorbable or non-absorbable suture (many use PDS or vicryl).
- Start posteriorly and work anteriorly so that last few stitches to be placed are in centre of anterior wall.
- Knots are placed internally on the posterior aspect of the anastomosis and then externally on the anterior aspect.
- Sutures can be placed and tied, or placed, left loose and oesophagus parachuted down and all knots tied sequentially.
- When nearly complete, do not tighten last few stitches until sutures inspected to ensure they pass through all layers—cut stitches out, rather than place rescue sutures.
- Do not tie sutures too tight—oesophagus swells post-operatively and will cut out.
- Gently rotate to inspect anastomosis at end.

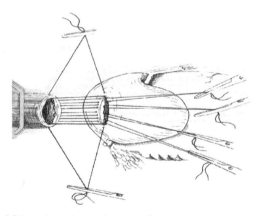

Fig. 8.8 Sutured oesophagogastric anastomosis.
Reproduced from *The Oxford Specialist Handbook of Operative Surgery*, eds. McLatchie & Leaper, copyright 2006 with permission of Oxford University Press.

Replacement conduits

Stomach

General

First choice of conduit when available.

- Well-vascularized.
- Only one anastomosis required.
- Simple to mobilize into thorax or neck.
- Good functional results.
- Posterior mediastinal/pre-vertebral route to pass stomach up to anastomosis site.
- Anterior mediastinal (retro-sternal) and subcutaneous (pre-sternal) routes can be used, but longer and non-anatomical.

Procedure

- Supine position.
- Upper midline incision.
- Exclude distant or unresectable disease.
- Use 3/0 or 2/0 vicryl to tie vessels.
- Divide greater omentum from transverse colon and gastrocolic omentum below right gastroepiploic vessels to enter lesser sac.
- Dissect towards gastric fundus and left gastroepiploic vessels.
- Divide cross-over vessel to middle colic vein.
- Dissect inferiorly to origin of right gastroepiploic vein.
- Dissect hepatic flexure from duodenum and kocherize duodenum to provide maximum gastric length.
- Divide lesser omentum close to liver, preserving right gastric artery as it emerges from common hepatic inferiorly.
- Divide hepatic branch of the vagus as it can have a large associated vessel (preserve other aberrant hepatic vessels).
- Divide gastrosplenic ligament and ligate short gastric arteries to free fundus.
- Divide lesser sac adhesions from pancreas and lift stomach.
- Divide and tie left gastric artery and vein separately.
- Perform lymphadenectomy of left gastric, common hepatic, splenic artery, and coeliac territories, and skeletonize abdominal aorta up to diaphragmatic hiatus.
- Stomach is now completely mobile.
- Perform pyloroplasty if favoured and skeletonize lesser curve by dividing lesser omentum and left gastric tissue above right gastric pedicle once specimen removed, draw fundus superiorly to neck or apex of thorax.
- Excise a portion of lesser curve and proximal stomach (depending upon extent of gastric involvement) with linear stapler to form gastric tube.
- Perform hand-sewn or stapled anastomosis with over-sew (2/0 PDS).
- Anastomosis should be performed in posterior fundus at high point of stomach and well away from resection line (to ensure no vascular compromise). If stapling device to be used, ensure that spike of the gun passes through fundus at least 2cm from suture or staple line.
- Place feeding jejunostomy via Witzel tunnel if favoured.
- Close abdomen as routine.

Colon

General

- Second most common conduit following stomach.
- Most favour pre-vertebral route for reconstruction.
- *Used only in certain situations:*
  - Absent or damaged stomach, e.g. caustic injury, ischaemia.
  - Where site and size of tumour requires total gastrectomy.
  - For extra-anatomical bypass where extra length needed, e.g. anterior mediastinal or subcutaneous routes.
  - Surgical preference.

Pre-operatively

- *Colonoscopy:* rule out significant disease, e.g. inflammatory bowel disease, severe diverticulosis, multiple polyps, malignancy.
- *Mesenteric angiogram:* assess pattern and sufficiency of blood supply and identify part of colon to be used (usually iso-peristaltic left colonic segment based upon left colic vessels).
- *Colonic preparation:* Picolax, fleet phosphosoda, Klean-prep.

Procedure

- Place patient in supine position.
- Perform long midline incision.
- Exclude distant or unresectable disease.
- Dissect greater omentum from transverse colon.
- Mobilize hepatic and splenic flexures, ascending and descending colon so that whole colon is mobile on its mesentery.
- Divide middle colic pedicle below its bifurcation close to origin in-line (to preserve any arcade).
- Divide transverse mesocolon and then divide right colon with a linear stapler.
- Draw left colon carefully up to anastomotic site (usually within a bowel bag or other atraumatic device), once specimen has been removed.
- Ensure colon not twisted and anchor it to diaphragm.
- Perform hand-sewn or stapled proximal anastomosis.
- Divide distal colon with a linear stapler according to position of vessels.
- If vagotomy performed, better functional outcome achieved by additional proximal 2/3 gastrectomy and end–end cologastric anastomosis to the antrum (2/0PDS), with pyloroplasty (Fig. 8.9).
- If vagal-preserving procedure performed, stomach can be retained with posterior end–side cologastric anastomosis, using circular stapling device through a small anterior gastrotomy.
- Insert NGT and pass through proximal anastomosis.
- Restore colonic continuity with end–end colocolic anastomosis (two layers of 2/0 PDS).
- Place feeding jejunostomy via Witzel tunnel.
- Close abdomen as routine.

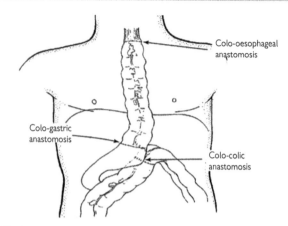

Fig. 8.9 Right colonic interposition from cervical oesophagus to antrum with colocolic anastomosis.
Reproduced from *The Oxford Specialist Handbook of Operative Surgery*, eds. McLatchie & Leaper, copyright 2006 with permission of Oxford University Press.

Jejunum
General
- Jejunum rarely used as a conduit.
- Can be used after pharyngo-laryngo-oesophagectomy for tumours in proximal cervical oesophagus and hypopharynx.
- Usually passed retrocolically.
- Can perform anastomosis in neck or apex of thorax.
- Can be hand-sewn or stapled anastomosis.

Procedure
- Supine position.
- Long midline incision.
- Isolate a long jejunal segment based upon second or third jejunal artery.
- Divide the jejunal segment with a linear stapler to form free conduit.
- Draw divided end superiorly through oesophageal diaphragmatic hiatus to site of anastomosis.
- Perform gastrojejunal anastomosis by stapling or suturing the caudal end of the jejunal segment to the gastric remnant.
- Restore jejunal continuity by performing jejo-jejunal anastomosis.

Post-operative care and complications

Post-operative care

- *ICU or HDU:* meticulous fluid balance and respiratory support as necessary.
- *Inotropes/vasoconstrictors:* used with caution particularly if concerns regarding conduit vascularity.
- *Pain relief:* epidural or PCA—also assist with respiration.
- *Nausea and vomiting:* regular anti-emetics often required.
- *NGT:* monitor output amount and type.
- *Nutritional support:* early enteral nutrition is important and feeding via jejunostomy can be commenced on the first or second post-operative day. Ongoing nutrition support is often required until patient is eating normally. Patients may continue to lose weight initially and should be advised that this will settle once they recommence a normal diet.
- *Chest drains:* monitor output amount and type.
- *Physiotherapy support:* respiratory (particularly following thoracotomy) and mobility support are crucial (early mobilization is key to prevent DVT and pulmonary embolism (PE)).
- *Mouth care and washes:* patients often complain of a bad taste in their mouth and good care also allows earlier feeding.
- *Bowel disturbances:* constipation and diarrhoea are both common.
- *Depression:* emotional and/or psychological support.

Complications

Early

- Haemorrhage.
- *Recurrent laryngeal nerve injury:* more common during dissection of the cervical and upper oesophagus. Majority unilateral and transient. Left nerve is at risk during mediastinal lymphadenectomy, and if cervical anastomosis to take place at the same time. Perform it on the left side so that both nerves are not at risk. Injury impairs the ability to cough and protect the airway in early post-operative period—can be an important contributor to pulmonary morbidity. In most patients there should be adequate compensation from contralateral side; if not, tracheostomy considered to protect airway and improve pulmonary toilet. Thyroplasty or vocal cord injections are rarely required.
- *Atelectasis:* very common, 2° to pain and can lead to pneumonia and respiratory failure.
- Pneumonia.
- *Acute pulmonary oedema:* 2° to extensive pulmonary lymphadenectomy and poor lymphatic drainage of the alveoli.
- ARDS.
- Pleural effusions.
- Pneumothorax.

- *Chylothorax:* occurs in 2–3% of thoracic oesophagectomies, and may be higher with transhiatal techniques. Recognized by milky discharge from chest drain.
- Diagnosis of chylothorax is based on the presence of chylomicrons in the pleural fluid. Chylomicrons are molecular complexes of proteins and lipids that are synthesized in the jejunum and transported via the thoracic duct to the circulation. They are only found in circulation post-prandially with a peak 3h after eating.
- Pleural fluid triglyceride of >110mg/dL 1% chance of being non-chylous and that a triglyceride of <50mg/dL 5% chance of being chylous.
- Pleural fluid triglyceride levels >1.24mmol/L (110mg/dL) with a cholesterol <5.18mmol/L (200mg/dL) is diagnostic of chylothorax.
- A triglyceride level <0.56mmol/L (50mg/dL) with a cholesterol >5.18mmol/L (200mg/dL) is found in pseudochylothorax. Cholesterol crystals are also often seen in this condition.
- Prolonged conservative treatment has high mortality due to hypo-albuminaemia and leucocyte depletion. If chyle production >10mL/kg/day on the fifth post-operative day—indication for re-operation and ligation of the thoracic duct (Fig. 8.10).
- Short and medium chain fatty acid feed/TPN and ocreotide.
- Operatively thoracic duct generally found at T10 and can be clipped or ligated. Perioperative lipid feed can assist identification.
- *Thrombo-embolism:* DVT and PE.
- *Anastomotic leak:* most bowel has serosa that forms fibrinous adhesions and seals small leaks, but oesophagus has no serosa except upon anterior aspect of abdominal segment. If leak occurs within 72h, usually represents technical failure. If general condition of the patient is good, exploration and repair is advisable. Majority of leaks occur at 2 weeks and probably represent anastomotic tension ± local ischaemia. Diagnosed by clinical suspicion and confirmation with water-soluble contrast studies/CT/OGD.
- Majority minor, managed conservatively with NG suction, local drainage, antibiotics, and jejunal feeding (Fig. 8.11).
- Major thoracic leaks require early recognition (may present with AF) and exploration for a good outcome.
- Leak rate should not exceed 5% (associated mortality 20%) and no evidence for difference in leak rates between hand-sewn and stapled anastomoses.
- Neck leaks are more common than thoracic, but have less severe consequences.
- *Conduit necrosis:* very rare with open procedures, but reportedly up to 13% laparoscopic cases in some series. Presents with devastating chest sepsis.
- Requires thoracotomy, excision of conduit, proximal diversion with oesophagostomy, distal conduit closure, drainage, and jejunostomy. Prolonged ITU support in most cases. Prolonged nutritional support and sepsis followed by reconstruction using colon or jejunum.
- *Gastric outlet obstruction:* particularly if no pyloroplasty, may respond to balloon dilatation.

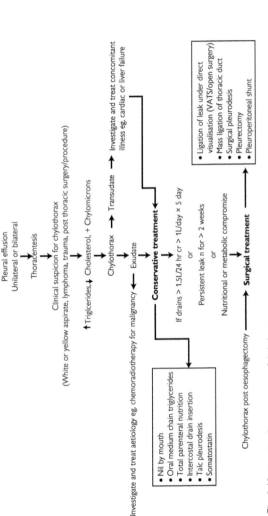

Fig. 8.10 Algorithm for management of chylothorax.

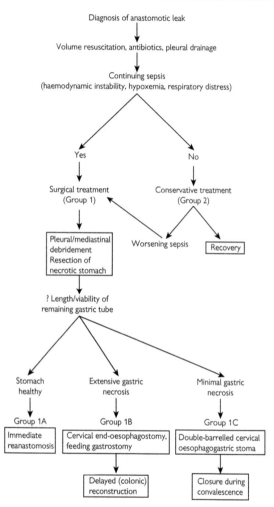

Fig. 8.11 Algorithm for managing patients with anastomotic leak following oesophagectomy

Reproduced from 'Surgical treatment of anastomotic leaks after oesophagectomy', Richard D. Page, Michael J. Shackcloth, Glenn N. Russell et al., *European Journal of Cardio-thoracic Surgery* **27** 337–343, copyright 2005 with permission of Oxford University Press.

Late
- *Anastomotic stricture:* particularly with small, circular stapling devices and cervical anastomoses. Benign strictures can occur in first few months and usually relate to post-operative fibrosis. Later strictures are often due to reflux—differentiating from recurrence is difficult and endoscopic assessment and biopsy is ∴ required. Early strictures are easily treated by endoscopic dilatation, although multiple sessions may be required.
- Reflux, dumping syndrome, post-vagotomy diarrhoea.
- Post-thoracotomy pain.
- *Cancer recurrence:* loco-regional, metastatic, or both.

Adjuvant therapy

General
- The rationale is to attempt to prevent local recurrence.
- Should be considered for T2 tumours and above.
- Patients with advanced tumours (T3/N1) should be considered for randomized controlled studies to assess role of novel multimodal therapies in conjunction with surgery.
- The majority of clinical studies evaluating the effectiveness of adjuvant therapy have dealt with SCC, which is slowly being overtaken by adenocarcinoma as commonest tumour. Data ∴ becoming less relevant.
- Surgical excision remains standard treatment and effectiveness of adjuvant therapies are still under evaluation.
- Oesophageal adenocarcinoma tends to be radio-resistant.
- GOJ tumours should generally be considered as gastric tumours and there is little evidence to support role of adjuvant or neo-adjuvant therapies.

Radiotherapy
This should be considered in SCC, particularly when the proximal level of the tumour is high.

External
- Given as short daily sessions.
- Length of course depends upon type and size of cancer.
- Skin is initially tattooed/marked to indicate direction of therapy.
- Often require PEG insertion prior to treatment as radiotherapy can make swallowing very painful, and also leads to decreased saliva production.
- Often need anti-emetics for nausea and vomiting.
- Other side-effects include depression, lethargy, hair loss.

Internal
- *Brachytherapy:* insertion of a radioactive metal rod, as a source of radiotherapy, into oesophagus.
- Radioactive source contained within protective tubing.
- Inserted by upper GI endoscopy or via NGT, which is left in situ with source inside it.
- Removed via endoscopy or by removing NGT.
- Left for between 30min to a few days depending upon amount of radiation required.
- Provides more focused treatment within a shorter time.
- Causes dysphagia so often need PEG and liquid analgesics.
- Leads to less systemic side-effects such as nausea, lethargy, hair loss.
- Often remain in hospital during their period of treatment.

Chemotherapy
- The use of post-operative chemotherapy is complicated in oesophagectomy by prolonged recovery period and conflicts with aims of adjuvant therapy.
- Trials usually include variations of ECF regimen.
- Side-effects include decreased resistance to infection, bone marrow suppression, bruising or bleeding, anaemia, nausea, mouth sores and ulcers, hair loss, diarrhoea, lethargy, soreness of hands and feet.

Chemoradiotherapy

See Table 8.5.
- Only used in the context of clinical trials.
- *McDonald NEJM 2001:* 556 patients' surgery or surgery + FU/ folinic acid (FA).
- Median overall survival 27/12 vs. 36/12.
- 3-year relapse free survival 48 vs. 31%.

Table 8.5 Chemoradiotherapy regimes

Treatment stage	Options currently in use
Neo-adjuvant chemotherapy	FU/cisplatin
	Taxane
Neo-adjuvant or definitive chemoradiation	FU/cisplatin
	Taxane-based
	Irinotecan-based
Adjuvant chemoradiation	FU/FA
	FU/cisplatin
Adjuvant chemotherapy	Epirubicin/cisplatin/FU
	Taxane-based
Advanced metastatic disease	FU-based
	Oxaliplatin-based
	Cisplatin-based
	Irinotecan-based
	Taxane-based

Follow-up and surveillance protocols

General
- Usefulness of surveillance is still largely unknown—rapid disease progression means majority are having active treatment with only a minority attending for symptomatic review.
- The development of clinical nurse specialist roles in follow-up should be encouraged—they have a crucial role to play in continuity of care between 1° and 2° care, and their role should include follow-up to reduce need for medical review.

Aims
- Detection of functional disorders related to complications of treatment.
- Detection of recurrence at the earliest opportunity.
- Assessment and management of nutritional requirements.
- Provision of psychosocial support to patients and carers, including liaison with palliative care where appropriate.
- Facilitation of treatment and outcome audit.

Format
- There is no evidence that intensive follow-up improves speed of detection of recurrence. Subsequently, there is no consensus for the mode, duration, or intensity of follow-up.
- Local protocols should be agreed upon—follow-up may be in the hospital or primary care setting. However, first follow-up should always be in hospital setting with MDT input, and patient then consulted and their wishes respected.
- When follow-up occurs in the hospital, it must be in multi-disciplinary setting to avoid investigation duplication, and wasting time and money.
- General practices taking part in follow-up should do so according to protocols and should be able to communicate effectively with hospital teams. They should take part in joint audit protocols, and should be guaranteed access to specialist services when necessary.
- Patients should be able to access services between appointments as and when necessary, and a named member of MDT as contact helps to facilitate this.
- Nutritional support is crucial following radical treatment and palliative therapy, and all patients should be offered dietary advice.

Palliative chemotherapy in oesophageal cancer

The majority of oesophageal tumours are only diagnosed at a stage at which curative treatment is not an option.

- Relapse after surgery or radical chemoradiotherapy is high. Survival of patients with recurrent or metastatic disease is low and ∴ palliative treatment of oesophageal cancer should primarily be aimed at QoL.
- Important to consider non-drug palliative measures alongside chemotherapy.
- 4 RCTs show gastric cancer palliative chemotherapy benefit over Best Supportive Care (BSC) mean survival: from 3–4 months to 7–10 months.
- Similar benefits in advanced oesophageal and GOJ cancer.

UK standard of care

- Epirubicin, oxaliplatin, capecitabine (EOX) is treatment of choice. Previously ECF.
- *REAL2 trial in 2008*: this trial randomized patients with adenocarcinomas or SCCs of oesophagus, GOJ, or stomach in a four-arm study investigating modifications of ECF regime.
- Multicentre randomized phase III trial for advanced oesophagogastric cancer.
  - 30% oesophageal.
  - 1002 patients—adenocarcinoma, SCC, undifferentiated all included.
- Regimes epirubicin, cisplatin, FU (ECF), epirubicin, oxaliplatin, FU (EOF), ECX, and EOX.
- Median follow-up 17.1 month. Response rate 41–48% for regimes, no significant difference. No survival advantage, but improved QoL.
- No significant HRQL differences between the four arms.

US standard of care

Triplet regime of docetaxel, cisplatin, and FU in medically fit patients.

V325 trial (van Cutsem, 2006)

- Docetaxel, cisplatin and fluorouracil combination chemotherapy regimen (DCF) superiority over the doublet of cisplatin and FU.
- Notable for also investigating health related quality of life prospectively.
- Statistically significant improvement in OS (9.2 vs. 8.6 months; $P = 0.020$) at the cost of significantly more toxicity, including febrile neutropenia.
- DCF vs. ECF.
- DCF resulted much higher neutropenia (41 vs. 18%).
- Docetaxel-containing regimens not currently approved in UK for this indication.
- Patients with adequate performance status with inoperable oesophagogastric cancer considered for EOX or ECX.

ToGA trial (2010)
- Patients with adenocarcinomas of the GOJ should be screened for over expression of HER2 and if positive (3+ on FISH) considered for HCX (trastuzumab, cisplatin, and capecitabine) chemotherapy.
- The augmented response rate of combination regimes is around 40–50%, but the median survival remains poor at around 9–11 months.
- Progression-free survival (6.7 vs. 5.5 months; $P = 0.0002$) and median OS (13.8 vs. 11.1 months; $P = 0.0046$).
- Toxicity of these regimes is high and only patients with performance status 0 or 1 should be considered for combination chemotherapy.
- There is no proven benefit to second line chemotherapy, but re-challenge with platinum-based regimes can be tried if an initial response was seen. Irinotecan-based regimes may also be considered.

Palliative radiotherapy, including brachytherapy, for oesophageal cancer

The aim of any palliative measure is symptom control and improvement in health-related QoL. For inoperable or metastatic oesophageal cancer the most common symptom that requires treatment is dysphagia. Localized pain, due to infiltration of the tumour in the mediastinum, and bleeding can also be helped by radiotherapy.

DXT advantages
- *Over palliative chemotherapy:* systemic toxicities are relatively mild.
- *Over stenting:* of controlling bleeding, as well as dysphagia.
- 70% of patients will experience an improvement in their dysphagia and for many maintained until death.

DXT disadvantages
- Slower onset of improvement in swallowing than a stent.
- Initial deterioration of swallowing 2° to oesophageal mucositis, during and shortly after treatment.
- Fatigue that can persist for several weeks after completion of treatment.

Palliative radiotherapy planning
- Simpler than for a radical course of treatment.
- Dose that can be safely administered is limited by the effect on surrounding normal tissues, in particular the spinal cord.
- Commonly used doses are 30Gy in 10 fractions over 2 weeks, or 20Gy in five fractions over 1 week.
- No evidence that adding external beam radiotherapy to stenting improves symptoms or life expectancy, but could reduce risk of bleeding.

Brachytherapy
- Radiation treatment given within tissues, most commonly within body cavities, using radioactive sources.
- Range of the radiotherapy given this way is limited to just a few centimetres around radioactive source so systemic toxicities are minimal.
- Brachytherapy for oesophageal cancer is usually given using iridium 192 placed within oesophagus via NGT or endoscopically. Dose is prescribed at 10mm from source circumferentially and whole length of tumour is treated with a craniocaudal margin of 2–3cm.
- Dose can be 10–12Gy as a single application or a course of 2 or 3 smaller doses at weekly intervals.

Studies comparing brachytherapy to stenting
SIREC multicentre RCT
- 12Gy brachytherapy vs. stent insertion.
- 209 patients in The Netherlands with inoperable oesophageal cancer.
- Primary outcome relief of dysphagia.

- Secondary outcomes were complications, treatment for persistent or recurrent dysphagia, HRQL, and cost.
- *Stent:* time to improvement in dysphagia is shorter.
- *Brachytherapy:* prolonged improvement.
- HRQL better overall, but deteriorated over time in both groups.
- *Conclusion:* if life expectancy of several months then brachytherapy could be considered, depending on availability of equipment and expertise.
- Combination of brachytherapy + DXT not better than either modality alone and evidence of increased risk of complications such as fistula formation when brachytherapy is given after high dose radiotherapy.

Oesophageal stenting

- Dilatation alone is unlikely to be effective in malignant strictures and is usually followed by some form of stenting (Fig. 8.12).
- Self-expandable metallic endoprostheses are available covered and uncovered, some of which have anti-reflux valves.
- Over 95 % of patients with inoperable oesophageal strictures can be palliated successfully with these devices (Fig. 8.12).
- Principally used to palliate dysphagia due to 1° tumour or anastomotic recurrence. May be used for extrinsic mediastinal compression.
- Retrievable oesophageal stents available if stenting is required as a bridge to future surgery or when complications occur as a result of surgery.
- Self-expanding metallic stents are inserted using small calibre delivery systems and often do not require pre-dilatation.
- Tracheo-oesophageal fistulae and oesophageal perforation.
- Covered stents used success rates of 80–100%.
- Stent insertion may not preclude further treatment with either chemoradiotherapy or more definitive surgery.
- Large bore stents (20–25mm) often necessary to adequately cover fistulae or perforation in patients following attempted recanalization of malignant strictures. To ensure adequate anchorage of the stent a temporary plastic balloon-expandable oesophageal stent (Wilson–Cook) placed endoscopically may be preferable to a metallic stent.
- *Early complications:* chest pain 90% (prolonged in 13%), bleeding, perforation, aspiration, fever, and fistula occur in 10–20% of patients, 30-day mortality is reported to be as high as 26%, incidence of stent migration for uncovered stents is low (0–3%), rising to 6% at cardia, but 30% covered stents particularly at cardia.
- *Late complications:* restenosis and tumour overgrowth 60%, haemorrhage (3–10%), oesophageal ulceration (7%), perforation or fistula (5%), stent torsion (5%), stent migration (5%), and stent fracture (2%).
- This may be a temporary measure allowing stabilization of patient prior to definitive surgery, or alternatively, in patients who are not surgical candidates, stent may provide adequate palliation.

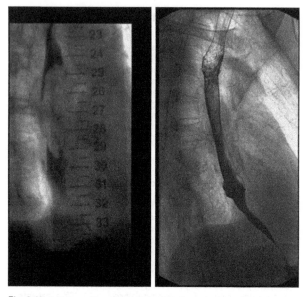

Fig. 8.12 A 26mm × 12cm self-expanding nitinol stent has been placed over a mid/distal oesophageal malignant stricture.

Further reading

Macdonald JS, Smalley SR, Benedetti J, et al. Chemoradiotherapy after surgery compared with surgery alone for adenocarcinoma of the stomach or gastroesophageal junction. *N Engl J Med* 2001; **345**(10): 725–30.

Van Cutsem E, Moiseyenko VM, Tjulandin S, et al. Phase III study of docetaxel and cisplatin plus fluorouracil compared with cisplatin and fluorouracil as first-line therapy for advanced gastric cancer: a report of the V325 Study Group. *J Clin Oncol* 2006; **24**(31): 4991–7.

Gastric cancer

Epidemiology

Gastric cancer (ICD code 151)

- Current UK incidence 16/100,000, male:female 2:1. Age 50–7.
- 6th commonest cancer in males and 9th in females in UK.
- 8000 new cases each year.
- UK AUGIS National Oesophagogastric (OG) Cancer Audit 2012: 1- and 3-year survival 78 and 46% (includes Siewert 3).
- Male to female ratio 5:3.
- Occurs mainly in elderly. Less than 8% of cases below age 55.
- Steadily increases with age and peaks in 8th decade.
- Incidence halved in UK over last 20 years.
- Worldwide decline in incidence of distal gastric cancer.
- *Most dramatic fall:* 8-fold in the last 50 years. Affluent Western countries, predominantly Caucasian population, and low population density, such as USA, Canada, Australia, and New Zealand.
- Western Europe significant, but less dramatic decline.
- Far East (Japan/China) and South America still affected by high incidence rates thought to be due to continuing high rates of *H. pylori* infection, adverse dietary factors, and genetic predisposition.
- Marked increase in incidence of GOJ cancer over last 30 years.
- Downward migration of oesophageal tumours and proximal shift of gastric tumours.
- GOJ cancer: fastest increasing solid malignancy of adult life in the West, with increasing incidence of 3–4% per annum.
- Adenocarcinoma is most common.
- Incidence of distal oesophageal adenocarcinoma could increase if more tumours at or near GOJ identified as arising from oesophagus, rather than stomach.
- Only specialist oesophagogastric surgical centres can accurately classify whether tumour of GOJ is arising in distal oesophagus, gastric cardia or subcardinal stomach.
- Siewert and Stein proposed a classification system of gastro-oesophageal cancers in an attempt to simplify conundrum (Box 9.1, Fig. 9.1).

The suggestion from an epidemiological standpoint is that adenocarcinoma of the oesophagus and gastric cardia are the same disease and the incidences of adenocarcinoma at the two locations should be combined. This is consistent with the two cancers having a similar phenotype and prevalence of the *p53* gene mutation. This has recently also been adopted by the surgical community.

Box 9.1 Siewert's classification of GOJ adenocarcinomas

- *Type 1:* adenocarcinoma of distal oesophagus arising in Barrett's segment, which may infiltrate GOJ from above.
- *Type 2:* true junctional carcinoma of the cardia.
- *Type 3:* subcardinal carcinoma, which may infiltrate GOJ from below.

Reproduced from 'Classification of adenocarcinoma of the oesophagogastric junction', Siewert JR, Stein HJ, *Br J Surg*, **85**: 1457–9, copyright 1998 with permission of John Wiley and Sons.

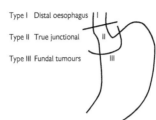

Fig. 9.1 Siewert's classification of GOJ adenocarcinomas.

Degree of differentiation and site

Gastric adenocarcinoma are divisible into two subtypes. The natural history and aetiology are distinct.

- Subtype that remains endemic in Far East, parts of South America, and Eastern Europe is principally a disease of distal stomach associated with chronic gastritis, intestinal metaplasia, and atrophy of mucosa.
- Increasingly occurring subtype found in Western countries is commonly found near GOJ and is not associated with significant gastritis.

Pathophysiology

Pathogenesis of gastric cancer

The pathogenesis of gastric cancer is complex and multifactorial (Correa hypothesis). Environmental factors are required to effect multistage progression to malignant transformation.

Risk factors

- Low socio-economic group.
- *Diet:* nitrosamines—dye, cured meat, fish, alcohol, and tobacco.
- Blood group A.
- *Obesity:* 2-fold increase in risk of gastric cancer.
- *Genetic predisposition:* E Cadherin mutations/ hereditary diffuse gastric cancer (HDCG; associated with lobular breast cancer).

Precursors

Chronic atrophic gastritis (40% >60 years)

- *H. pylori* (micro-aerophilic, Gram negative, spiral micro-organism, see 🕮 *Helicobacter pylori*, p. 96) classed by WHO as Group 1 carcinogen (100% infection results in 6-fold increase in incidence of cancer). Causes cell loss due to urease, ammonia, acetaldehyde activity, resulting from chemotactic effect of inflammatory cells releasing oxygen metabolites. Resulting loss of fundic glands leads to hypochloridia and proliferation of *H. pylori*.
- Chemical irritants (reflux/ingested).
- *Autoimmune disease:* pernicious anaemia.

All cause inflammatory damage to the gastric mucosa, resulting in atrophic gastritis and intestinal metaplasia.

Gastric polyps (7% >80 years)
- *Hyperplastic:* no increased risk of cancer.
- *Fundic gland:* no increased risk of cancer (hyperproliferative hamartomas).
- Associated with familial adenomatous polyposis, but more commonly sporadic.
- *Neoplastic:* adenomas. Malignant change in 40% >2cm.
- *Gastroduodenal:* associated with familial adenomatous polyposis (usually fundic or hyperplastic). Increased risk of malignant transformation (duodenal and peri-ampullary carcinoma).

Gastric remnant
Previous gastrectomy: there is a 2% increase risk of gastric cancer, usually found at the stomal site. There is a higher risk for the first 40 years post-resection, highest 15–20 years. Alkalinity may play a role.

Menetrier's disease
A hypertrophic rugal gastropathy resulting in hypochloridia and a protein losing enteropathy with a 10% association.

Chronic peptic ulcer
<1% undergo malignant change.

Gastric epithelial dysplasia
- *Mild/moderate/severe:* natural history is not a relentless march to carcinoma. There is regression to normal in 60–70% of mild to moderate cases; regression less common in severe cases with 50–80% progressing to invasive carcinoma.
- Vienna Classification of Epithelial Neoplasia is described in Box 9.2

Note: Low-grade dysplasia can be confused with inflammatory atypia, which can regress with acid suppression. ∴ a first diagnosis of LGD on endoscopy should receive full acid suppression for 3/12 prior to re-examination.

Box 9.2 Vienna classification of epithelial neoplasia
1. Negative for neoplasia.
2. Indefinite for neoplasia.
3. Non-invasive low grade neoplasia.
4. Non-invasive high grade neoplasia.
4.1. High grade adenoma.
4.2. Non-invasive carcinoma.
4.3. Suspicious for invasive carcinoma.
5. Invasive carcinoma.
5.1. Intramucosal carcinoma.
5.2. Submucosal carcinoma or beyond.

Reprinted by permission from Macmillan Publishers Ltd: 'The Vienna classification of gastrointestinal epithelial neoplasia', Schlemper RJ, Riddell RH, Kato Y et al., *Gut* 2000 Aug; **47**(2): 251–5.

Early gastric cancer
- Malignant tumour confined to mucosa (T1a) or submucosa (T1b) independent of lymph node metastases.

- Penetration of muscularis mucosae allows subdivision into intramucosal or submucosal types.
- Early tumours often tattooed with indigo carmine (blue dye). Local staging undertaken with endoscopic ultrasound to decide if amenable to local EMR, avoiding need for radical curative resection.
- EMR pioneered by Japanese who have unique experience of large numbers of very early carcinomas.
- Criteria used by most Japanese units have included:
  - Size < 2cm.
  - Morphological type I or II. *Or*
  - No associated ulceration.
  - No definitive invasion of the submucosa.

Advanced gastric cancer
- 90% of malignant tumours of the stomach are adenocarcinomas (Fig. 9.2).
- Others include lymphoma and smooth muscle tumours.
- In the western world there is a falling incidence of distal gastric cancer, but rising incidence of junctional tumours and tumours of the gastric cardia. There is an association with blood group A.

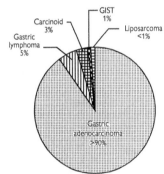

Fig. 9.2 Breakdown of tumours affecting the stomach.

Borders' classification
- Developed in 1942 and is original classification.
- Classifies gastric carcinoma on degree of cellular differentiation, independent of morphology.
- Ranges from type 1 (well differentiated) to type 4 (anaplastic).

Lauren classification (microscopic appearance) 1965
- *Intestinal type (53%):*
  - Typically arises in presence of precancerous conditions, such as gastric atrophy or intestinal metaplasia.
  - More common in men than women.
  - Incidence increases with age.
  - Dominant type in areas in which gastric cancer is epidemic, usually well differentiated, and tends to spread haematogenously to distant organs.

- Diffuse type (30%)—associated with mucin secreting signet ring cells (poorer prognosis):
  - Poorly differentiated, lacks gland formation.
  - Clusters of small uniform cells, tends to spread submucosally and metastasizes early by transmural extension and via lymphatics.
  - Poor prognosis.
  - More common in women and younger age groups.
  - Associated with blood type A and familial cases suggesting genetic aetiology.
- Mixed type.

Borrmann classification (macroscopic appearance) 1926
- *Type 1:* fungating (polypoid).
- *Type 2:* excavating (ulcer).
- *Type 3:* ulcerating and raised.
- *Type 4:* linitis plastica (diffusely thickened).

These tumours tend to be large (6–10cm), 40% occurring in the antrum, 40% body, 15% at gastric cardia, and 5% affecting entire stomach.

WHO classification 1990
- Based on morphological features. Divides gastric cancer into five types.
- Adenocarcinoma, adenosquamous cell carcinoma, squamous cell carcinoma, undifferentiated carcinoma, and unclassified carcinoma.
- Adenocarcinoma subdivided into four types according to growth pattern. Papillary, tubular, mucinous, and signet ring. Each type further subdivided by degree of differentiation.
- Widely used system, but offers little in terms of patient management.

Mode of spread
- *Direct extension:* into adjacent viscera.
- *Lymphatic spread:* high propensity towards loco-regional nodal spread, rarely ever metastasizing via bloodstream before spreading to numerous local nodes. Lateral spread occurs in submucosal/subserosal plexuses then to perigastric lymph nodes and, subsequently, along lymphatics that follow arteries to coeliac trunk.
- *Peritoneal spread:* high propensity once it has breached serosa to spread via peritoneal surfaces, shedding miliary metastatic nodules in a fashion that renders patient incurable.
- *Haematogenous spread:*
  - Portal venous drainage arrangement can ultimately facilitate liver metastases.
  - Despite the stomach's rich blood supply, liver metastases rare at presentation.
  - Evidence from studies of early gastric cancers from japan suggest that well-differentiated cancers may metastasize more frequently to liver and poorly-differentiated tumours to lymph nodes.

Clinical presentation

Frequently presents late due to the non-specific nature of the symptoms, with >80% patients presenting with >T1 disease.

Referral pathways
- *2-week rule:* UK national initiative 1996.
- General practitioner.
- *Endoscopy unit:* open access.
- Radiologist.
- Other consultants.
- Emergency.

Acute presentation
- Acute UGI bleed (haematemesis/melaena).
- Gastric outlet obstruction.
- Abdominal pain/mass.

Sub-acute presentation
- Dyspepsia.
- Anorexia/weight loss.
- Iron deficiency anaemia.
- Nausea and vomiting.
- Abdominal bloating/early satiety.
- Fatigue.
- Epigastric mass.
- Metastatic disease.

BSG guidelines for referral of suspected gastric cancer
Dysphagia
Dyspepsia is combined with one or more of these alarm symptoms: weight loss, anaemia, and anorexia.

Dyspepsia in a patient aged 55 years or older, with at least one of the following 'high risk' features:
- Onset of dyspepsia <1 year ago.
- Continuous symptoms since onset.
- Dyspepsia combined with at least one of following known risk factors:
  - Family history of UGI cancer in more than one first degree relative.
  - Barrett's oesophagus.
  - Pernicious anaemia.
  - Peptic ulcer surgery over 20 years ago.
  - Known dysplasia.
  - Atrophic gastritis.
  - Intestinal metaplasia.
  - Jaundice.
  - Upper abdominal mass.

Physical signs
- Develop late.
- Most commonly associated with locally advanced or metastatic disease.
- Findings may include:
  - Palpable abdominal mass.
  - Palpable supraclavicular (Virchow's) or peri-umbicular (sister Mary Joseph's) nodule.
  - Jaundice.
  - Ascites.
  - Cachexia.
- Succussion splash on examination.
- *Acanthosisnigricans:* velvety skin changes around axilla associated with plantar tylosis.

Screening and early diagnosis

- As gastric cancer begins as epithelial proliferation and disorganization, it has no features that either stimulate pain receptors or significantly influence function making it inherently difficult to diagnose at early stage.
- Aim to detect gastric cancer in its earliest stages when prognosis is better, as only 40% of early gastric cancer associated with symptoms.
- Annual mass population screening in high incidence countries: Japan, Korea, Venezuela, and Chile).
- Screening methods and intervals vary in different settings.

Japan

Gastric cancer is the leading cause of cancer death—50,562 in 2004.

- Nationwide screening for all individuals >40 years since 1983.
- *Initial pilots:* photofluorography, endoscopy, serum pepsinogen testing, and *H. pylori* Ab testing compared.
- *Standard approach:*
  - Simple risk interview and barium studies.
  - Double contrast barium meal with photofluorography or digital fluorography adopted.
  - OGD if any abnormality.
- *Case–control studies:* 40–60% decrease in mortality with photofluorography screening.
  - Tsubonometa-analysis 3 Japanese case-control studies.
  - Mortality reduction from gastric cancer (male OR: 0.47, 95% CI: 0.29–0.52; female OR: 0.50, 95% CI: 0.34–0.72).
  - Significantly decreased mortality in males (RR: 0.54, 95% CI: 0.41–0.70) reduction in mortality was not significant in females (RR: 0.74, 95% CI: 0.52–1.04).
  - Incidence and mortality of gastric cancer decreased in last decade, but remain high overall.
  - Screening rate has plateaued.
- Endoscopic screening suggested as alternative strategy to radiography. No Japanese studies have evaluated effectiveness in gastric cancer mortality reduction sensitivity compared with radiography is unclear.
  - *Chinese study*—Linqu County, 1989–1999, endoscopic screening 4394 residents. Incidence and mortality from gastric cancer monitored until 2000.
  - *85 gastric cancers detected*—29 early cancers. Compared with overall population mortality for Linqu County, standard morality ratio was 1.01 (95% CI: 0.32–1.37).
  - Mortality reduction associated with endoscopic screening remains unclear. RCT may delineate this in future.

Korea

- Individuals aged 40 years and older.
- Screening every 2 years contrast studies or OGD.
- Retrospective cohort study of 2485 patients gastric adenocarcinoma.
- *Chance of detecting advanced cancer:* 1 year screening vs. 4- or 5-year intervals (4-year interval OR 2.5, 95% CI 1.4–4.5, 5-year interval OR 2.2, 95% CI 1.3–3.7), but 2- or 3-year intervals similar to 1-year.
- *Subgroup analysis:* family history of gastric cancer or age >60 years, higher stage at detection if OGD 3-yearly annually compared with (family history of gastric cancer OR 2.68, 95% CI 1.3–5.7, gastric cancer in 60s OR 2.09, 95% CI 1.0–4.3).
- In high incidence populations, screening 2-yearly is appropriate for over 60s or if family history of gastric cancer, every 3 years for other individuals.

UK referral guidelines

- Patients are referred via their general practitioner, to be seen by 2° hospital specialist within 2 weeks of referral. Despite best efforts in this referral pathway, detection rates of oesophagogastric cancer remain at 3%.
- Mass screening not indicated for UK with current diagnostic modalities due to relatively low incidence (see Box 9.3).

Box 9.3 Criteria for OGD in UK

1. Dyspepsia, at any age, and chronic GI bleeding.
2. Dyspepsia, at any age, and weight loss.
3. Dyspepsia, at any age, and iron deficiency anaemia.
4. Dyspepsia, at any age, and dysphagia.
5. Dyspepsia, at any age, and vomiting (persistent).
6. Dyspepsia, at any age, epigastric mass.
7. Dyspepsia, at any age, suspicious contrast meal.
8. Dyspepsia, >55 years, symptomatic onset < 1 year.

Clinical evaluation

Diagnosis and pre-operative staging
- Flexible upper endoscopy.
- Modality of choice once gastric cancer is suspected.
- Multiple biopsies (seven or more required) from ulcer edges.
- Avoid biopsying ulcer crater (may reveal necrotic debris only).
- Note the size, location, and morphology of the tumour.
- Blood test should be carried out once gastric cancer is confirmed.
- *FBC:* may reveal anaemia.
- *LFT:* abnormal in advanced disease and sign of liver metastasis.
- *Coagulation:* abnormal in advanced disease.

Double-contrast barium swallows
- Cost effective and 90% diagnostic accuracy.
- However, unable to distinguish benign from malignant lesions.
- Used in Japanese screening programme, but seldom used in West.
- Endoscopy preferable.

Endoscopic ultrasound scan
- Can assess the extent of gastric wall invasion and nodal status.
- Better accuracy for T1 and T3 lesions, but poor for T2 (cannot assess invasion of the muscularis propria).
- Superior to CT for T1 and T3 tumours.
- Cannot reliably distinguish tumour from fibrosis, thus not suitable for evaluating response to therapy.
- Good for evaluating lymph nodes and have added advantage of fine-needle aspiration.
- Overall staging accuracy is about 80%.
- Complimentary to CT and not a substitute.

CT (computed tomography)
- Chest, abdomen, and pelvis should be scanned.
- Stomach should be well distended to increase accuracy.
- Cannot distinguish T1 and T2 tumour (i.e. early gastric cancers that may be suitable for endoscopic mucosal resections).
- Cannot detect small (<5mm) metastasis in liver or peritoneal disease.
- Nodal detection relies on size and is poor predictor of involvement particularly in chest.

Positron emission tomography (PET)-CT
- May improve detection of distant metastasis. Not routine exam in UK. Mainly used in follow-up and where there is suspicion of progression.
- Overall accuracy of 80–85%.

Diagnostic laparoscopy
- Due to the inherent inaccuracies of CT and EUS, laparoscopy indicated for evaluation of patients with locoregional disease.
- Can detect metastatic disease in 30% of patients who are judged to be resectable on CT and EUS.
- Addition of laparoscopic ultrasound may improve detection of liver and peritoneal metastasis, though highly operator dependent.
- *Cytology of peritoneal fluid:* obtained at laparoscopy may reveal presence of free intraperitoneal gastric cells, but errors in reporting (false positive and negative) decrease sensitivity of this method.
- *Immunostaining of peritoneal fluid:* and reverse transcriptase polymerase chain reaction for carcino-embryonic antigen messenger RNA may provide better and more accurate detection in the future.

Patient pathway and selection for gastric surgery
- Tissue confirmation of diagnosis (usually on OGD and biopsy).
- Staging CT scan (thorax/abdomen and pelvis).
- Discussion of diagnosis and stage with patient and assessment of fitness for Rx/palliation.
- Clinical nurse specialist (CNS) co-ordinates information giving to the patient and family and information providing to the specialist oesophagogastric multi-disciplinary team (MDT).
- MDT discussion.
- Evaluation of history, stage, intent of possible treatment, patient fitness and choice:
  - Endoscopic vs. radical surgery.
  - New therapeutic and neoadjuvant regimes.
  - Patient selection and assessing outcomes.
- Discussion with patient to outline management options and an informed, realistic discussion regarding the implications of surgery and future QoL.

Despite multimodal therapy and adequate surgery only 30% of gastric cancer patients are alive at 3 years.

Multi-disciplinary team membership
Cancer nurse specialists, gastroenterologists, surgeons, radiologists, anaesthetist/intensivist., oncologists, pathologists, palliative care team, physiotherapists/occupational therapists, dieticians, data collection/MDT coordinator.

Considerations
See Chapter 7.
- *Clinical assessment (eyeball test):* throughout process, this is best time to assess patient and recommend an honest, realistic opinion about most appropriate future management strategy. Walk your patient—can they manage a flight of stairs?

- Blood investigations (FBC, U&E, LFT, clotting).
- Simple radiology (*Note*: staging CT).
- Pulmonary function testing/echocardiography (ECHO) cardiography (static).
- CPET (dynamic).
- Formal anaesthetic assessment.

Other evaluators of fitness for radical surgery

- ASA grading.
- Physiological and Operative Severity Score for the Enumeration of Mortality and Morbidity (P-POSSUM).

Specific considerations

- *Nutrition:* BMI <20 or >30 increases risk of post-operative complications, e.g. ARDS, infection, and impaired wound healing. Consideration to peri-operative nutritional support is mandatory in each case. Dieticians should be involved at an early stage to ensure nutritional requirements are met, e.g. oral supplements, nasojejunal feeding, feeding jejunostomy, TPN. Enteral route should be used at all times if possible.
- *Mono-amine oxidase inhibitors (MAOI):* should be stopped 4 weeks pre-operatively.
- *Oral contraceptive pill (OCP):* should be stopped 2 weeks pre-operatively due to increased venous thrombo-embolic (VTE) risk.
- *Smoking:* patients should be encouraged to stop at all times. Ideally, cessation should occur to minimize respiratory complications, a minimum of 8 weeks pre-operatively. There is good evidence that even stopping 48h pre-operatively improves oxygen carrying capacity of blood.
- *GORD:* consider pre-operative acid suppression and rapid sequence induction (RSI) of anaesthesia.
- *Blood transfusion:* if required should be given >24h pre-operatively to allow optimization of oxygen carrying capacity.
- *Recent myocardial infarction:* elective surgery should ideally be deferred 6 months following acute MI. In case of gastric malignancy, this is not feasible, but formal cardiology input should be sought, with deferment of surgery for 6 weeks post-event.
- *Coronary artery bypass grafting (CABG)/angioplasty:* following re-vascularization, there is increased risk of peri-operative complications if good left ventricular (LV) function remains. Consult cardiology and anaesthetic colleagues.
- *Beta-blockers:* frequently a contentious issue. Current recommendations are if patient is already commenced on beta-blockers then continue, if not do not start.

Principles of staging

Ideally, no patient should be subjected to an exploratory operation or trial dissection. Initial staging investigations are vital in management algorithm (Fig. 9.3) of gastric cancer.

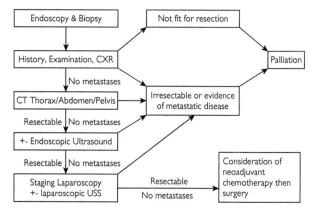

Fig. 9.3 Algorithm for the clinical staging of gastric cancer. CXR, chest X-ray; USS, ultrasound scan.

Staging tumour, node, and metastasis (TNM; internationally unified system)

In all cases microscopic proof of malignancy is required. Once staging investigations are complete, the patient is discussed at Specialized MDT, to propose an individually tailored management plan.

TNM

See Box 9.4.

T: tumour size.

N: assessment of regional lymph node metastases.

M: presence/absence of distant metastases.

- *cTNM:* clinical and pre-operative staging.
- *pTNM:* final pathological staging.
- *ypTNM:* final pathological staging following multimodal therapy i.e. neoadjuvant chemotherapy.

UICC TNM 7: Stomach (2009)

A tumour with its epicentre within 5cm of GOJ and extending into the oesophagus is classified and staged according to the oesophageal scheme. All other tumours with their epicentre in the stomach >5cm from the GOJ or those within 5cm of GOJ without extension into the oesophagus are staged using the gastric scheme.

See also Fig. 9.4.

Box 9.4 TNM 7 classification of gastric cancer

T1: invades lamina propria or submucosa.
T1a—invades lamina propria or muscularis mucosae.
T1b—invades submucosa.
T2: invades muscularis propria.
T3: invades subserosa.
T4: invades serosa.
T4a—perforates serosa.
T4b—invades adjacent structures.
N0: no involved regional lymph nodes.
N1: 1–2 regional lymph nodes involved.
N2: 3–6 regional lymph nodes involved.
N3a: 7–15 regional lymph nodes involved.
N3b: >15 regional lymph nodes involved.
M0: no distant metastases.
M1: distant metastases.

Reproduced from *The TNM Classification of Malignant Tumours* 7th edn., eds. Leslie H. Sobin, Mary K. Gospodarowicz, and Christian Wittekind, copyright 2009 with permission of Wiley-Blackwell.

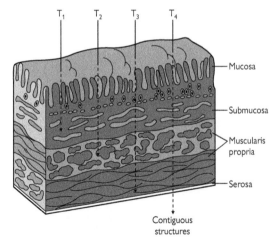

Fig. 9.4 Gastric wall cross-section.
Reproduced from *The Oxford Specialist Handbook of Surgical Oncology*, eds. Chaudry and Winslet, copyright Oxford University Press 2009, with permission of Oxford University Press.

Staging
See Box 9.5. Final pathological stage, following curative surgery assists in determining prognosis. Survival is significantly poorer among patients with pathological stages II, IIIa and IV.

Box 9.5 TNM 7 staging of gastric cancer

Stage 0: Tis, N0, M0.
Stage IA: T1, N0, M0.
Stage 1B:
- T1, N1, M0.
- T2, N0, M0.
Stage IIA:
- T3, N0, M0.
- T2, N1, M0.
- T1, N2, M0.
Stage IIB:
- T4a, N0, M0.
- T3, N1, M0.
- T2, N2, M0.
- T1, N3, M0.
Stage IIIA:
- T4a, N1, M0.
- T3, N2, M0.
- T2, N3, M0.
Stage IIIB:
- T4b, N0, N1, M0.
- T4a, N2, M0.
- T3, N3, M0.
Stage IIIC:
- T4a, N3, M0.
- T4b, N2, N3, M0.
Stage IV: Any T, Any N, M1.
5-year survival rates
Stage 0: greater than 90%.
Stage IA: 60–80%.
Stage IB: 50–60%.
Stage II: 30–40%.
Stage IIIB: 20%.
Stage IIIC: 10%.
Stage IV: less than 5%.

Reproduced from *The TNM Classification of Malignant Tumours* 7th edn., eds. Leslie H. Sobin, Mary K. Gospodarowicz, and Christian Wittekind, copyright 2009 with permission of Wiley-Blackwell.

R status
Used to describe the tumour status after resection.
- *R0:* microscopically negative margin.
- *R1:* microscopically positive margin.
- *R2:* gross residual disease.

Japanese classification of gastric carcinoma

- Designed to describe the anatomic locations of nodes removed during gastrectomy (Fig. 9.5).
- 16 distinct anatomic stations of lymph nodes.
- Grouped into three groups (N1, N2, and N3).
- Nodal basin dissection dependent on the location of the 1°.
- Not used in Europe and in America.

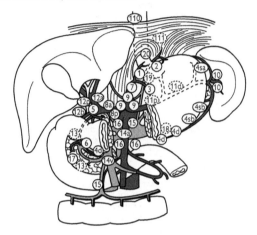

Fig. 9.5 Anatomic lymph node stations.
Reproduced from *The Oxford Specialist Handbook of Surgical Oncology*, eds. Chaudry and Winslet, copyright Oxford University Press 2009, with permission of Oxford University Press.

Neoadjuvant treatment for gastric adenocarcinoma

Peri-operative chemotherapy for gastric cancer
- Standard of care in UK and most of Europe for localized gastric cancer (and type II and III GOJ adenocarcinoma).
- Accepted perioperative regimens are ECF or ECX.
- MRC MAGIC trial of peri-operative chemotherapy published in 2006.
- 503 patients randomized. Three cycles ECF chemotherapy before and three cycles after surgery, or to surgery alone.
- Survival at all time points was increased in chemotherapy arm, with a hazard ratio for overall survival of 0.75 in favour of peri-operative chemotherapy.
- 5-year survival rate was increased from 23 to 36%.
- Similar results were achieved in French study of perioperative cisplatin and FU published by Ychou (2011) (Fédération Francophone de Cancérologie Digestive (FFCD)/ Fédération Nationale des Centres de Lutte Contre le Cancer (FNCLCC)), with the 5-year survival increasing from 24 to 38%. Perioperative chemotherapy is currently standard treatment for resectable gastric cancers in UK and Europe.

'MAGIC' regime
Epirubicin 50mg/m², cisplatin 60mg/m² (with hydration), FU 200mg/m²/day by continuous infusion on days 1–21 for three cycles followed by surgery.
- *ECX completion rates:* 54% any of the planned post-operative treatments. Only 41% completed all 6 cycles.
- MAGIC trial randomized 503 patients with the following characteristics:
  - All patients had WHO performance status 0 or 1.
  - 79% male/21% female.
  - *Tumour distribution*—74% gastric, 12% junctional, and 14% lower oesophageal adenocarcinoma.
- Surgery scheduled 3–6 weeks after completion of chemotherapy.
- *Resection rate was high:* 91% vs. 96% surgery only.
- *Higher proportion of resections in treated group were considered curative by surgeon:* 79% after chemotherapy vs. 73% for surgery alone.
- Rate of R0 resections was increased from 74 to 87% in French trial.
- No increase in 30-day mortality, which was less than 6% in both arms.
- Post-operative complication rates were not increased at 45%.
- Hazard ratio for overall survival was 0.75 in favour of peri-operative chemotherapy. The 5-year survival rate was increased from 23 to 36%.
- Toxicities include nausea, neutropenia, thrombocytopenia, anaemia, cardiac dysfunction, fatigue, neuropathy, nephropathy, diarrhea, and mucositis.
- Patients should be fit, WHO performance score 0 or 1. They should have adequate cardiac function as determined by multigated acquisition scan (MUGA) or ECHO, with left ventricular ejection fraction (LVEF) >50%, and normal renal function.
- Regime usually modified by replacing infusional FU with oral capecitabine at a dose of 625mg/m² bd continuously throughout each 3-week cycle.

MAGIC criticism

- *Heterogenous tumour location:* gastric/lower oesophagus.
- Poor rate of completion of adjuvant chemotherapy in 'perioperative chemotherapy' trial.
- All patients WHO PS 0/1.
- Lack of well-designed RCTs with HQRL outcomes comparing perioperative treatment strategies for tumours of stomach or GOJ: MRC STO3 incorporates comprehensive assessment of HRQL.

MRC ST03 trial

- *Two-arm randomized 1:1 Phase II/III trial:* comparing ECX and bevacizumab with ECX alone for cancer of the stomach, oesophagus, or junction of stomach and oesophagus.
- Recruitment November 2007 to November 2013.
- History confirmed gastric or Type III GOJ adenocarcinoma considered to be TNM 6 stage Ib (T1 N1), II, III, or stage IV (T4, N1 or N2 M0).
- Chemotherapy in three cycles over 9 weeks. 5–6 weeks break then surgery.
- Outcomes:
  - *Stage I safety and feasibility of ECX/bevacizumab (Bv)*—perforations at 1° tumour, cardiac toxicity, wound healing complications, GI bleeding.
  - *Feasibility*—acceptance of randomization and completion rate.
  - *Stage II*—1° outcome, overall survival.
  - *Secondary outcomes:* response rates to preoperative treatment, R0 rate, Rx morbidity, disease-free survival (DFS). QoL and cost-effectiveness.

Chemoradiation

- Non-randomized studies show substantial pathological response (downstaging of tumour) to preoperative chemoradiation.
- Trials currently underway to assess usefulness of this regime.
- In UK, this is only available as part of a trial.

Radiotherapy alone

- Recent randomized trials from China revealed a survival benefit with preoperative radiotherapy (30 vs. 20%).
- Currently trials under way in the west to try and replicate this.
- In the UK pre-operative radiotherapy is not standard.

Surgical management

The 1° objective of surgery is to excise 1° tumour with clear longitudinal and circumferential resection margins (R0 resection), then safely restore intestinal and biliary continuity to allow adequate nutritional intake.

A loco-regional disease?

- *Gunderson and Sosin:* gastric cancer is a loco-regional disease.
- 80% Recurrence rates in patients with T4 serosal positive disease.
- Majority of recurrences locally either in gastric bed, retroperitoneum or anastomosis, rather than distant metastases.
- Median time to recurrence 2 years.
- *T1/2 serosal negative disease:* fewer recurrences as expected, but those that did recur recurred later and more frequently. Distant failure (liver metastases) potentially due to a sub-set that micro-metastasizes early.
- Radical surgery in T4 disease produces little benefit.

Strategies to minimize loco-regional recurrence

- Complete resection of 1° lesion, including extending resection line in continuity with adjacent structures if safe/feasible, i.e. *en bloc* resection. Attempt to prevent gastric bed recurrence.
- Meticulous surgical technique with *en bloc* resection of stomach, affected adjacent organs and intact gastric lymphatic chains to prevent iatrogenic cell spillage. This would attempt to prevent peritoneal dissemination.
- In reality, large multicentre randomized controlled trials i.e. MRC MAGIC trial have recommended neoadjuvant/adjuvant chemotherapy in conjunction with adequate surgery (multimodal therapy) to improve outcomes in gastric cancer.
- However, neoadjuvant and adjuvant therapies are no substitute for inadequate surgery.
- *Pragmatic approach:* is excision of *all* neoplastic tissue/cellular material feasible? In this patient? Only likely in early gastric cancer (EGC) and early T2s with radical resection, beyond this, multimodal treatment essential. Preoperative chemotherapy may, however, increase proportion of tumours for whom this is possible.

Types of gastrectomy

- Depends on site of the primary tumour (Fig. 9.6).
- *Resection margin:* aim = minimum 5cm from palpable edge of tumour.
- Diffuse type tumours more prone to lateral spread, some advocate total gastrectomy for all diffuse types. May not be necessary for distal tumours as long as adequate staging. Mapping biopsies, careful radiological review, on-table OGD ± frozen section.

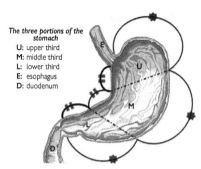

The three portions of the stomach
U: upper third
M: middle third
L: lower third
E: esophagus
D: duodenum

Fig. 9.6 Stomach divided into proximal (U), middle (M), and distal (L) thirds.
Reproduced from 'EORTC-ROG expert opinion: Radiotherapy volume and treatment guidelines for neoadjuvant radiation of adenocarcinomas of the gastroesophageal junction and the stomach', Oscar Matzinger, Erich Gerber, Zvi Bernstein et al., *Radiotherapy and Oncology*, Aug; **92**(2): 164–75, copyright 2009 with permission of Elsevier.

Distal 1/3 cancers: tumours of the gastric antrum

- Subtotal (80%) gastrectomy, including division of left gastric artery and vein, and excision of regional lymphatic tissue.
- Total gastrectomy only when large tumour or when submucosal tumour infiltration to within 7–8cm of GOJ.

Middle 1/3 cancers: tumours of the gastric body

- Total or subtotal gastrectomy depending on proximal margin of tumour.
- Total gastrectomy often necessary. This depends on amount of stomach remaining below GOJ (minimum necessary = 2cm).
- *Serosa negative cancer:* requires 7cm margin from GOJ.
- *Serosa positive cancer:* requires 8cm margin from GOJ.
- Smaller margins acceptable in elderly patients especially if intestinal type.

Proximal 1/3 cancers: tumours of the gastric cardia

- Siewert 3 GOJ tumours may be amenable to total gastrectomy, if enough proximal clearance is possible. True junctional tumours (Siewert 2) should be treated with extended total gastrectomy or cardio-oesophagectomy.
- All patients with proximal gastric tumours, should be made aware that at time of dissection/resection, it may be necessary to proceed to cardio-oesophagectomy with possible thoracotomy, so as not to compromise resection margins.

Extent of lymphadenectomy

Surgical lymph node tiers
- *N1:* peri-gastric nodes closest to 1°.
- *N2:* distant peri-gastric nodes and nodes along main arteries supplying stomach.
- *N3:* nodes outside normal lymphatic pathways from stomach, involved in advanced stages or by retrograde lymphatic flow due to blockage of normal pathways.

Lymphadenectomy definitions

- *D1:* all N1 nodes removed *en bloc* with the stomach (limited).
- *D2:* all N1 and N2 nodes removed *en bloc* with stomach (systematic).
- *D3:* more radical *en bloc* resection including N3 nodes (extended). This more commonly includes only some lymph node stations, e.g. D2 lymphadenectomy and station 12 (hepatoduodenal).
- *Note:* Current European description of D2 lymphadenectomy involves removal of >15 lymph nodes, irrespective of node stations.

Japanese recommendations
- *D1 total gastrectomy:* stations 1, 2, 3, 4, 5, 6, and 7 resected.
- *D2 total gastrectomy:* stations 8a, 9, 10, 11, and 12 added.
- *D1 subtotal gastrectomy:* stations 1, 3, 4, 5, 6, and 7 resected.
- *D2 subtotal gastrectomy:* stations 8a, 9, 11p, and 12a added.

Historical considerations

- Much debate still exists between West and East as to what is achieved by performing more radical lymphadenectomies.
- *Japanese view:* radical systematic D2 lymphadenectomy. Increased survival benefit following observation gastric cancer commonly remained localized to stomach and adjacent LN.
- Excision of 1° lesion with omenta, and N1 and N2 LN that drain affected area of stomach can cure patients even in presence of LN metastases.
- Originally, *en bloc* clearance of perigastric nodes, all LN along main branches of coeliac axis, with routine resection of spleen and distal pancreas during total gastrectomy to ensure full nodal clearance along splenic artery.
- *Western non-radical view:* more radical lymphadenectomy only gives more accurate pathological staging, rather than confer improved survival benefit.
- Much of the stage-specific improvement in survival after D2 resection likely to be a result of better pathological staging stage migration factor, particularly stages II and IIIa.
- Japanese view based on large observational studies compared with western RCTs (German Gastric Cancer Study Group, Dutch Gastric Cancer Trial, MRC Gastric Cancer Surgical Trial), which are smaller, but more powerful.

MRC D1 vs. D2 lymphadenectomy
- Final results 1999 (pre-perioperative chemotherapy era).
- *737 patients:* 337 patients ineligible by staging laparotomy due to advanced disease—400 were randomized.

- *5-year survival:* 35% for D1 resection and 33% for D2 resection (difference −2%, 95% CI = −12% to 8%).
- No difference in overall survival between two arms (hazard ratio (HR) = 1.10, 95% CI 0.87–1.39, where HR >1 implies a survival benefit to D1 surgery).
- Survival based on gastric cancer death similar (HR = 1.05, 95% CI 0.79–1.39) as was RFS (HR = 1.03, 95% CI 0.82–1.29).
- *Multivariate:* stages II and III, old age, male sex, and removal of spleen and pancreas independently associated with poor survival (30 vs. 50% 3 years).
- *Morbidity:* 46 vs. 28%; *P* < 0.001 D2 vs. D1.
- *Conclusion:* classical Japanese D2 no survival benefit over D1.
- However, D2 resection without pancreaticosplenectomy may be better than standard D1.
- *Criticism:* trial surgeons on steep learning curve at low volume centres, and difficulty of ensuring patients receive assigned surgery, poor training by videos, poor quality control.

Dutch D1D2 trial: 15-year results 2010

- *1989–1993:* 1078 patients, 996 eligible. 711 randomized (380 D1 group 331 D2). 285 had palliative treatment.
- Prospectively data. Follow-up 15.2 years (range 6.9-17.9 years).
- 174 (25%) alive, all but one without recurrence.
- Overall survival 15 years 21% D1, 29% D2 group (*P* = 0.34).
- *Gastric cancer-related death rate:* significantly higher in the D1 group 48% vs. D2 group 37%.
- Local 22% D1 group vs. 12% D2, and regional recurrence was 19% D1 vs. 13% D2.
- *Operative mortality:* D2 significantly higher 10 vs. 4%.
- *Complication rate:* 43 vs. 25%, D2 vs. D1.
- *Reoperation rate:* 18 vs. 8%, D2 vs. D1.
- 20% of D2 group with N2 nodes were still alive at 11 years; this was unlikely to have been the case if D1 alone performed.
- *Overall D2:* lower locoregional recurrence and gastric cancer-related death rates. D2 has significantly higher post-operative mortality, morbidity, and reoperation rates. Spleen-preserving D2 resection recommended for resectable gastric cancer.
- Smaller series from specialized European centres have shown equivalent results to Far East operative mortality <5% and corresponding survival.
- Uptake of radical resections remains poor in West due to relative technical difficulty of achieving nodal clearance due to adiposity and lack of formalized training in systematic lymphadenectomy. In practice, many centres perform inadequate D2, despite intent leading to results equivalent to D1 and claim of futility of D2.
- Practice likely to change as training increasingly centralized at high volume centres with lower operative mortality and lower failure to recue rates due to astute management of complications.
- Future trend towards lymphadenectomy tailored to individual preoperative and operative staging, age, and fitness.

Western radical: AUGIS/BSG/BASO guidelines 2011

Staging

TNM criteria Minimum 15 LN resected and examined histologically.

EGC

- Not suitable for endoscopic resection—proximal or distal partial resection + limited lymphadenectomy.
- *Japanese data:*
  - Mucosal disease—N1 tier LN + left gastric (station 7) and anterior hepatic nodes (station 8a) (D1a).
  - Submucosal—N1 tier with left gastric, anterior hepatic and coeliac axis nodes (station 9) (D1b) for submucosal.

Distal (antral) tumours

- Should be treated by subtotal gastrectomy with oncological adequacy whilst maintaining HRQL.
- Limited gastric resections only for palliation or in very elderly.
- Distal pancreas and spleen should not be resected for a cancer in distal 2/3 of stomach.

Proximal tumours

- *Cardia, subcardia, some type II GOJ:* extended total gastrectomy.
- *Oroesophagogastrectomy:* if adequate proximal margin compromised:
  - Transhiatal vs. left thoraco-abdominal extended total gastrectomy.
  - Sasako RCT 2006.
  - TH—5-year overall survival 52.3% (95% CI 40.4–64.1).
  - Left thoraco-abdominal oesophagectomy (LTA)—37.9% (26.1–49.6) hazard ratio of death for LTA compared with TH was 1.36 (0.89–2.08, p = 0.92) increased morbidity due to thoracotomy. TH also better HRQL.
- *Overall aim:* adequate local clearance, appropriate lymphadenectomy and an uncomplicated anastomosis with low morbidity.
- *Ex vivo* proximal margin of >3.8cm of normal oesophagus (5cm in vivo) associated with minimal risk of anastomotic recurrence and independent predictor of survival.
- Intraoperative frozen section suggested as standard.
- *Lymphadenectomy:* formal D2 and posterior mediastinal, peri-oesophageal nodes.
- *Splenic and hilar node resection:* should only be considered in patients with tumours of proximal stomach located on greater curvature/ posterior wall of stomach close to splenic hilum where incidence of splenic hilar nodal involvement is likely to be high.

D1 vs. D2

- Extent of lymphadenectomy should be tailored to age and fitness of patient together with location and stage of the cancer.
- Long-term *Dutch (Songun (2010))* and Japanese *(Sasako (2008)* and *Yonemura (2008))* data: significant proportion of patients with N2 disease survive for >5 years after a D2 resection. Unlikely that they would survive as long after lesser lymphadenectomy. D2 recommended as standard of care for stage II and III cancer in fit patients.

Extended lymphadenectomy
- No advantage D3 vs. D2, but D3 vs. D1 improved overall survival (Wu 2006).
- *D2 + para-aortic lymphadenectomy (PAND) for advanced cancer:* two multicenter randomized trials in Japan comparing D2 with D4 (Sasako 2008; Yonemura 2008).
- *D4 resection:* no improved survival, but increased surgery related complications—20.9 vs. 28.1%.

Laparoscopic resection of gastric cancer
- Totally laparoscopic or laparoscopic-assisted safe in trials.
- Oncological equivalence of D2 lymphadenectomy achievable.
- Most published studies from Asia with T1 or T2 cancers.
- Open vs. laparoscopic-assisted distal gastrectomy (LADG) Memon meta-analysis 2008—few suitable RCTs with small sample sizes and limited follow-up.
- Reduced blood loss, longer operating time and reduced nodal yield in LADG, trend to faster post-operative recovery and discharge after LADG.
- *Kim (2008):* randomized trial of laparoscopy-assisted or open distal gastrectomy in EGC, HRQL advantages to minimal access surgery.

HRQL
- Lack of multicenter randomized trials in gastric cancer with comprehensive patient-completed assessments of HRQL.
- *Avery (2010):* D1 vs. D3 lymphadenectomy, nurse administered questionnaires—similar HRQL.
- Risk of observer bias in trials high—non-blinded observers, patients self-assessment preferable.
- Prospective patient reported outcomes evaluating impact of gastrectomy on HRQL show there is marked HRQL deterioration after surgery, and total gastrectomy has greater long-term HRQL deficit than subtotal surgery.

Reprinted by permission from Macmillan Publishers Ltd: 'Guide-lines for the management of oesophageal and gastric cancer', Allum WH, Blazeby JM, Griffin SM, et al.; Association of Upper Gastrointestinal Surgeons of Great Britain and Ireland, the British Society of Gastroenterology and the British Association of Surgical Oncology. Gut 2011 Nov; 60(11): 1449–72.

Other historic controversies

Total gastrectomy 'de principle'
- During the 1970s, enthusiasts in West suggested concept of total gastrectomy as appropriate radical surgical management of gastric cancer—total gastrectomy 'de principle'.
- They argued there was less risk of positive proximal resection margin, that gastric cancer is multicentric disease, with gastric mucosal field change, and with subtotal gastrectomy there was inadequate lymphadenectomy (miss left cardia group).
- In Japan, however, total gastrectomy was only carried out when required to allow R0 resection to be achieved, whilst subtotal gastrectomy was carried out for many antral tumours with satisfactory results.

- Several RCTs were subsequently carried out, including French and Italian studies, which showed no difference in post-operative morbidity or mortality, or difference in 5-year survival. Indeed, some showed that 5-year survival after subtotal was better than after total gastrectomy.
- Theoretically, oncological gain provide by total over subtotal gastrectomy lies in reduction in risk of positive resection margins, removal of missed second primaries and increased extent of lymphatic clearance.
- Extent of nodal dissection is increased with dissection of left cardiac, short gastric, splenic hilum, and distal splenic artery nodes.
- Pattern of lymphatic spread in antral cancers would indicate that removal of these node groups unlikely to improve outcome (5% involved and, if positive, poor prognostic sign).
- Issue of positive margins mainly due to inaccurate diagnosis of proximal extent of tumours.

Operative technique: staging laparoscopy

Indication

Staging laparoscopy is an important part of the staging process for advanced gastric cancer (T2 disease or greater) due to gastric cancer's propensity for peritoneal seeding with individual nodules below the size resolution of CT currently.

- Allows direct visualization of tumour, peritoneal cavity, assessment of tumour bulk, fixity, and longitudinal extension into contiguous structures (Fig. 9.7). Opportunity for peritoneal lavage and cytology.
- Often combined with on-table OGD for surgeon to re-evaluate proximal and distal extent of tumour.
- Affords trial of anaesthesia and anaesthetic assessment prior to major resection, which can highlight further preoperative investigations that maybe required, and facilitate additional patient information with regard to risks of major surgery.

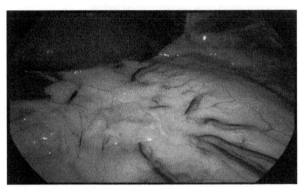

Fig. 9.7 Staging laparoscopy: direct visualization of stomach and associated viscera.

Pre-operative

Satisfactory clinical evaluation, counselling, MDT discussion, informed consent.

Procedure

- GA, supine, hair removal.
- *Ports variable:*
  - Trans- or peri-umbilical under direct vision (11mm).
  - Left flank, upper abdomen (5mm).
  - Right flank, upper abdomen (5mm) or single sub-xiphisternal (5mm).
- Standard 12mmHgCO_2 insufflation to establish pneumoperitoneum.
- *30-degree laparoscope:* atraumatic graspers, e.g. Johan.

- Formal laparoscopy surveying the peritoneal surfaces, liver, small bowel, colon, omentum, and pelvic organs with biopsy of any suspicious tissue.
- Reverse Trendelenberg, and formal assessment of stomach and tumour looking specifically for signs of serosal disease, fixity, and general signs of irresectability.
- Sub-xiphisternal port/retractor assists retraction of left lobe of liver to carefully inspect area of GOJ/lesser curve/omentum.
- If serosal disease or ascites visualized, aspiration of ascitic fluid or peritoneal washings can be performed for cytological evaluation.
- Review OGD.

Complications
Bleeding, infection, wound complications, inadvertent visceral injury, thrombo-embolism, shoulder tip pain.

Immediate post-operative period
- Routine ward observations.
- Surgical/specialist nurse review to outline findings.
- Prophylactic LMWH prior to day case discharge.

Future
- Await histology/cytology if biopsies or peritoneal washings taken.
- Further discussion at MDT. Preliminary discussion with patient.
- Referral for consideration of perioperative chemotherapy.

Operative technique: D2 total gastrectomy

Indication
Gastrectomy is rarely indicated for benign disease of the stomach these days. For proximally advanced tumours or large tumours a total gastrectomy is performed. For distally-located tumours that don't involve the proximal 1/3 of the stomach a subtotal gastrectomy is preferred.

Principles
Complete resection of the stomach with at least a 5-cm resection margin and lymphadenectomy stations 1–7, 8a, 9–12.

Pre-operative
Subject to a satisfactory clinical evaluation, counselling, MDT discussion, and informed consent.

Procedure
- GA with epidural, hair removal, abdomen prepped with povodine iodine, and draped. Antibiotic prophylaxis.
- *Incision:* rooftop ± mercedes (cranial) extension or upper-midline.
- It is now commonplace that majority of dissection is performed with harmonic scalpel.
- formal laparotomy to ensure resectability.
- Two folded swabs may be placed behind spleen in attempt to prevent capsular avulsion.
- It is the author's preference to start by dividing lesser omentum close to liver and perform hiatal dissection by dividing adipose tissue and thick nerve structures on crura surrounding oesophagus and reduce any HH to confirm resectability.
- Complete omentectomy with resection of anterior leaf of mesocolon is performed. This can be difficult when approaching pancreas.
- Dissection on duodenal side is continued until accessory right colic vein is identified and followed proximally where it joins with right gastroepiploic vein forming Henlé's surgical trunk, which flows into superior mesenteric vein.
- Right gastroepiploic vein, once identified, is ligated and divided at its origin.
- Plane of dissection now changes to anterior surface of pancreas.
- Several vessels coming from behind pancreas towards anterior leaf of mesocolon controlled at inferior border of pancreas.
- Capsule of pancreas now dissected from parenchyma until gastroduodenal artery is recognized.
- By following this artery, origin of right gastroepiploic artery is found.
- Following ligation and division of this artery, stomach is then lifted up to divide back surface of proximal duodenum from pancreas and gastroduodenal artery is followed cranially until bifurcation of the common hepatic artery is recognized. Common hepatic artery can be slung to aid nodal clearance at stations 5 and 8a.
- Stomach then returned to normal position and continued division of lesser omentum near lateral segment of liver ensues. Lesser omentum now divided from left edge of hepatoduodenal ligament to oesophageal hiatus (Fig. 9.8).

- This resection line is extended on hepatoduodenal ligament to left side of common bile duct where line is turned caudally towards duodenum.
- Supra-duodenal vessels (usually numbering 3 or 4) are controlled close to duodenal wall.
- This creates window above duodenum, through which gastroduodenal artery can clearly be seen.
- Connective tissue containing lymph nodes in hepatoduodenal ligament, left of common bile duct, is dissected from right to left, from duodenum towards liver hilum along gastroduodenal then hepatic artery.
- Right gastric artery will now be clearly visible, and can be ligated and divided at its base.
- At this point, duodenum is divided with linear stapler, a couple of centimetres from pylorus and over-sewn.
- With assistance, stomach is now distracted right to left and/or cranially, supra-pancreatic, common hepatic, coeliac, left gastric, and splenic artery nodes are dissected starting from nodal tissue on left side of portal vein, moving towards nodal tissue around splenic artery.
- Downward pancreatic traction by assistant useful at this point.
- During this dissection, left gastric vein and artery are encountered. They should be carefully found, ligated, and dived near origins.
- Hiatal and splenic artery nodal dissection can now be completed. Care should be made to identify, haemostase/ligate, and divide posterior gastric artery. During this procedure, remaining short gastric vessels should also be haemostased/ligated and divided.
- Both vagal nerves are divided 2–3cm proximal to cardia and once a sufficient length of intra-abdominal oesophagus has been revealed it can be transected below 3-stay sutures and specimen removed for histological examination.

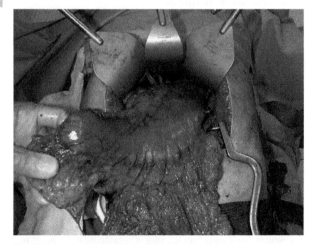

Fig. 9.8 Intraoperative image during D2 total gastrectomy.

Reconstruction

There are several methods of restoring intestinal continuity post-total gastrectomy. Simplest and most commonly used is Roux-en-Y reconstruction (Fig. 9.9):

- Convenient loop of proximal jejunum is prepared. Care should be taken to ensure apex will reach transected oesophagus.
- Mesentry then divided vertically with ligation and division of traversing vessels and jejunum divided with further firing of linear stapler.
- Biliary limb over-sewn.
- Incision made in transverse mesocolon, taking care to avoid colic vessels and alimentary limb of jejunum led up in retrocolic fashion.
- Hand-sewn or stapled end-to-side oesophagojejunal anastomosis then fashioned.
- It is the author's preference to perform a stapled anastomosis.
- Oesophagealprolene purse-string is performed and tightened around anvil of circular stapler. Previously created jejunal staple line is excised and main body of circular stapling device inserted 4–5cm into jejunum.
- Once gun has been fired, open jejunum is closed (either with linear stapler and over-sewn, or sutures) and four buttress sutures inserted to reinforce anastomosis.
- 30–40cm distal to oesophagojejunal anastomosis, a side-to-side jejuno-jejunal anastomosis is created between biliary and alimentary limbs.
- *Drains*: if used, tube drain left in sub-hepatic space (duodenal stump) and led up to oesophagojejunal anastomosis.
- A NJ tube is left on free drainage distal to oesophagojejunal anastomosis, which may be secured with septal bridle.
- *Closure*: two-layer PDS and skin clips.

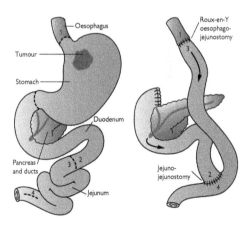

Fig. 9.9 (a) Total gastrectomy. (b) Roux-en-Y oesophagojejunostomy.
Reproduced from *Emergencies in Clinical Surgery*, eds. Chris Callaghan, J. Andrew Bradley, Christopher Watson, copyright 2008 with permission of Oxford University Press.

Complications

Complications include bleeding, infection, wound complications, chest complications (atelectasis/pneumonia), cardiovascular complications, venous thromboembolism, anastomotic leak, and duodenal stump leak.

Immediate post-operative period

- Extubation/HDU.
- Post-operative doses of antibiotics.
- Intensive physiotherapy. Early mobilization.
- Nil by mouth (NBM) for 3 days. Then incremental oral intake.
- Judicious fluid management.
- Prophylactic LMWH.
- Contrast swallow at day 5 if favoured.

Future

- Careful clinical follow-up.
- Referral for consideration of adjuvant chemotherapy.

Operative technique: D2 sub-total gastrectomy

Indication

For distally located tumours that do not involve the proximal 1/3 of the stomach, a subtotal gastrectomy is preferred (Fig. 9.10). Many of the steps are common to both total and subtotal gastrectomy.

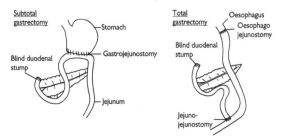

Fig 9.10 (a) Subtotal gastrectomy. (b) Roux-en-Y gastrojejunostomy.
Adapted from *Handbook of Surgical Consent*, eds. Rajesh Nair, David J. Holroyd, copyright 2011 with permission from Oxford University Press.

Pre-operative

Subject to satisfactory clinical evaluation, counselling, MDT discussion, and informed consent.

Procedure

- GA with epidural, supine with arms out to facilitate omnitract, hair removal, abdomen prepped with povodine iodine (betadine) and draped. Antibiotic prophylaxis.
- *Incision:* extended right subcostal or rooftop or upper midline.
- Now commonplace that majority of dissection is performed with harmonic scalpel.
- Formal laparotomy to ensure resectability.
- Two-folded swabs may be placed behind spleen in attempt to prevent capsular avulsion.
- Extensive mobilization of duodenum and head of pancreas should be performed to allow visualization and palpation of para-aortic area.
- If suspicious non-regional lymph nodes encountered (∴ potential M1 disease) should be sampled and sent for frozen section. If negative, subtotal gastrectomy begins.
- Complete omentectomy with resection of anterior leaf of mesocolon performed.
- Dissection on duodenal side is continued until accessory right colic vein is identified and followed proximally where it joins with right gastroepiploic vein forming Henlé's surgical trunk, which flows into superior mesenteric vein.

- Right gastroepiploic vein, once identified, is ligated and divided at its origin.
- Plane of dissection now changes to anterior surface of pancreas.
- Several vessels coming from behind pancreas towards anterior leaf of mesocolon should be haemostased or ligated, and divided at inferior border of pancreas.
- Capsule of pancreas is now dissected from parenchyma until gastroduodenal artery recognized.
- By following this artery, origin of right gastroepiploic artery is found.
- Following ligation and division of this artery, stomach is then lifted up to divide back surface of proximal duodenum from pancreas and gastroduodenal artery is followed cranially until bifurcation of common hepatic artery is recognized.
- Stomach then returned to neutral position and lesser omentum is divided near lateral segment of liver from left edge of hepatoduodenal ligament to oesophageal hiatus.
- Resection line extended on hepatoduodenal ligament to left side of common bile duct where line turned caudally towards duodenum.
- Supra-duodenal vessels (usually numbering 3 or 4) controlled close to duodenal wall.
- Creates window above duodenum through which gastroduodenal artery can clearly be seen.
- Connective tissue containing lymph nodes in hepatoduodenal ligament, left of common bile duct, is dissected from right to left, from duodenum towards liver hilum along gastroduodenal then hepatic artery.
- Right gastric artery will now be clearly visible, and can be ligated and divided at its base.
- At this point duodenum is divided with linear stapler a couple of centimetres from pylorus and over-sewn.
- With assistance, stomach is now distracted right to left and/or cranially, supra-pancreatic, common hepatic, coeliac, left gastric, and proximal splenic artery nodes are dissected starting from nodal tissue on left side of portal vein and moving towards nodal tissue around splenic artery.
- Downward pancreatic traction by assistant is useful at this point.
- During this dissection, left gastric vein and artery are encountered and should be carefully found, ligated, and dived near their origins.
- Remaining short gastric vessels and tissue of the lesser curve are haemostased/ligated and divided to facilitate a minimum of 5cm proximal clearance from palpable edge of tumour.
- Stomach can then be distracted downwards and divided with one or more firings of a linear staple. Distal stomach can then be removed for histological evaluation and staple line is over-sewn.

Reconstruction

The simplest and most commonly used is Roux-en-Y reconstruction:

- Convenient loop of proximal jejunum prepared. Care should be made to ensure apex will reach gastric remnant.
- Mesentery is then divided vertically with ligation and division of traversing vessels and jejunum divided with further firing of linear stapler.
- Biliary and alimentary limbs are over-sewn.
- Incision made in transverse mesocolon, avoiding colic vessels and alimentary limb of jejunum is led up in retrocolic fashion.
- Hand-sewn or stapled posterior end-to-side gastrojejunal anastomosis is then fashioned.
- 30–40cm distal to gastrojejunal anastomosis, side-to-side jejunojejunal anastomosis is created between biliary and alimentary limbs.
- *Drains:* Wallace–Robinson tube drain left in sub-hepatic space (duodenal stump) and led up to gastrojejunal anastomosis if favoured.
- NJ tube is left on free drainage distal to gastrojejunal anastomosis which is secured with septal bridle.

Complications

Complications include bleeding, infection, wound complications, chest complications (atelectasis/pneumonia), cardiovascular complications, venous thromboembolism, anastomotic leak, and duodenal stump leak.

Immediate post-operative period

There is no clear standardized protocol, typical approach may include:

- Extubation/HDU.
- Two post-operative doses of antibiotics.
- Intensive physiotherapy. Early mobilization.
- NBM for 3 days, then incremental oral intake.
- Judicious fluid management.
- Prophylactic LMWH.

Follow-up

- Careful clinical follow-up.
- Referral for consideration of adjuvant chemotherapy.

Operative technique: laparoscopic gastrectomy

The first description was given by Kitano, Korea, in 1994.

Guidance (NICE 2008)

Current safety and efficacy evidence suggests adequate support for the use of this procedure for cancer, providing normal arrangements are in place for clinical governance, consent, and audit.

The procedure is technically demanding. Surgeons performing the procedure should have specific training and special expertise in laparoscopic surgical techniques, and should perform their initial procedures with an experienced mentor.

Patient selection and management should be carried out in the context of a MDT with established experience in the treatment of gastric cancer.

Note: A patient who is 'unfit' for an open procedure does not become 'fit' for a laparoscopic procedure.

Indications

- NICE guidance only extends to adenocarcinoma. For patients whose gastric cancer is diagnosed at a stage that is amenable to surgical treatment, options include open or laparoscopic gastrectomy.
- Initially indicated only for EGC patients with a low risk LN metastasis.
- *The Japanese Gastric Cancer Association guidelines 2004:* EMR or ESD for stage Ia (cT1N0M0) diagnosis; patients with stage Ib (cT1N1M0 and cT2N0M0) referred for LG.
- *Western patients relatively obese:*
  - Increased risk of bleeding if lymphadenectomy performed.
  - *Technically difficult operations than normal weight*—reduced visibility, difficulty retracting tissues, dissection plane hindered by adipose tissue, and difficulty with anastomosis.
  - *Open gastrectomy*—obesity not a risk factor for survival of patients with gastric cancer, although it is independently predictive of post-operative complications.
- *Noshiro et al. (2005):* LG for obese patients results in longer operative times, delayed recovery of bowel activity, and greater rate of extension of mini-laparotomy incision or conversion to laparotomy.
- Careful approach needed, especially for male patients with high BMI.

Principles

The same principles that govern open surgery should be applied to laparoscopic surgery:

- *Commonly five operative ports are used:* one 10–12-mm port peri-umbilically, three 10–12-mm ports in the right and left flank, and wide left flank, with further 5-mm port at epigastric level. Positions and sizes are open to local preference (Fig. 9.11).

- The series of steps described in open gastrectomy are identical in laparoscopic gastrectomy, except performed through much smaller incisions with specialized laparoscopic equipment. Liver retractor, e.g. Nathanson's, gastric retraction maintained by combination of elevation with atraumatic graspers, e.g. Johan's, and 'tenting' stomach from lesser sac. Vascular pedicles divided using vascular haemostatic staplers, ligaclips, haemolocks, or laparoscopic ligation.
- *Laparoscopic anastomosis* (Fig. 9.12):
  - *Total gastrectomy*—Orvill anvil useful (introduced orally).
  - *Partial gastrectomy*—laparoscopic linear staplers.
- Larger incision may facilitate a hand being introduced into peritoneal cavity for hand-assisted gastrectomy or laparoscopically-assisted subtotal gastrectomy depending on the site of the tumour.
- Removal of the draining lymph nodes is integral part of procedure.
- Slightly larger incision may be required in order to remove diseased stomach (through wound protector), but location of this can be cosmetic and less likely to cause pain/respiratory complications.
- Laparoscopic pylorus preserving gastrectomy advocated in Korea and Japan for early tumours with minimal risk of station 5 LN metastasis i.e. minimally 6cm from pylorus.

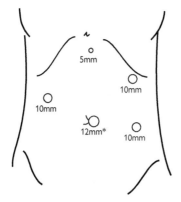

Fig. 9.11 Trocar placement for totally laparoscopic gastrectomy (*extended to 3.5cm long when retrieving specimen).

Reproduced from 'Laparoscopic distal gastrectomy with regional lymph node dissection for gastric cancer', Tanimura, S. *Surgical Endoscopy*, Sep; **19**(9): 1177–81, copyright 2005 with kind permission of Springer Science and Business Media.

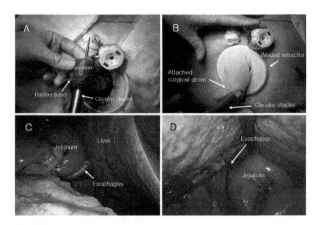

Fig. 9.12 Laparoscopic oesophagojejunal anastomosis. (a) Circular stapler is inserted into jejunum, which is tied with rubber band to prevent slippage of jejunum from circular stapler. (b) Circular stapler is introduced into abdomen, sealing off laparotomy wound with attached surgical glove. (c) After pneumoperitoneum is established, double-stapling oesophagojejunostomy is performed under direct laparoscopic view. (d) After completion of anastomosis, jejunal stump is closed with an endoscopic linear stapler.
Figure 5 from ♪ http://www.springerimages.com/Images/MedicineAndPublicHealth/1-10.1007_s00464-009-0461-z-4

Efficacy

- Multicentre case series have reported 5-year disease-free survival rates for early gastric cancer treated with laparoscopic gastrectomy as 99.8, 98.7, and 85.7% for stage IA, IB, and II, respectively.
- *Advanced disease:* 5-year overall survival 59% and DFS 57%.
- *Conversion from laparoscopic to open surgery:* 2–3% reasons include anatomical constraints, bleeding, and mechanical problems.
- Early results suggested lower lymph node harvest, particularly in laparoscopic subtotal gastrectomy group compared with open surgery.
- Key efficacy outcomes include 30-day mortality, cancer-free survival rates, adequate surgical margins, and number of lymph nodes removed.
- *Adachi (2000) comparative study of LG vs. OG:* laparoscopy-assisted distal gastrectomy (LADG) for EGC: reduced surgical trauma, improved nutrition, reduced post-operative pain, rapid return of GI function, shorter hospital stays, and no reduction in curability.
- *Usui (2005):* laparoscopy-assisted total gastrectomy (LATG) vs. conventional open total gastrectomy (OTG). LATG successful in 20 patients, operating time equal, reduced blood loss in LATG vs. OTG time to ambulatory status, first flatus, and first oral intake significantly shorter in LATG group, as was the length of the post-operative hospital stay. The frequency of analgesics given in LATG group was lower than that in OTG group.

- *KLASS trial (Korea):* phase III multicentre prospective RCT. LADG vs. ODG: 342 patients randomized (LADG, 179 patients; ODG, 161 patients) 2006–2007, no significant differences age (20–80) gender, and comorbidities.
  - *Post-operative complications*—LADG and ODG groups were 10.5% (17/179) and 14.7% (24/163).
  - *Reoperations*—three cases each group.
  - *Post-operative mortality*—1.1% (2/179) and 0% (0/163) in LADG and ODG groups ($P = 0.497$).
  - Currently recruiting further patients.

Safety

- Meta-analysis have shown fewer complications overall following laparoscopic subtotal gastrectomy compared with open gastrectomy. However, there was no difference between groups with respect to mortality, anastomotic leak, stricture, or wound infection.
- Pulmonary complications were surprisingly non-significantly higher in the open gastrectomy group.
- Post-operative ileus was significantly reduced following laparoscopic gastric resection.

Complications of gastric surgery

Major oesophagogastric surgery has inherent risks and complications. In the UK, following the Clinical Outcomes Group (COG) guidance, it was recommended that oesophagogastric cancer services were centralized to regional units, where high volumes of cases were dealt with by experts, both to improve outcomes and manage complications.

- Expected mortality/major morbidity should be <5% and 5–10%, respectively; however, we should continually strive to reduce these rates further.
- *'Failure to rescue' is a significant cause of mortality:* critical complications are recognized early and managed proactively.
- Overt signs of sepsis, failure to progress as expected, or subtle signs, such as new onset cardiac arrhythmias should heighten suspicion of complication and require investigation in first instance with contrast-enhanced CT (with oral contrast).

Early complications

- *Haemorrhage:* managed by surgery, supportive care, or radiological embolization.
- *Duodenal stump leak:* usually due to technical error, distal obstruction, or ischaemia. *Aim of management*—create a controlled fistula.
  - *Early leak*—surgical re-exploration.
  - *Delayed leak*—in absence of overwhelming sepsis, possible to manage non-operatively; adequate drainage with existing drains or radiologically-guided percutaneous drains.
  - Contrast study should be considered via drain to ensure no distal obstruction at BP limb anastomosis.
  - Gentle suction can be applied to drain.
  - TPN is often not necessary but should be considered, as a minimum an elemental diet should be recommended. Somatostatin analogues (octreotide) and high dose PPI may suppress residual acid and pancreaticobiliary secretions.
  - As drainage volumes reduce, drain can slowly be retracted. Again, if output remains > 200mL/24h a technical problem should be sought with further contrast studies.
- *Anastomotic leak:* usually a consequence of technical error, ischaemia, or tension. Recommended that drains are left next to high-risk anastomoses.
  - *Early leaks*—if apparent within 72h of surgery, surgical re-exploration is warranted with either taking down of anastomosis, 1° repair if feasible (but often futile) or creation of controlled fistula with, in all cases, washout, drainage, and insertion of feeding jejunostomy.
  - *Delayed leaks*—decision lies between radiological drainage vs. surgical re-exploration. If, on contrast study and patient not unwell, can be managed conservatively with either distal feeding or TPN, and serial contrast studies to ensure resolution.

- *Intra-abdominal sepsis:* if occurs within 2 weeks of surgery, usually a result of complication from anastomosis, duodenal stump, or pancreatitis. Again, management revolves around surgical vs. radiological drainage in conjunction with antibiotics and attention to nutrition.
- *Pancreatic fistula:* if it is felt at time of surgery that injury to pancreatic tail could have occurred, surgical drain should be left.
  - *If controlled*—commence a somatostatin analogue (octreotide) and allow to close spontaneously.
  - *If uncontrolled*—surgical drainage and debridement of necrotic pancreatic tissue in conjunction with somatostatin analogue.
- Post-splenectomy infections:
  - *If planned*—preoperative vaccines (H. influenza, meningococcal and pneumococcal vaccines). Consult local haematological policy with regard to long-term penicillin V. Subsequent annual influenza and 2–3-yearly Pneumovax®II.
  - *If unplanned*—triple vaccines should be given on recovery from surgery after 2 weeks.

Late complications
Close multidisciplinary follow-up with surgeons, specialist nurse, and dieticians is crucial following oesophagogastric surgery to optimize both physical and psychological QoL.

Side effects and post-prandial sequelae
Early satiety

Caused due to loss of reservoir function of the stomach. It is important to obtain good early dietary advice and limit meal size. Early dumping can result. There is a defect of normal peristalsis in the long jejunal limb resulting in voluntary and involuntary regurgitation.

Early dumping
- Results from rapid filling of proximal small intestine with hypertonic food leading to rapid movement of fluid into gut from extracellular space resulting in diarrhoea.
- Can lead to food avoidance with reduced QoL and malnutrition. More troublesome following subtotal gastrectomy or where pylorus is destroyed or bypassed.
- Patients who have undergone total gastrectomy are more 'fortunate' as they cannot tolerate a large load.
- Dietician should be involved at early stage and patients encouraged to complete a dietary record along with symptoms experienced.

Reactive hypoglycaemic attacks
- Complex neurohumoral response produces unpleasant GI and cardiovascular symptoms.
- Hypoglycaemic attacks, blackouts, and seizures 2h following meal.
- Dietetic input crucial. Involves reducing amount of carbohydrate in main meals with regular glucose in-between (glucose tablets).

Diarrhoea

Causes include truncal vagotomy, early dumping, and bacterial overgrowth.

- Due to combination of loss of gastric acid and formation of blind loops resulting in accumulation of aerobic and anaerobic organisms only normally found in colon.
- Faecal bacteria release toxins that destroy brush borders vital to digestion and consume B vitamins. They deconjugate bile acids, which are essential for normal fat absorption in proximal small intestine, increasing faecal fats, resulting in steatorrhoea and weight loss.
- Investigation involves ^{14}C glycoholate breath test.
- *Treatment:* metronidazole/neomycin and probiotics (fresh unpasteurized yoghurt, to inhibit recolonization with and after antibiotics).

Steatorrhoea

- Relative pancreatic insufficiency results in fat malabsorption, large bowel colic, flatus and greasy stools.
- Once bacterial overgrowth is excluded, treatment commences with pancreatic enzyme supplementation (Creon®).

Bile reflux (alkaline)

- *Symptoms:* epigastric discomfort, heartburn, and vomiting. Persistent reflux can lead to structuring and dysphagia.
- *Investigation:* OGD and Tech ^{99}M HIDA scanning. Bilitec®.
- Treatment options limited, but can include revisional surgery if symptoms are unremitting (change reconstruction/lengthening of Roux loop).

Nutritional problems

General

- Malabsorption is a rare cause of malnutrition.
- Usually, due to failure to ingest sufficient calories (especially in case of total gastrectomy patients).
- Carbohydrate absorption is usually satisfactory, protein and particularly fat absorption is reduced resulting in weight loss.
- Bacterial overgrowth, early satiety, dumping, and relative pancreatic insufficiency should be excluded then close dietetic follow-up should ensue.

Vitamins and minerals

- *Vitamin B12:*
  - Virtually no absorption of B12 post-gastrectomy.
  - B12 is bound to intrinsic factor in stomach and absorbed via terminal ileum.
  - All gastrectomy patients require 3-monthly hydroxocobalamin injections.
  - Methyl-methionine testing is more accurate than B12 in presence of PPI use.
- *Other B vitamins:* frequently consumed with bacterial overgrowth and, ∴ patients should be supplemented with vitamin B during and after treatment.

- *Vitamin D:* malabsorption of vitamin D results in osteomalacia, especially in post-menopausal women. All patients >70 years should receive calcium supplements and undergo 5-yearly assessments for metabolic bone disease.

Iron (Fe^{2+}): iron malabsorption not normally an issue unless vegetarian or vegan, as small intestine takes over absorption. Iron and vitamin C supplements should be considered for first post-operative year.

Follow-up and surveillance

As mentioned previously, following gastrectomy, close clinical follow-up with surgeons, cancer nurse specialists and dieticians is mandatory to ensure physical and psychological QoL.

- No quality evidence to suggest optimal follow-up regime.
- Follow-up frequently combined between surgeons and oncologists.
- One approach is to routinely review with clinical and haematological testing 8 weeks post-discharge, then 3-monthly for the first year, 6-monthly thereafter for 5 years in total then discharge at that time if satisfactory.
- Large degree of flexibility built into any follow-up regimes should specific problems arise.
- Patients and 1° care physicians may be given direct telephone access via cancer nurse specialists should specific problems or queries arise. Similar pathway exists to access dietetic service.
- Imaging (CT) and endoscopy reserved for time when clinically warranted as symptoms dictate.

Adjuvant chemoradiotherapy

- The US Intergroup 0116 trial (MacDonald) randomized 556 patients to surgery followed by chemoradiotherapy (radiotherapy 45Gy in 25 fractions for 5 weeks plus bolus FU/leucovorin before, during, and after radiotherapy to stomach and nodal bed + 2-cm margins to proximal and distal resection margins, kidney also included in field) or surgery alone.
- 71% male, 94% WHO performances score 0 or 1, 31% T1 or T2, 62% T3, 84% had nodal involvement.
- Only 46% D1 or D2 dissections.
- Significant benefit in both median overall survival (36 vs. 27 months; $P = 0.005$) and local control rates (30 vs. 19 months; $P < 0.001$) reported.
- Post-operative chemoradiation standard of care in USA.
- Longer-term (>11 years) follow-up, both overall survival and DFS benefit maintained (overall survival, 35 vs. 27 months, $P = 0.005$; DFS, 27 vs. 19 months, $P < 0.001$).
- *UK and Europe:* less enthusiasm.
- *Toxicity abdominal chemoradiotherapy:* nausea and vomiting, myelosuppression including neutropenia, fatigue, mucositis, and diarrhoea. 54% of patients had grade 3 or 4 haematologic toxicity and 33% had grade 3 or 4 GI toxicity. Three patients (1%) died of toxic effects of treatment. (*Note:* DXT planning much improved since INT0116 and capecitabine now used).
- Uncertain benefit post-'optimum' surgery.
- *Considered in patients at high risk of recurrence:* no neoadjuvant therapy and/or suboptimal surgery, e.g. in emergency context.
- The UK (MAGIC) strategy of perioperative chemotherapy was adopted by Europe and is now also recommended option in NCCN guidelines.
- Post-operative chemoradiotherapy remains option for selected patients after an R0 resection and is recommended in USA for all patients with positive resection margins.

Adjuvant chemotherapy

- Several meta-analyses suggest small survival benefit for adjuvant chemotherapy.
- Considerable variation between treatment regimens used and outcomes between Western and Asian populations.
- Japanese ACTS-GC (Adjuvant Chemotherapy Trial of TS-1 for Gastric Cancer) trial: significant benefit in overall survival: 12 months of S-1 (an oral fluoropyrimidine) monotherapy vs. observation post-curative D2 gastrectomy (3 year overall survival of 80.1% vs. 70.1%; $P - 0.0024$).
- Applicability to Western population uncertain.
- Adjuvant chemotherapy alone may confer a survival benefit and should be considered in patients at high risk of recurrence who have not received neoadjuvant therapy.

Nutrition during chemotherapy and radiotherapy

- Chemotherapy and radiotherapy side effects including: dysphagia, mucositis, sore mouth, nausea, and diarrhoea can impinge on appetite and dietary intake.
- *Dietician review essential:* aim to maintain weight and nutritional status to reduce effect of malignancy and therapy.
- Prolonged oral supplementation or retention of feeding adjuncts, such as jejunostomy tubes vital. Evidence of improved HRQL-related to weekly dietetic input.
- Prolonged benefit in adjuvant setting for colorectal patients receiving chemoradiation.
- Consider removable stents (e.g. polyflex) in patients with persistent dysphagia.

Palliative chemotherapy in gastric cancer

- Gastric cancer commonly presents with locally advanced or metastatic disease. In many patients, curative surgery not an option. In 2010, the UK national audit found that only 34% of newly-diagnosed patients have curative treatment plan.
- Without surgery all treatment is palliative, directed at improving quality and duration of life.
- *Early clinical trials:* patients with WHO performance score of 0, 1, or 2 combination chemotherapy—increased median survival, from 3–9 months, and improved QoL, compared with best supportive care alone.
- Response rates for combination chemotherapy regimens are between 40 and 50%.
- Up to 15% of gastric cancers over-express the HER2 receptor. All tumours in medically fit patients should be assessed for HER2 status and, if positive, should be offered trastuzumab in combination with chemotherapy.
- ECF became standard palliative chemotherapy in the UK after the publication in 1997 of Cunningham's paper comparing it with FAMTX. Median survival increased from 5.7 to 8.9 months and QoL was better in ECF arm.
- More recently, REAL 2 trial of 1002 patients demonstrated equivalent efficacy for EOX regime (epirubicin, oxaliplatin and capecitabine) with an improved side effect profile.
- In 2006, van Cutsem published the results of trial comparing TCF to CF (with the addition of docetaxel to cisplatin and FU) showing improved median survival (9.2 vs. 8.6 months) with three-drug regime. This now standard of care in USA.
- Second line chemotherapy after tumour progression of uncertain benefit. RR up to 30% seen with regimens which include irinotecan. Trials of chemotherapy vs. best supportive care in progress.
- Palliative chemotherapy offered alongside best supportive care to patients with locally advanced or metastatic gastric or GOJ cancer if medically fit and with WHO performance score of 2 or better. Combination regimes are more effective, but more toxic than single agents. Second line chemotherapy remains investigational, but irinotecan-containing regimes can be considered.

First line regimes

- *ECF:* epirubicin 50mg/m², cisplatin 60mg/m², infusional FU 200mg/m²/day days 1–21, every 3 weeks.
- *EOX:* epirubicin 50mg/m², oxaliplatin 130mg/m², oral capecitabine 625mg/m² bd days 1–21, every 3 weeks.
- *TCF:* docetaxel 75mg/m², cisplatin 75mg/m², infusional FU 750mg/m²/day days 1–5, every 3 weeks.

Toxicities include nausea and vomiting, neutropenia, cardiac failure, neuropathy, alopecia, diarrhoea, and hand and foot syndrome.

Targeted therapies in gastric cancer

- Approximately 15% of gastric and oesophageal junctional adenocarcinomas over-express human epidermal growth factor receptor-2 (HER2) on the cell membrane.
- HER2 receptor can be targeted by the monoclonal antibody trastuzumab.
- When combined with chemotherapy, this drug can increase response rate over chemotherapy alone and has been used to treat HER2 positive breast cancer for over 10 years.
- HER2 is involved in signalling mechanism for cell proliferation and survival. HER2 is a tyrosine kinase receptor and dimerization of HER2 receptors on the cell surface activates the intracellular signalling cascade.
- Trastuzumab prevents dimerization of the HER2 receptor. The small molecule tyrosine kinase inhibitor, lapatinib, targets intracellular domain of the same receptor.
- In the ToGA trial, published in 2010, 596 patients randomized to receive either chemotherapy alone or a combination of trastuzumab and chemotherapy.
- Increased response rate of 47 vs. 34% in chemotherapy alone arm.
- Median survival in combination arm was 13.8 months compared with 11.9 months with chemotherapy alone.
- Strength of expression of HER2 antigen predicts likelihood of response and when only those tumours, which had a score of 3+ (looking at strength of membrane staining using immunohistochemistry) were included in analysis median survival increased to 16 months.
- Trastuzumab is now recommended for first line treatment of locally advanced or metastatic gastric and gastro-oesophageal cancer, which is HER2 3+ positive.
- Trastuzumab can be cardiotoxic and monitoring of LVEF is recommended. It cannot be used in combination with anthracycline chemotherapy, such as epirubicin, which is also cardiotoxic.

Regime

- Trastuzumab 8mg/m² IV loading dose (given over 90min and monitoring patient carefully for up to 6h for allergic reactions) then 6mg/m² every 3 weeks (over 30min) with IV cisplatin 80mg/ m², with hydration, every 3 weeks and oral capecitabine, either 1000mg/m² bd days 1–14 or 625mg/m² continuously.
- After completing six cycles of chemotherapy trastuzumab is continued as a single agent until disease progression.
- Trials with other targeted agents including bevacizumab and lapatinib are ongoing.

Palliation

- Over 50% of oesophagogastric cancers are inoperable or metastatic at the time of presentation.
- Survival rates from incurable gastric cancer are miserable despite best efforts, with 50% mortality at 6 months and remainder dead within 2 years.
- Palliative resection or bypass has in recent years been superseded by self-expanding metal stents (SEMS; Fig. 9.13) for obstruction (Fig. 9.14), and advances in endoscopic ablative therapies and radiological embolization techniques for haemorrhage, hence reducing need for surgical intervention.

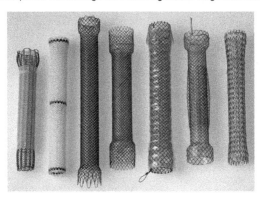

Fig. 9.13 Currently available self-expanding metal and plastic stents (from left to right): Ultraflex (Boston Scientific, Natick, MA, USA); Polyflex (Boston Scientific); Wallflex (Boston Scientific); Evolution (Cook Medical, Limerick, Ireland); SX-Ella esophageal HV (ELLA-CS, s.r.o., Hradec Kralove, Czech Republic); double-layered Niti-S (TaeWoong Medical, Seoul, Korea); and Alimaxx-E (Merit Medical, South Jordan, UT, USA).
Figure 1 from ℬ http://www.springerimages.com/Images/MedicineAndPublicHealth/1-10.1007_978-1-4614-3746-8_13-0

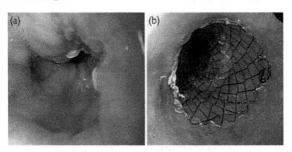

Fig. 9.14 (a) Endoscopic view of extrinsic compression caused by mediastinal lymphadenopathy in the mid-oesophagus. (b) Successfully deployed self-expanding metal stent.
Figure 1 from ℬ http://www.springerimages.com/Images/MedicineAndPublicHealth/1-10.1007_s10620-007-9967-1-0

Self-expanding metal stents

- Median survival <3/12 at insertion.
- Frequently inserted for obstructive issues either radiologically or endoscopically, alone or in conjunction with biliary stenting.
- Despite satisfactory position and confirmation of patency on contrast studies, gastroparesis in diseased stomach can persist and becomes difficult problem to manage.
- Close working with palliative care teams with use of analgesia, prokinetics, and anti-emetics frequently via subcutaneous syringe driver is essential.

Complications (mortality 2%)

Early (0–40%)

- Malposition.
- Incomplete expansion.
- Pain.
- Perforation (5–10%).
- Upper GI bleeding.
- Migration.
- Aspiration pneumonia.

Late (20%)

- Migration.
- Tumour in/overgrowth.
- Food bolus obstruction.
- Reflux.
- Late perforation resulting in fistulation.
- Disintegration.
- Stent torsion.
- Bleeding.
- Continued eating difficulties.

Endoscopic/radiological palliation

- *Endoscopic haemostasis:* APC, diathermy, or clips can be useful in some circumstances of haemorrhage, as can radiological embolization in conjunction with PPI therapy and tranexamic acid.
- For obstructive symptoms, laser recannulation or dilatation is possible.

Surgical palliation

Palliative resection

- Palliative resection has a limited role to play in the modern management of gastric cancer.
- Benefits include prolonging survival, although survival range for R2 resection is 6–24 months and must be weighed up against increased morbidity/mortality associated with surgery.
- Major haemorrhage if not amenable to embolization may warrant resection if massive and life-threatening, but anaemia without overt bleeding can often be treated with repeated transfusion.
- Palliative resection does little to improve other symptoms, e.g. nausea, vomiting, anorexia, or cachexia.

Other palliative surgery

- Conventional palliative option for gastric cancers, which cannot be resected has been gastroenterostomy, but reported outcomes are very poor.
- Median survival is only 3–6 months, operative mortality is around 25% and fewer than half patients having undergone this procedure leave hospital.

Gastrointestinal stromal tumours

- Mesenchymal tumours of the gastrointestinal tract. Those tumours that express true smooth muscle or neural differentiation are excluded from the gastrointestinal stromal tumours (GIST) subgroup, i.e. leiomyomas, neurofibromas.
- Clinical behaviour of GISTs is difficult to predict. 10–30% are malignant. Stomach is the most common site (50–60%). Size <1–20cm.

There are three groups of mesenchymal stomach tumours on immunohistochemistry (see Table 9.1).

- 60% Submucosal, 30% subserosal, 10% intramural.
- Assigned very low/low/intermediate/high risk of malignant potential.
- However, 10% are still unpredictable.

Table 9.1 Categories of mesenchymal gastric tumours based on immunohistochemistry

Leiomyomas	Positive staining for Desmin and Actin Negative staining for CD34
Neurofibroma	Positive staining for S100 Negative staining for other markers
GIST	Positive staining: CD34, CD117, cKIT, DOG 1 Negative for other markers

Sites

- 52% Stomach.
- 25% Small bowel.
- 11% Colon.
- 5% Oesophagus.
- Overall survival best for oesophagus and worst for small bowel. Male > female. Mean age 50–60 years. Increased risk of malignant GIST <40 years of age. All GISTs should be considered to have malignant potential which can be stratified.

Miettinen classification (GIST risk stratification)

See Table 9.2.

- *Overtly metastatic GIST and radical resection:* 18-month median survival.
- *Prognostic features:* site, size, mitotic rate.

Table 9.2 GIST risk stratification by tumour size and mitotic rate

Tumour parameters		% Patients with progressive disease during long-term follow-up			
Size	Mitotic rate	Gastric (n = 1055)	Jejunal/ileal (n = 629)	Duodenal (n = 144)	Rectal (n = 111)
≤2cm	≤5/50 HPFs	0 None	0 None	0 None	0 None
>2cm, ≤5cm	≤5/50 HPFs	1.9% V. low	4.3% Low	8.3% Low	8.5% Low
>5cm, ≤10cm	≤5/50 HPFs	3.6% Low	24% Moderate	34%* High	57%*† High
>10cm	≤5/50 HPFs	12% Moderate	52% High		
≤2cm	>5/50 HPFs	0†	50%†		54% High
>2cm, ≤5cm	>5/50 HPFs	16% Moderate	73% High	50% High	52% High
>5cm, ≤10cm	>5/50 HPFs	55% High	85% High	86%* High	71%* High
>10cm	>5/50 HPFs	86% High	90% High		

HPFs, high powered fields.

* Combined data due to small patient numbers.

† Calculated using small patient numbers.

Reproduced from 'Gastrointestinal stromal tumors: pathology and prognosis at different sites', Miettinen M, Lasota J, *Semin. Diagn. Pathol.*, **23**: 70–83, copyright 2006 with permission of Elsevier.

Presenting features
- 60% Symptomatic, 40% asymptomatic.
- GI bleed (70%).
- Abdominal pain.
- Bowel obstruction.
- Weight loss.
- Abdominal mass.

Investigation
- Endoscopy (proximal and distal GISTs).
- *EUS and fine needle aspiration (FNA):* (Fig. 9.15) cytology and immunohistochemistry.
- *Staging CT:* (Fig. 9.16) no percutaneous biopsy.
- Staging laparoscopy and review OGD (if deemed resectable).
- *?Magnetic resonance imaging (MRI)/selective mesenteric angiogram:* acute GI bleed.

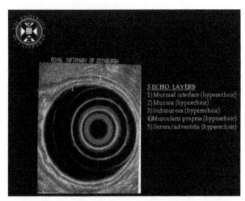

Fig. 9.15 Labelled view at endoscopic ultrasound. Echo layers: (1) mucosal interface (hyperechoic); (2) mucosa (hypoechoic); (3) submucoa (hyperechoic); (4) muscularis proposa (hypoechoic); (5) serosa/adventitia (hyperechoic).

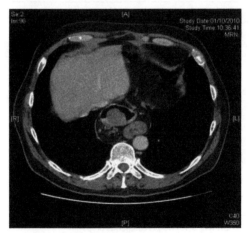

Fig. 9.16 CT image of gastric GIST in a hiatus hernia.

GIST syndromes

- *Familial:* multiple small bowel GISTs. Due to mutation in kinase domain of KIT.
- *Carneys Triad:* 85% female. Two out of three required for diagnosis.
  - Stromal stomach tumours.
  - Extra-adrenal paraganglioma.
  - Pulmonary chondroma.
- *Von Recklinghausen's disease:* GISTs reported in neurofibromas.

Dissemination

- *Haematogenous:* liver > pulmonary.
- *Lymphatic:* nodal metastases (1%).
- *Transcoelomic:* peritoneal deposits (14%).
- *Direct invasion:* adjacent structures (13%).

Management

All cases should be managed in the setting of the specialized MDT.

Resectable disease

- Assessment for fitness for surgery/risk:benefit of surgery.
- Staging laparoscopy and review OGD.
- *Surgical resection:* laparoscopic vs. open wedge excision of GIST ± gastrectomy.

Irresectable/metastatic disease

Options

- Imatinib 400mg daily. Monitor response/disease progression (3-monthly CT).
- If relapse/disease progression, double dose (800mg daily).
- *If progression:* 2nd line chemotherapy, sunitinib.
- Embolization if acute GI bleed.

Systemic therapy of GISTs

- 90% of GISTs have mutations in the *KIT* gene leading to an over-expression on cell surface of protein KIT (or CD117), which is receptor tyrosine kinase.
- When growth factors bind to EC domain of KIT proteins, they cause them to dimerize and this lead to activation of intracellular signalling pathways. These pathways are involved in cell proliferation and apoptosis, cell differentiation, adhesion, and motility.
- Around 50% of GISTs are unresectable or metastatic at presentation, and for these patients surgery is not curative.
- KIT protein is also over-expressed in chronic myeloid leukaemia (CML) and small molecule tyrosine kinase inhibitor, imatinib, was developed for treatment of this disease.
- Imatinib binds to KIT and prevents activation of signalling pathway. Initial trials of imatinib in metastatic GIST were very successful and achieved responses that had never previously been achieved in this tumour type, as GIST's are resistant to most conventional chemotherapeutic agents. Because response was so impressive traditional phase III trials comparing imatinib with standard treatment, or against best supportive care, never performed.
- Standard dose of 400mg daily of oral drug established after trial by Demetri:
  - 147 patients comparing 400mg and 600mg of imatinib daily.
  - Long term results were published by Blanke in 2008.
  - Response rates same at both dose levels—67% of patients achieving at least a partial response, a further 15% experiencing disease stability.

- Median time to progression 24/12 and median overall survival 5yrs (57/12).
- Patients who initially progressed despite imatinib had a much worse prognosis with 5-year survival of only 9%.
- Response to first line imatinib should be assessed after 12 weeks and monitored throughout treatment.
- PET CT scanning has been shown to demonstrate early response to treatment with a marked reduction of uptake of 18-fluorodeoxyglucose (FDG). On CT scanning there may be little reduction in size of tumour, but this is coupled with a reduction in density.
- Standard Response Evaluation Criteria In Solid Tumors (RECIST) criteria underestimate response as they demand a 25% reduction in size. The following definition of response has been proposed by Choi:
  - 10% decrease in size or tumour density (Hounsfield unit (HU)) of 15% on CT, no new lesions and no obvious progression of non-measurable disease.
  - *Imatinib well tolerated*—adverse events include oedema, fatigue, myalgia, muscle cramps, rash, abdominal pain, diarrhoea, and nausea.
  - Side effects managed with dose reduction, but occasionally omission.
  - *Multiple interactions*—including warfarin review of other medication necessary when commencing imatinib.
- Further work on genetics of GISTs performed and a relationship has been identified between particular genetic abnormalities and chance of a response to imatinib.
- *Most mutations in KIT exon 11:* tumours respond well to imatinib.
- Mutations in exon 9 less frequent, found predominantly in intestinal GISTs, and associated with lower RR to imatinib.
- Some gastric GISTs have mutations in platelet-derived growth factor-alpha (PDGFRA) and these tumours are less aggressive, may not be KIT positive on immunohistochemistry, but may still respond to imatinib. Most GISTs with a PDGFRA mutation stain for DOG1: now included routinely in diagnostic assessment of GISTs.
- Eventually, all GISTs will develop new mutations that lead to them becoming resistant to imatinib. Some responses have been seen on increasing dose to 800mg daily. Second-line therapy with the tyrosine kinase inhibitor sunitinib can be offered, with increase in progression-free survival from 6 to 27 weeks over placebo.

Adjuvant treatment of GISTs

- After complete resection of GIST, risk of recurrence and metastatic potential of tumour can be estimated by considering size, location, and mitotic rate of the tumour.
- Gastric GIST's have lower malignant potential than those arising in small or large bowel.
- Risk of recurrence can be reduced by use of adjuvant imatinib. One trial showed that recurrence-free survival at 1 year was 98% with imatinib compared with 83% in control arm. Optimal duration of adjuvant treatment remains uncertain, although improved survival was seen with longer duration in trial comparing 1–3 years of treatment.

Operative technique: laparoscopic or open resection of gastric GIST

- Small stalked GISTs on greater curve are most amenable to laparoscopic wedge excision.
- GISTs close to or abutting GOJ frequently require an open procedure so as to ensure narrowing of GOJ does not occur.

Indication Resectable gastric GIST.

Pre-operative Satisfactory clinical evaluation, counselling, MDT discussion, informed consent.

Procedure
GA, supine (with epidural or local anaesthetic infiltration catheters (PainBuster®) if open, hair removal, abdomen prepped with povidone iodine and draped. Antibiotic prophylaxis.
- Ports:
  - *Peri-umbilical open cut down*—most frequently supra-umbilical just off centre to the right (11mm camera port).
  - Left paramedian, upper abdomen (11mm working port).
  - Right paramedian, upper abdomen (11mm working port).
  - Epigastric (5mm)—Nathanson liver retractor.
  - Left flank (5mm)—assistant retraction.
- Standard 11mmHgCO$_2$ insufflation to establish pneumoperitoneum.
- 30-degree laparoscope.
- *Incision:* left subcostal (if open or open/assisted procedure).
- Formal laparoscopy/laparotomy surveying the peritoneal surfaces, liver, small bowel, colon, omentum, and pelvic organs with biopsy of any suspicious tissue.
- Reverse Trendelenberg, operator between legs and formal assessment of stomach and tumour looking specifically for general signs of irresectability.
- For GISTs on greater curve, lesser sac is opened just outside gastroepiploic arcade with harmonic scalpel.
- As only a 1-cm resection margin is needed and formal lymphadenectomy is not indicated, only limited gastric mobilization is required.
- Once GIST is isolated, gastroepiploic vessels can be divided close to stomach and wedge excision performed.
- In either a laparoscopic or open procedure this commonly requires single or multiple firings of a linear stapler with care taken not to narrow gastric lumen and, in particular, GOJ unnecessarily.
- For GISTs arising from posterior wall of stomach, an anterior gastrotomy can be performed between stay sutures and GIST prolapsed out of anterior wall of stomach. Excision is performed with firings of linear stapler and anterior gastrotomy closed.

- Specimen (Fig. 9.17) can then be removed through wound or an extended port site (with wound protector) and staple line over-sewn.
- NGT placement secured with septal bridle.
- *Closure:* 1/0 PDS to 1°/extended port site/laparotomy wound (two layers) and skin clips.

Complications
Bleeding, infection, wound complications, inadvertent visceral injury, thrombo-embolism, shoulder tip pain, intra-abdominal sepsis (usually as a result of leak from gastrotomy site).

Immediate post-operative period
- Routine ward observations.
- Sips orally from 1st post-operative day.
- Two post-operative doses of antibiotics.
- Prophylactic LMWH.

Future Discussion of histology at MDT to decide follow-up requirements.

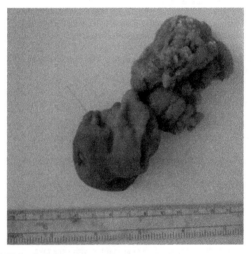

Fig. 9.17 Pathological specimen of excised gastric GIST.

Gastric lymphomas

MALT lymphoma accounts for 3–6% of gastric malignancies. The stomach is the commonest site for GI lymphoma.

Pathology

- The majority are B-cell non-Hodgkin's lymphomas, others include T-cell and Hodgkin's lymphoma.
- Arise from lymphoid tissue in mucosa and are associated with *H. pylori* and *H. heilmanni* infections.
- Most occur > 50 years of age.
- Subgroup of marginal zone lymphomas (MZL), a heterogeneous group that includes nodal MZL and splenic MZL, as well as gastric and non-gastric MALT lymphomas.
- Other gastric lymphomas generally diffuse large B-cell lymphomas staged and treated as other high grade non-Hodgkin's lymphomas (NHLs) with chemotherapy. R-CHOP is standard first line regime— rituximab (an anti-CD-20 monoclonal antibody), cyclophosphamide, doxorubicin, vincristine, and prednisolone.
- Spread is usually to regional lymph nodes, but uncommonly can occur to peripheral lymph nodes. Spread can also occur to other mucosal sites, e.g. ileum. Microscopic appearances are characterized by intense mononuclear cell infiltration.

Diagnosis

- OGD and biopsy (Fig. 9.18). *H. pylori* confirmed on histology, urea breath test, stool antigen test, or blood antibody test.
- Staging CT (neck, thorax, abdomen and pelvis).
- Bone marrow aspirate and biopsy, EUS, and blood tests including FBC, biochemical profile and lactate dehydrogenase (LDH).
- Genetic analysis with fluorescent in situ hybridization (FISH) or polymerase chain reaction (PCR) should be done as the presence of the translocation t(11;18) confers a poorer prognosis to the possibility of resistance to antibiotic treatment.

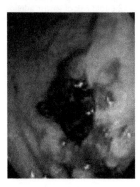

Fig. 9.18 Gastric lymphoma with superficial ulceration and bleeding.

Differential diagnosis
- *H. pylori* associated gastritis.
- Sjogren's disease.
- Hashimoto's disease.

Management
- Most gastric MALT lymphomas are localized at time of diagnosis, stage I or II. Some have involved regional nodes, but systemic disease is rare.
- Mainstay of treatment of *H. pylori*-associated gastric MALT lymphoma is the eradication *H. pylori* with antibiotics and PPI.
- Any standard double or triple therapy can be used. Response to treatment can be slow so re-evaluation with repeat endoscopy should only be done after an interval of 3 months. A further biopsy should be taken at this stage and repeat assessment for ongoing infection with *H. pylori* is required to determine further Rx.
- If complete remission is found after 3 months and *H. pylori* no longer present—surveillance endoscopy every 3/12.
- If evidence of response to treatment, or if disease is stable, but *H. pylori* still present, then second line eradication therapy with further course of antibiotics is given. If persistent disease is identified, patients can be safely monitored for between 12 and 18 months, if asymptomatic before proceeding to active treatment with either involved field radiotherapy or systemic chemotherapy.
- Tumours that have the *t*(11;18) translocation are less likely to respond to *H. pylori* eradication so early consideration should be given to radiotherapy or chemotherapy.
- If progressive or symptomatic disease in absence of active *H. pylori*, then either DXT or systemic chemotherapy used for follicular lymphoma. If diffuse large B-cell lymphoma found on repeat endoscopy and biopsy then re-staging and use of systemic treatment indicated.
- The radiation doses needed for lymphoma are moderate, usually around 30Gy to stomach and involved regional nodes.
- Complete remission frequently achieved from antibiotic therapy alone, but late relapse common. *Follow-up*—OGD every 3–6 months for 5 years, then annually. 6-fold risk of gastric adenocarcinoma in patients treated for MALT lymphomas, cf. general population.

Further reading

Bang YJ, Van Cutsem E, Feyereislova A, et al. Trastuzumab in combination with chemotherapy versus chemotherapy alone for treatment of HER2-positive advanced gastric or gastro-oesophageal junction cancer (ToGA): a phase 3, open-label, randomised controlled trial. Lancet 2010; **376**: 687–97.

Blanke CD, Demetri GD, von Mehren M, et al. Long-term results from a randomized phase II trial of standard- versus higher-dose imatinibmesylate for patients with unresectable or metastatic gastrointestinal stromal tumors expressing KIT. J Clin Oncol 2008; **26**: 620–62.

Capelle LG, de Vries AC, Looman CW, et al. Gastric MALT lymphoma: epidemiology and high adenocarcinoma risk in a nation-wide study. Eur J Cancer 2008; **44**: 2470–6.

Casali PG, Blay J-Y. On behalf of the ESMO/CONTICANET/EUROBONET Consensus Panel of Experts. Gastrointestinal stromal tumours: ESMO Clinical Practice Guidelines for diagnosis, treatment and follow-up. Ann Oncol 2010; **21**(Suppl. 5): v98–102.

Choi H, Charnsangavej C, Faria SC, et al. Correlation of computed tomography and positron emission tomography in patients with metastatic gastrointestinal stromal tumor treated at a single institution with imatinibmesylate: proposal of new computed tomography response criteria. J Clin Oncol 2007; **25**: 1753–9.

Cunningham D, Allum WH, Stenning SP, et al. Perioperative chemotherapy versus surgery alone for resectable gastroesophageal cancer. N Engl J Med 2006; **355**: 11–20.

Cunningham D, Starling N, Rao S, et al. Capecitabine and oxaliplatin for advanced esophagogastric cancer. N Engl J Med 2008; **358**: 36–46.

Jansen EPM, Boot H, Saunders MP, et al., A Phase I–II study of postoperative capecitabine-based chemoradiotherapy in gastric cancer. Int. J. Radiation Oncology Biol. Phys. 2007; **69**: 1424–8.

MacDonald JS, Smalley SR, Benedetti J, et al., Chemoradiotherapy after surgery compared with surgery alone for adenocarcinoma of the stomach or gastroesophageal junction. N Engl J Med 2001; **345**: 725–30.

Miettinen M, Lasota J. Gastrointestinal stromal tumors: pathology and prognosis at different sites. Sem Diag Pathol 2006; **23**(2): 70–83.

Sasako M, Sano T, Yamamoto S, et al. D2 lymphadenectomy alone or with para-aortic nodal dissection for gastric cancer. N Engl J Med 2008; **359**(5): 453–62.

Songun I, Putter H, Kranenbarg EM, et al. Surgical treatment of gastric cancer: 15-year follow-up results of the randomised nationwide Dutch D1D2 trial. Lancet Oncol 2010; **11**(5): 439–49.

Stathis A, Chini C, Bertoni F, et al. Long-term outcome following Helicobacter pylori eradication in a retrospective study of 105 patients with localized gastric marginal zone B-cell lymphoma of MALT type. Ann Oncol 2009; **20**: 1086–93.

Van Cutsem E, Moiseyenko VM, Tjulandin S, et al. Phase III study of docetaxel and cisplatin plus fluorouracil compared with cisplatin and fluorouracil as first-line therapy for advanced gastric cancer: a report of the V325 Study Group. J Clin Oncol 2006; **24**: 4991–7.

Ychou M, Boige V, Pignon J-P, et al. Peri-operative chemotherapy compared with surgery alone for resectable gastroesophageal adenocarcinoma: an FNCLCC and FFCD multicenter phase III trial. J Clin Oncol 2011; **29**: 1715–21.

Yonemura Y, Wu CC, Fukushima N, et al. Randomized clinical trial of D2 and extended paraaortic lymphadenectomy in patients with gastric cancer. Int J Clin Oncol 2008; **13**(2): 132–7.

Zucca E, Dreyling M. On behalf of the ESMO Guidelines Working Group: Gastric marginal zone lymphoma of MALT type: ESMO Clinical Practice Guidelines for diagnosis, treatment and follow-up. Ann Oncol 2010; **21**(Suppl. 5): v175–6.

Bariatric surgery

Indications for bariatric surgery

- BMI imperfect, but commonest method of measuring obesity (Table 10.1).
- Body weight (kg)/height (m) squared.
- *Adult BMI 25–29.9*: overweight and BMI of 30 or over obese.
- NICE guidelines (2006) recommend bariatric surgery as a treatment option for people with morbid obesity (BMI > 40kg/m²) or who have lower BMI (35kg/m²) + other significant disease.
- Surgery only offered when all appropriate non-surgical measures unsuccessful.
- Adults with BMI >50kg/m² may be offered surgery as a first line treatment option, and should be part of a comprehensive package of obesity services provided by an MDT.
- *UK*: financial constraints, patients from some regions subject to more restrictive referral criteria—considered if BMI >50Kg/m² + comorbidity or 55kg/m² without.
- 2010 25% of UK adults obese (BMI> 30kg/m²).
- By 2050, 60% of adult males and 50% of adult females will be obese in the UK, if nothing is done to curb current trend.
- *2011*: US Food and Drugs Administration (FDA) approved use of a specific gastric band in patients BMI 30–34kg/m² + weight-related comorbidity as a preventative measure.
- NHS-commissioned bariatric procedures performed in England increased from 1317 in 2006/7 to 3642 procedures in 2009/10: represents <2% of all morbidly obese adults.
- Recognition that bariatric surgery has such a profound effect on metabolism has increased its potential repertoire of indications.
- Include management of type 2 diabetes in patients with BMI <35, patients with non-alcoholic steatosis hepatitis (NASH) progressing to cirrhosis and in the algorithm in the management of infertility investigations for patients with BMI >35.

Table 10.1 Classification of obesity based on BMI

Classification	BMI (kg/m²)
Normal	18.5–24.9
Overweight	25–29.9
Obese	30–34.9
Severely obese	35–39.9
Morbidly obese	40–49.9
Super morbidly obese	50+

Note: With every 10 units of BMI above 50 prefix classification with another 'super'. Table based on European population and ethnicity must be taken into consideration.

NICE 2006
Consider surgery for people with severe obesity if:
- BMI of 40kg/m^2 or more.
- 35–40kg/m^2 and other significant disease (e.g. type 2 diabetes mellitus (T2DM), high blood pressure (BP)) that could improve if they lost weight.
  - All appropriate non-surgical measures have failed to achieve or maintain adequate clinically beneficial weight loss for at least 6 months.
  - They are receiving or will receive intensive specialist management.
  - They are generally fit for anaesthesia and surgery.
  - They commit to the need for long-term follow-up.
- Consider surgery as a first-line option for adults with a BMI >50kg/m^2 in whom surgical intervention is considered appropriate; consider or list at before surgery if the waiting time is long.

Metabolic syndrome

- A combination of medical disorders that, collectively, increase risk of cardiovascular disease and DM.
- Association of visceral fat to insulin resistance.
- Highly prevalent in West USA, ~25% of population increases with age.
- *Synonyms:* metabolic syndrome X, cardiometabolic syndrome, syndrome X, insulin resistance syndrome, Reaven's syndrome, and coronary artery disease, hypertension, atherosclerosis, obesity, and stroke (CHAOS).
- Obesity is a multisystem chronic pro-inflammatory, prothrombotic disorder associated with increased morbidity and mortality.
- *Adipocytes more than lipid storage vessels:* secrete a large number of physiologically active adipokines—lead to inflammation, vascular and cardiac remodelling, airway inflammation, and altered microvascular flow patterns, attract and activate inflammatory cells, such as macrophages.
- Changes collectively lead to organ dysfunction particularly cardiovascular and pulmonary systems.
- *Mechanisms:*
  - ? *Hepatic dysfunction*—ectopic liver fat correlates with dysfunctional insulin dynamics from which metabolic syndrome derived.
  - *Liver*—1° metabolism for trans-fats, branched-chain amino acids, ethanol, and fructose all associated with obesity and metabolic syndrome.
  - *All*—(1) are not insulin regulated and (2) deliver metabolic intermediates to hepatic mitochondria without a depletion mechanism for excess substrate, enhancing lipogenesis, and ectopic adipose storage.

- Excessive fatty acid derivatives interfere with hepatic insulin signal transduction.
- Reactive oxygen species accumulate, which cannot be quenched by adjacent peroxisomes; reactive oxygen species reach endoplasmic reticulum, leading to a compensatory process termed the 'unfolded protein response', driving further insulin resistance and eventually insulin deficiency.

Definitions See Box 10.1, Box 10.2, and Box 10.3.

Box 10.1 The World Health Organization criteria (1999)

DM, impaired glucose tolerance, impaired fasting glucose or insulin resistance, *and* two of:
- *Blood pressure*: ≥140/90mmHg.
- *Dyslipidemia*: triglycerides (TG): ≥1.695mmol/L and high-density lipoprotein cholesterol (HDL-C) ≤0.9mmol/L (male), ≤1.0mmol/L (female).
- *Central obesity*: waist: hip ratio >0.90 (male); >0.85 (female), or body mass index >30kg/m².
- *Microalbuminuria*: urinary albumin excretion ratio ≥20 micrograms/min or albumin:creatinine ratio ≥30mg/g.

Reproduced from 'Definition, diagnosis and classification of diabetes mellitus and its complications. Part 1: diagnosis and classification of diabetes mellitus provisional report of a WHO consultation', Alberti KG, Zimmet PZ, *Diabet Med* Jul; **15**(7): 539–53, copyright 1998 with permission of John Wiley and Sons.

Box 10.2 International Diabetes Federation consensus worldwide definition of the metabolic syndrome (2006)

Central obesity (increased waist circumference; ethnicity-specific) *and* any two:
- *Raised triglycerides*: >150mg/dL (1.7mmol/L), or specific treatment for this lipid abnormality.
- *Reduced HDL cholesterol*: <40mg/dL (1.03mmol/L) in males, <50mg/dL (1.29mmol/L) in females, or specific treatment for this lipid abnormality.
- *Raised BP*: systolic BP >130 or diastolic BP >85mmHg, or treatment of previously diagnosed hypertension.
- *Raised fasting plasma glucose (FPG)*: >100mg/dL (5.6mmol/L), or previously diagnosed T2DM.
- If FPG is >5.6mmol/L or 100mg/dL, an oral glucose tolerance test is strongly recommended, but not necessary to define presence of the syndrome.
- If BMI is >30kg/m², central obesity can be assumed and waist circumference does not need to be measured.

Reproduced from *International Diabetes Federation (IDF) Worldwide Definition of the Metabolic Syndrome*, Copyright 2006 International Diabetes Federation.

Box 10.3 European Group for the Study of Insulin Resistance (1999)

Insulin resistance defined as the top 25% of the fasting insulin values among non-diabetic individuals, and two or more of the following:
- *Central obesity*: waist circumference ≥94cm (male), ≥80cm (female).
- *Dyslipidemia*: TG ≥2.0mmol/L and/or HDL-C <1.0mmol/L or treated for dyslipidaemia.
- *Hypertension*: BP ≥140/90mmHg or antihypertensive medication.
- Fasting plasma glucose ≥ 6.1mmol/L.

Reproduced from 'Comment on the provisional report from the WHO consultation. European Group for the Study of Insulin Resistance (EGIR)', Balkau B, Charles MA, *Diabet Med* May; **16**(5): 442–3, copyright 1999 with permission from John Wiley and Sons.

Bariatric surgery for diabetes management

- *Prevalence of T2DM and obesity rising*: 2010, global prevalence 8.3% of adults. WHO suggest it will be 9.9% by 2030 and this poses costly public health challenge.
- *20% and 25% morbid obesity patients*: T2DM and complications.
- Less than half of patients with moderate to severe T2DM on medical treatment achieve and maintain adequate glycaemic control.
- *Observational studies level two meta-analyses*: bariatric surgery in obese and non-obese patients with leads to rapid and sustained glycaemic control.
- *Administrative datasets*: overall cost of surgery fully offset by reduced expenditure on anti-diabetic drugs within 26 months.
- International Diabetes Federation recommended bariatric surgery as adjunct.

Severely obese patients with T2DM

Laparoscopic Roux-en-Y gastric bypass

- *Schauer: Pittsburgh 2003*: 1160 patients laparoscopic Roux-en-Y gastric bypass results in significant weight loss (60% percent of excess body weight loss BMI 50 to 34) and resolution (83%) of T2DM. Patients with the shortest duration and mildest form of T2DM have higher rate of resolution post-operative. Early surgical intervention increases likelihood of euglycaemia.
- HbA1C normalized (83%) or markedly improved (17%) in all patients. A significant reduction in use of oral anti-diabetic agents (80%) and insulin (79%) followed surgical treatment. Patients with the shortest duration (<5 years), the mildest T2DM (diet controlled), and greatest weight loss after surgery were most likely to achieve complete resolution of T2DM.

Bariatric surgery vs. medical Rx
- Bariatric surgery results in better glucose control than medical therapy and overwhelmingly leads to disease remission.
- *Mingrone:* Rome, NEJM 2012:
  - Single-centre, non-blinded, RCT.
  - 60 patients 30–60 years BMI >35, DM >5 years and glycated haemoglobin (Hb) >7.0%.
  - Conventional medical therapy vs. gastric bypass or BP diversion.
  - *Primary end point:* DM remission at 2 years (defined as a fasting glucose level of <100mg/dL [5.6mmol/L] and glycated Hb <6.5% in absence of pharmacological therapy).

Results at 2 years
- *Medical cohort:* DM remission 0%.
- *Gastric bypass group:* 75%.
- *BP-diversion group:* 95% (*P* < 0.001).
- Age, sex, baseline BMI, duration of DM, and weight changes not predictors of remission at 2 years or improvement in glycaemia at 1 and 3 months. Average baseline glycated Hb (8.65 ± 1.45%) decreased in all groups, patients in surgical group's greatest improvement (7.69 ± 0.57% in the medical-therapy group, 6.35 ± 1.42% in the gastric-bypass group, and 4.95 ± 0.49% in the BP-diversion group).

Lap Sleeve gastrectomy
- Evidence to suggest laparoscopic sleeve gastrectomy as good as bypass surgery to induce T2DM remission.
- *Adamo 2010, UCL:* 85% T2DM patients have normalized HbA1C at 3/12 post-laparoscopic sleeve gastrectomy. Mean BMI 53 reduced to 44 at 3/12.

BMI <35 with T2DM post-bariatric surgery
- *Scopinaro 2010—systematic review:* 1979–2009, 343 patients, 6–216/12F/U. 85.3% patients off T2DM medications with fasting plasma glucose approaching normal (105.2mg/dL, –93.3), and normal glycated haemoglobin, 6% (–2.7).
- *Subgroup comparison:* BMI reduction and T2DM resolution greatest following malabsorptive/restrictive procedures, and in the preoperatively mildly obese (30.0–35.0) vs. overweight (25.0–25.9).
- Operative mortality 0.29%.

General considerations and the multidisciplinary team

General considerations
Obesity is an all-encompassing chronic illness affecting patients physically, psychologically, emotionally, and sexually. Their needs are multifactorial and often complex. They remain a vulnerable patient group, are high users of the health service and have a significantly lower life expectancy compared with normal weight patients. All hospitals should have in place policies and protocols to look after such patients that are found within all wards and departments. The provision of care is not the sole responsibility of the bariatric team.

Looking specifically at the bariatric patient, their needs can be organized into different hospital departments.

Outpatients
- Large chairs.
- Large BP cuffs.
- Scales that can take a large weight and accommodate wheel chairs.
- Consulting room doors wide enough to accept wheel chairs.
- Appropriate toilet facilities.

The Ward
Space is needed for:
- Bariatric beds (note that the average NHS bed can accommodate most bariatric patients with a maximum load of between 30 and 35 stone (180–210kg), large chairs, commodes, gowns, wheelchairs.
- Appropriate meals from the kitchen, TED stockings, hoists, scales.

Theatre
- Operating table and accessories, hoist.
- Hover mattresses, appropriate operating instruments, e.g. long ports.
- Ensure that the bariatric bed can be transported to all departments without hindrance (Theatre/ward/HDU/ITU).

Endoscopy
Adequately-sized trolley.

The multidisciplinary team
The management of the obese patient (see NICE Clinical Guideline 43) requires multidisciplinary effort, and a bariatric MDT discussion should precede all cases of bariatric surgery when possible.

Members of the MDT
- *Surgeon:* patient selection for appropriate procedure.
- *Endocrine/metabolic physician:* acts as a gate keeper in many services having worked the patient up for referral to surgeons. Follow-up to ensure metabolic well-being of the patients.
- *Anaesthetist:* stratification of operative risk and formulation of plan for optimization.

- *Dietitian:* pre-operative assessments advise pre-operative liver reduction diets and post-operative diet regimes.
- *Psychologist:* explore trigger factors for abnormal eating behaviour. Teach coping/control mechanisms using cognitive behavioral therapy.
- *Specialist nurses:* instrumental in the delivery of the service seeing both pre- and post-operative patients.
- *Pharmacist:* advice on ability to absorb certain medications and help in suggesting alternative drugs and or routes.

The extended MDT includes anaesthetists, respiratory physicians, the ward sister, the theatre sister, managers of the community weight management programmes, and child protection office.

MDT discussion
- *Structured assessment of each patient:*
  - *Bariatric history/eating habits*—input from dietitian and if required the psychologist.
  - Current status vis a vis NICE guidelines, BMI, comorbidities.
  - Screening blood tests reviewed and acted on.
  - Relevant correspondence from all professionals involved with the patient are checked and if not available requested.
- Patients considered appropriate, showing good motivation, willing to make behavioural changes and showing pre-operative weight loss assessed by surgeon for consideration of surgery.
- Patients discovered to have outstanding issues, e.g. emotional eating habits or awaiting formal sleep studies are patients in progress. Appropriate referrals made and patient discussed at later MDT meeting to assess progress.
- Patients considered having no insight into their eating habits, not fit for anaesthetic, current self-harmers, and those showing no inclination to make behavioural changes are discharged from the service at the next outpatient screening with appropriate follow-up.
- Post-operative patients whose weight loss is less than expected are also discussed at MDT meeting to revisit both dietetic and psychological reasons why their weight loss is sub-optimal.

Risk management in obese surgical patients

Risk reduction strategies occur at all points of patient contact.

Outpatients
- Assessment of anaesthetic and operative risk. High risk patients may benefit from a lesser procedure, e.g. gastric band over bypass.
- Men over 45 years old with BMI >55kg/m² and comorbidity have significant operative risks. Patient selection is fundamental.

Preoperative assessment
Respiratory system
- All bariatric patients screened for obstructive sleep apnoea (OSA) using the Epworth sleepiness score.
- Score 11/24 referred to a respiratory physician for formal sleep studies.
- *OSA requiring treatment:* treated for a minimum of 6 weeks prior to surgery and are asked to bring their continuous positive airway pressure (CPAP) machine in with them to hospital.
- *Obese patients have a reduced functional residual capacity:* can lead to airway closure and desaturation in the supine position. If difficulty occurs in intubating the trachea then rapid desaturation can occur.
- *Room air pulse oximetry:* useful screening tool—supine SpO₂ <96% on room air may indicate investigation (spirometry, arterial blood gas analysis (ABG)).
- Morbidly obese patients with co-existing asthma/COPD at risk of peri-operative respiratory complications. Referral to a respiratory physician allows optimization of these conditions prior to surgery.
- Chest X-rays can be difficult to interpret due to poor penetration.

Cardiac disease
- *Increased prevalence cardiovascular disease:* hypertension, hyperlipidaemia, IHD, and heart failure.
- *If significant:* cardiology referral.
- Obese patients do not tolerate exercise tests well if at all and the practical problem of how to take an accurate BP will need to be addressed, e.g. using the forearm.

Metabolic Disease
- Screening of all obese patients for DM and hypothyroidism is mandatory and should be performed in 1° care.
- Assess the adequacy of control of each condition.
- *DM assess:* HbA1C, complications, cardiac disease, renal disease, and autonomic dysfunction.
- *Hypothyroid:* commence thyroxine and re-test post-replacement.
- *Screening for vitamin D deficiency also mandatory:* >70% obese population vitamin D deficient. Once discovered adequate vitamin D replacement should occur pre surgery and be part of the follow-up regime.

- Despite weight significant malnutrition prior to surgery. Complete biochemical and haematological profile essential.
- Malaborbative procedures may compound this.

Thromboprophylaxis
- Obese patients are at significantly greater risk of venous and pulmonary thromboembolism.
- All obese patients considered for mechanical (e.g. Flowtron boots) and pharmacological thromboprophylaxis.
- Patient specific weight adjusted dose of low molecular weight heparin is calculated and administrated prior to surgery and depending on the surgery up to 7–10 days post-surgery with patients being taught how to self-administer.
- Correct size thrombo-embolic stockings and calf compressors in theatre are required.

Day case/in-patient listing
- Endoscopic gastric balloon insertion and laparoscopic gastric band placement can be performed as day case procedures in suitable patients.
- Careful risk assessment essential.

Smoking cessation
- Single most important act in general a patient can do to improve their health and operative risk if >6 weeks pre-operative.
- *Respiratory and cardiovascular disease risk and surgery related complications:* ulceration of anastomotic/staple lines and wound infections reduced.

Liver reduction diet
- 10–14 days prior to surgery patients commenced on a low fat low carbohydrate diet to reduce fat content of liver.
- Aids liver retraction and laparoscopic approach overall.
- Most patients will lose weight on this restrictive diet which, in turn, makes operation easier and safer.

The Epworth Sleepiness Score
The Epworth Sleepiness Score sums the likelihood of a patient dozing or sleeping during each of eight activities of daily living. Patients scoring more than 11h are referred to a respiratory physician for formal sleep studies.

Use the following score to choose the most appropriate number for each situation:
- 0 = would never doze or sleep.
- 1 = slight chance of dozing or sleeping.
- 2 = moderate chance of dozing or sleeping.
- 3 = high chance of dozing or sleeping.

Bariatric anaesthetic considerations

- Previous anaesthetic histories and charts checked prior to surgery.
- *Peripheral IV access can be difficult:* a central line may be required with sonosite localization.
- Anaesthetic assistant must be familiar with the equipment to manage the difficult airway.
- Some patients may require awake intubation and such anaesthetic skills should be available.
- GORD common and a PPI is prescribed for each case.
- Post-operative patients nursed semi-erect.

SOBA guidelines 2011

Pre-operative evaluation

Sleep apnoea: predictor of airway problems after induction and should be anticipated (see Fig. 10.1 and Table 10.2).

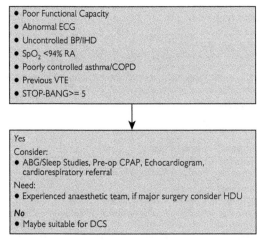

Fig. 10.1 Recommended peri-operative pathway according to pre-operative assessment.

Table 10.2 STOP-BANG (validated tool)

S: Snore	Have you been told that you snore?	Y/N
T: Tired	Are you often tired during the day	Y/N
O: Obstruction	Do you know if you stop breathing or has anyone witnessed you stop breathing whilst asleep	Y/N
P: Pressure	Do you have high blood pressure or are you on medication for high BP	Y/N
B: BMI	BMI >28	Y/N
A: Age	Age >50	Y/N
N: Neck	Male neck >17' Female neck >16'	Y/N
G: Gender	Male?	Y/N

Reproduced from 'STOP questionnaire: a tool to screen patients for obstructive sleep apnea', Chung F, Yegneswaran B, Liao P, et al., *Anesthesiology*, **108**: 812–21, copyright 2008 with permission from Wolters Kluwer Health.

Obesity type

Android obesity
- Most weight above waist.
- Difficult airway/ventilation problems more likely.
- Greater risk of CVS disease.
- *Increased risk of metabolic syndrome:* dyslipidaemia, insulin resistence, prothrombotic, pro-inflammatory.

Gynaecoid obesity
- Most weight below waist.
- Less co-morbidity.

Intra-operative anaesthesia

Premedication Consider PPI, pre-operative analgesia, DVT prophylaxis, Boehringer Mannheim test for blood glucose control.

Recommended equipment
- *>135kg:* suitable trolley/operating table.
- Gel padding, large BP cuff, ramping device (tragus level with sternum—improves laryngoscopy and ventilation), difficult airway equipment, ventilator capable of PEEP and pressure modalities, hover mattress, depth of anaesthesia monitoring.

Anaesthetic technique
- Self-positioning on table.
- Pre-oxygenate in ramped position.
- Minimize induction to ventilation interval to avoid desaturation.
- Avoid spontaneous ventilation.
- Tracheal intubation recommended.
- Use short acting agents, e.g. desflurane or propofol TCI, short-acting opioids, multimodal analgesia. Post-operative nausea and vomiting (PONV) prophylaxis.
- Monitor neuromuscular block, ensure full reversal.
- Extubate and recover in head up position.

Post-operative
Day case surgery
Avoid long-acting opioids, but use multimodal analgesia including local anaesthetic (LA). The patient may be discharged if baseline pulse oximeter oxygen saturation (SpO_2) is maintained on room air without stimulation, no apnoea and routine discharge criteria attained, consider LMWH 10–14/7.

OSA or obesity hypoventilation syndrome (OHS)
- Avoid sedatives/opioids. Reinstate CPAP if used pre-operatively.
- *Patients intolerant of CPAP at risk of hypoventilation:* need oximetry.
- Additional time in recovery needed only discharge to ward if apnoea free without stimulation.
- *In-patients:* multimodal analgesia, caution with long acting opioids and sedatives.
- Mobilize early.
- Ensure thromboprophylaxis administered.
- Admit to HDU/ITU if significant co-morbidity or if major surgery.

Thromboprophylaxis in bariatric surgery (SOBA guidelines 2012)
- DVT occurs in 3.5% of patients undergoing laparoscopic bariatric surgery.
- PE occurs in up to 1% of cases resulting in 30-day mortality up to 2%.
- *Traditional mechanical thromboprophylaxis:* TEDS/pneumatic compression unsuitable for some obese patients. Sequential calf compression devices—use throughout surgery and in the immediate post-operative period until patient is mobilized.
- Prevention by early mobilization and LMWH.

High risk for the development of DVT and PE
- Previous history of DVT or PE.
- *Positive thrombophilia screen (?Family history VTE):* FBC, activated protein C resistance, protein C%S, antithrombin, and lupus anticoagulant.
- Expected prolonged period of post-operative immobility.
- *High risk patients:* consider insertion of IVC filter, insert, 1–2 days pre-operatively remove 2–3 weeks post-operatively.

Early: mobilization
- Laparoscopic surgery, rather than open surgery.
- Adequate multimodal post-operative analgesia.
- Adequate multimodal post-operative anti-emesis.
- Early removal of urinary catheter.

LMWH
- Start peri-operative and continue for a min 1 weeks post- laparoscopic adjustable gastric band.
- *3 weeks:* more complex surgery or in the high risk patient.
- Dose related to weight, but increasing dose leads to increasing bleeding complications.

- Risk of thrombus formation extends into the post-operative period prolonged post-operative therapy for between 1 and 4 weeks depending on the type of surgery.
- *Typical regime:*
  - Dalteparin 2500U subcutaneously 1h pre-operatively.
  - Dalteparin 5000U subcutaneously od for 7 days post-gastric band surgery and 21 days following more complex surgery.

Surgical procedures: general

Open surgery

- Majority of bariatric surgery now performed laparoscopically, small percentage is still open and the laparoscopic surgeon must be comfortable if conversion to open surgery is required.
- An upper midline incision is made from the xiphoid to the umbilicus (rooftop incision is alternative).
- Dissection of the falciform ligament to the left of the patient allows access into the peritoneum with retraction of the fatty falciform ligament to the patient's right.
- Access to the GOJ in the morbidly obese with enlarged fatty livers restricted.
- Tilting the patient with their left side up helps control the liver and/or dividing the left triangular ligament of the liver and rolling the left lobe of the liver to the right and out of the way.
- Open surgery is associated with longer inpatient stay, higher wound infection rates and a higher incidence of incisional hernia. It is not the approach of choice.

Laparoscopic surgery

- Patient placed in cruciate position with abdomen and thorax at a 45° angle to horizontal. The operating surgeon is between patient's legs, the first assistant to patients left, and the second assistant and/or scrub nurse to patient's right. The monitor is midline or patients left.
- Once positioned and draped access to the peritoneum is achieved, direct open access difficult. Veress insufflation at Palmerer's point followed by blind or with use of optical port and a 0° camera.
- Standard pressure 12mmHg can be increased to 15mmHg.
- 30° laparoscope essential.
- The other working ports are then placed under vision.
- Liver retractor, e.g. Nathanson's retractor or similar is used to retract the left lobe of the liver.
- Adequate liver retraction essential to visualize diaphragm and GOJ.
- Left tilt and division of left triangular ligaments may help.
- Expensive consumable laparoscopic equipment should not be opened until this stage is completed. If the liver is too big and cannot be retracted consider abandoning at this stage with a view to encouraging more preoperative weight loss. Intra-gastric balloon may have a role.
- *Abdominal wall thickness may restrict a fulcrum of angulation for the ports:* longer ports may be of use, if still sub-optimal additional ports may be required.

Bariatric procedures

See Table 10.3.

Table 10.3 Bariatric operations categorized by primary mode of action

Principle of action	Procedure
Restrictive	Laparoscopic adjustable gastric band
	Sleeve gastrectomy
	Gastric balloon
	Vertical banded gastroplasty (VBG)
Restrictive and Malabsorptive	Roux-en-Y gastroduodenal bypass
	Bilio-pancreatic diversion (Scopinaro)
	Bilio-pancreatic diversion with duodenal switch

Outcomes of bariatric surgery

Operative intervention is proven to be more effective than conservative measures in the treatment of obesity. This is seen with absolute weight loss, excess weight loss, resolution of co-morbidities, and cost effectiveness (Table 10.4 and Table 10.5).

- At 1 year mean total % weight loss from all approaches is 20–21.6% vs. non-surgical of 1.4–5.5%.
- At 2 years this is 16–28.6% following surgery vs. weight gain of 0.1–0.5% for non-surgical.
- *Swedish Obesity Study (SOS):* weight loss maintained at 10 years with weight gain in the non-surgical arm.
- *No weight loss differences:* open vs. lap approach.

A 40% reduction of death over a 7-year period has been reported following surgery with a decrease in IHD of 56%.

Table 10.4 Weight loss and mortality

	Mean % excess wt loss	30-day mortality (%)
Gastric banding	47.5 (40.7–54.2)	0.1
Sleeve gastrectomy	57.6% (51.8–64.3)	0.3
Gastric bypass	61.6 (56.7–66.5)	0.5
Biliopancreatic diversion (BPD)/switch	70.1 (66.3–73.9)	1.1

Table 10.5 Resolution and improvement of co morbidities (as measured by a cessation or reduction in medication of any given condition along with a measurable clinical parameter)

	Resolved (%)	Resolved/improved (%)
T2DM	76.8	86
Hyperlipidaemia	70	79
Hypertension	61.7	78
OSA	83	85

Other clinical benefits

• Reduced pain associated with weight bearing joints.
• Increase in eligibility for major joint replacement surgery.
• Fertility of women of child bearing age and eligibility for assisted fertilization if required.
• GORD.
• NASH and potential progression to cirrhosis and hepatocellular carcinoma.
• Stress incontinence.
• Reduction in physical disability, depression, and increase in activity.

Economic benefits

• Cost of surgery balanced by benefits within 3 years.
• Patients' drug bill decreases with time.
• Increased economic contribution to society by work, tax revenue, and discontinuing long-term state welfare benefits.

In the UK the introduction of the National Bariatric Surgery Registry (NBSR) in 2009 and in the US the Bariatric Outcomes Longitudinal Database (BOLD) will lead to the collation of robust prospective data.

Bariatric surgical procedures

Laparoscopic gastric banding

Principle
- Restrictive.
- The stretching of a small gastric pouch above the band gives rise to early satiety, reducing the volume of food consumed, leading to weight loss.

Predicted weight loss Up to 50–60% of excess weight at 2 years.

Set up Preoperative LMWH, proton pump inhibitors, antibiotic, and a combination of anti-emetics.

Incisions See Fig. 10.2.

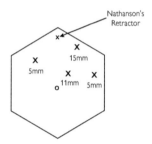

Fig. 10.2 Port sites for laparoscopic gastric banding.

Procedure
- Dissection of the angle of His.
- Division of pars flaccida to right of lesser curve.
- Identification of right crus and the point where fat crosses its lower margin. (This is a consistent laparoscopic finding.)
- Creation of a retrogastric tunnel to the angle of His.
- Introduction of the prepared prosthesis via 15mm port.
- Delivery of the prosthesis from behind stomach.
- Closing the prosthesis with its buckle.
- Securing the prosthesis anteriorly with 2–3 gastrogastric non-absorbable sutures. Plication of cardia over band with reduction in fundal volume recommended.
- Delivering the gastric band tubing.
- Creating a port placement site and tunnelling tubing to this site.
- Attaching tubing to port and securing port to fascia with non-absorbable sutures (Fig. 10.3).
- Re-laparoscoping to pull down excess tubing back into the abdomen.
- Skin closure.

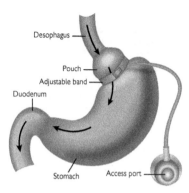

Fig. 10.3 The gastric band.

Post-operative care
Immediate
- Nurse upright in recovery with oxygen.
- Allow sips as tolerated.
- Discharge when oral intake satisfactory.

Follow-up
- The band is placed deflated.
- At first follow-up appointment, the first band fill takes place to a set regime depending on band used.
- A non-coring Huber type needle used to inject 3mL N saline.
- Regular initial follow-up every 4–6 weeks is associated with better weight loss.
- Patients asked to drink two cups of water before leaving department to ensure band is not too tight.

Considerations before band filling
- Patients initially lose 0.5–1kg a week following gastric band insertion.
- What is the degree of restriction.
- Is patient vomiting?
- Has patient got heartburn?
- Does patient suffer symptoms of aspiration?
- A positive answer to the last three questions suggests band too tight and inflation not indicated.
- Poor weight loss, despite adequate band filling and confirmation that the band is in the right place, suggest patient is non-compliant with post-operative instruction, and help of a dietitian and psychologist may help.

Complications
Immediate
Iatrogenic oesophageal and gastric injury is usually caused at the time the retro-gastric tunnel is created by too forceful a dissection.

Early
- *Acute dysphagia:* may be due to band being place around a large quantity of fat that compresses the stomach. Re-operation may be required to remove excess fat and replace same band.
- *Slippage:* post-operative vomiting may lead to early band slippage. Adequate dosage of anti-emetics given during surgery can avoid.
- *Infection:* port site infection (<5%) doesn't usually respond to antibiotics and removal of port recommended. Sometimes whole band needs removing as prosthesis becomes source of recurrent infections.

Late
- *Slippage:*
  - May present with vomiting that may respond to an emergency deflation.
  - Contrast swallow likely to show relatively transverse angle of band with possible dilation of cardia/proximal stomach.
  - If persistent and patient has abdominal pain an emergency laparoscopy with a view to a band removal is advised.
  - Risk of gastric ischaemia proximal to constricting band.
  - Late recognition may mandate emergency total gastrectomy.
- *Erosion:*
  - *Presentation*—weight gain, abdominal pain possible haematemesis.
  - Contrast study may suggest erosion confirmed on endoscopy with presence of a usually blackened band protruding into lumen.
  - *Management*—endoscopic removal using a band cutter or laparoscopic/open removal. Laparoscopy may be complicated by adhesions to abdominal wall and/or liver, associated collections and difficulty in closing gastric defect once eroded band excised.
- *Oesophageal dilatation:*
  - *Risk factors*—band overfilling, symptoms tolerance during adequate weight loss.
  - Reflux symptoms, vomiting, and aspiration are common.
  - Poor diet with nutritional exclusion due to excessive restriction.
  - *Rx*—band deflation, oesophageal damage may be permanent.
- *Leakage:*
  - Poor weight loss and expected fluid volume in the band not observed and patients not having restriction post-fill. This can be due to leaks in the port, tubing, and band itself or a disconnection of tubing (older prosthesis beginning to perish).
  - Investigation of choice is a band fill using an image intensifier to confirm diagnosis. If band itself is leaking (usually damaged when inserted) needs removal. If problem is with port or tubing adjacent to port, then this can be corrected by exchange or tubing excision and re-attachment depending on prosthesis. Performed under local anaesthetic.
- *The flipped port:* access is impossible as Huber hits metal port plate. Revision under local anaesthetic is recommended.
- *Intolerance:* if, despite band being in perfect position, patient cannot tolerate the restrictive nature of their eating behaviour, band will need removing.

Vertical banded gastroplasty (VBG)

Now largely a historic procedure (Fig. 10.4).

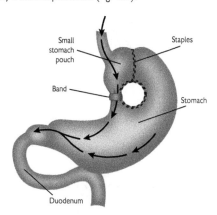

Fig. 10.4 The vertical banded gastroplasty.

Principle
- Restricts the volume of food ingested leading to early satiety and weight loss.
- This operation has been superseded by newer and more successful procedures. It is included as it was at one time a common procedure and patients who have undergone a VBG may be encountered.

Incisions Upper midline laparotomy.

Procedure
- Fashion a circular stapled opening in the stomach 5cm from the GOJ.
- A stapling device is used from this opening and angle of His to separate new pouch from fundus and body of stomach.
- A strip of polypropylene mesh sutured to itself or silastic ring is wrapped around gastrogastric outlet on lesser curvature.

Predicted weight loss 20–30% at 2 years.

Complications
- Erosion of the polypropylene mesh into the gastric lumen.
- Enlargement of the pouch.
- Stomal stenosis.
- Reflux oesophagitis.
- Vertical staple failure.

Sleeve gastrectomy

Principle

The excision of 80% of the stomach leads to reduced gastric volume resulting in early satiety and, hence, weight loss. Excision of fundus decreases circulating Ghrelin, reducing appetite. Originally advocated as first step in gastric bypass surgery, but extensive evidence since 2008 suggests outcomes similar to bypass when used primarily.

Set up Preoperative Tinzaparin, proton pump inhibitors, antibiotic, and anti-emetic administered. A 32–36FG oral gastric tube is place.

Incisions See Fig. 10.5.

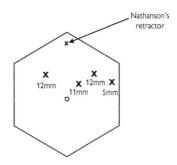

Fig. 10.5 Port sites for sleeve gastrectomy.

Procedure

- The lesser sac is entered by dividing branches of gastro-epiploic vessels with a chosen energy source, e.g. harmonic scalpel or equivalent.
- The greater curvature is fully mobilized to GOJ/angle of His remaining close to gastric wall.
- Dissection proceeds distally to within 5cm of the pylorus.
- Posterior adhesions are divided so stomach can be completely reflected anteromedially.
- 36F Bougie, orogastric tube or endoscope commonly used to size sleeve.
- Single firing of appropriate linear stapler to create a pouch distally.
- Oral gastric tube manipulated into pylorus and duodenum and pulled back to prevent excess tubing in stomach.
- Continual firings of stapler cutter using the intragastric oral gastric tube as a guide on the right.
- Oral gastric tube pulled back and methylene blue test performed to exclude leak from staple line.
- Excised stomach removed by enlarging left upper quadrant 12mm incision (Fig. 10.6).
- Haemostasis at patient's normal BP.
- Close the enlarged port defect.
- Skin closure.

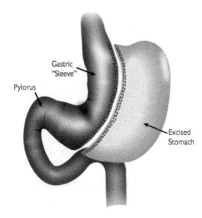

Fig. 10.6 Sleeve gastrectomy.

Post-operative care
- Nurse upright in recovery with oxygen.
- Allow sips as tolerates on the same day.
- Increase oral intake on the 1st post-operative day. Mobilize. Introduce soft diet.
- Home post-operative day 1–3.

Predicted weight loss The predicted excess weight loss at 2 years is 50–60%.

Complications Specific to this operation.

Immediate Splenic injury, bleeding from short gastrics.

Early
- *Staple line leaks:*
  - Failure to progress.
  - *Low grade sepsis*—pyrexia/tachycardia.
  - Contrast swallow may confirm a leak.
  - Chest X-ray may show a left-sided effusion.
  - Early laparoscopy washout, drainage, and placement of a feeding tube indicated. Double lumen NJ tube useful adjunct that allow feeding distal to the leak and drainage proximal and avoid formal feeding jejunostomy.
- *Vomiting:*
  - May be due to too tight a sleeve especially at incisura angularis.
  - If poor response despite liquid diet and balloon dilatation then consider converting to formal gastric bypass.
- *Reflux:*
  - *Despite resecting 80% of the stomach*—reflux due to increase in intraluminal pressure coupled with denervation around the gastro-oesophageal sphincter allowing for a lax tone.

• All patients are on PPI for first 6 months, but this may need to be continued. Persistent symptoms may require a revision to a bypass or placement of a gastric band.

Late
• *Weight gain:*
  • Progressive gastric dilatation allows increased portion size.
  • Re referral to a dietician and psychologist may help.
  • Contrast study may confirm a normal sized stomach and consideration of revisional surgery a sensible choice.
  • Sleeve revised, converted to a gastric bypass or the sleeve banded (Box 10.4).
• *B12 deficiency:* this is a possibility with 80% stomach resected and loss of intrinsic factor. Not universal, but consider B12 supplementation as standard and check blood levels annually as part of follow-up.

Box 10.4 International Sleeve gastrectomy expert panel consensus statement 2011

12,799 cases were examined by the panel. A percentage consensus was indicated.

Patient selection
• Laparoscopic sleeve gastrectomy (LSG) is a valid stand-alone procedure—90.
• LSG is a valid option for patients considered high risk—96.
• LSG is a valid option for transplant candidates (kidney and liver)—96.
• LSG is a valid option for morbidly obese patients with metabolic syndrome—91.
• LSG is a valid option in patients with BMI 30–35kg/m² with associated comorbidities—95.
• LSG is a valid option for patients with irritable bowel disease—86.
• LSG is valid for adolescent morbidly obese patients—77.
• LSG is valid for elderly morbidly obese patients—100.
• Barrett's oesophagus is an absolute contraindication for LSG—81.

Technique
Sizing sleeve
• Optimal bougie size is 32–36F—87.
• Invaginating staple line reduces lumen size—83.
Staple height
• It is not appropriate to use staples with closed height less than that of a blue load (1.5mm) on any part of sleeve gastrectomy—81.
• When using buttressing materials, surgeon should never use any staple with closed height less than that of a green load (2.0mm)—79.
• When resecting the antrum, surgeon should never use any staple with closed height less than that of a green load (2.0mm)—87.
• *First firing:* transection should begin 2–6cm from pylorus—92.
• *Last firing:* it is important to stay away from GOJ on last firing—96.
• *Mobilization:* important to completely mobilize fundus before transection—96.
• Reinforcement staple line to reduce bleeding along staple line—100.

Complications

Managing

- A chronic leak is a leak that has lasted 12 weeks—72.
- Leaks can be classified as acute, early, late, and chronic—73.
- In a patient in whom endoscopic dilation has failed for 6 weeks, reoperation indicated—80.
- Gastric bypass is always the last treatment option for leaks—83.
- A patient with uncontained, symptomatic leak requires immediate reoperation—86.
- Roux-en-Y reconstruction is treatment of choice after failed re-interventions for chronic stricture—88.
- Early leaks those observed 1–6 weeks from 1° procedure—89.
- Stenting has limited utility for chronic leaks—89.
- Patients with fever and tachycardia with normal UGI or other studies require immediate reoperation or re-intervention—90.
- Roux-en-Y reconstruction valid option in proximal chronic leaks—90.
- Stent use for acute proximal leak is a valid treatment option—93.
- The surgeon should wait 12 weeks of conservative Rx before re-operating to convert or revise proximal leak (assumes stable)—94.
- Staple line disruptions can be classified as proximal or distal and they behave differently—95.
- Staple line disruptions can be divided into early and late—95.
- The use of a stent is a valid treatment for an acute proximal leak that has failed conservative therapy—95.
- Staple line disruptions can be classified as proximal or distal—100.
- Staple line disruptions behave differently based on anatomic location—100.
- Acute leaks; those observed within 7 days of primary procedure—100.
- Late leaks are those observed after 6 weeks—100.
- Early strictures are symptomatic in first 6 weeks after surgery—100.
- The smaller the bougie size, the tighter the sleeve, the greater the stricture rate—78.

Avoiding

- The smaller the bougie size, the tighter the sleeve, the greater the incidence of leaks—70.
- When over-sewing, the surgeon should always over-sew with the bougie in place—78.
- Maintaining symmetric lateral traction while stapling will reduce the potential for strictures—75.

Reproduced from 'International Sleeve Gastrectomy Expert Panel Consensus Statement: best practice guidelines based on experience of >12,000 cases', Rosenthal RJ; International Sleeve Gastrectomy Expert Panel, Diaz AA, et al., *Surg ObesRelat Dis* Jan–Feb; 8(1): 8–19, copyright 2012 with permission of Elsevier.

Laparoscopic Roux-en-Y gastric bypass

Principle

The creation of a small stomach pouch leads to early satiety combined with the bypassing of the stomach, duodenum, and up to 200cm of jejunum leading to malabsorption. Release of distal gut hormones and changes in taste also have a role in the mechanism of action.

Set up Preoperative tinzaparin, proton pump inhibitors, antibiotic, and antiemetic administered. A 14–16FG NGT is placed orally.

Incisions See Fig. 10.7.

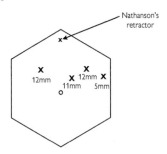

Fig. 10.7 Port sites for laparoscopic Roux-en-Y gastric bypass.

Procedure

- Access to the lesser sac is achieved by dissection of the lesser omentum from the lesser curvature of the stomach 5–6cm distal from the GOJ.
- A single firing of a stapler cutting device is made at right angles to the stomach.
- Continuous firings of stapler cutting device are made at right angles to the first firing up to and including angle of His to create a gastric pouch.
- An enterotomy is made at end of new stomach pouch.
- The greater omentum is retracted cranially and ligament of Trietz identified.
- Loop of proximal jejunum is mobilized with 'omega' configuration.
- Anastomosis is made between stomach pouch and omega loop of small bowel.
- NGT is placed under vision into stomach pouch before anastomosis is completed.
- Between 100–150cm of efferent jejunum is measured and a side to side anastomosis fashioned between efferent loop and afferent loop of jejunum within 15cm of gastrojejunal anastomosis.
- A methylene blue test is conducted to assess both anastomoses.
- Afferent limb between gastrojejunal anastomosis and jejuno-anastomosis divided completing laparoscopic Roux-en-Y (Fig. 10.8).
- Skin closure.

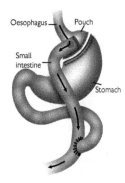

Fig. 10.8 Roux-en-Y gastric bypass.

Technical points
- Multiple approaches to performing operation. Anastomoses can be all stapled, hand-sewn or a mixture of both. Staplers used can be linear or for gastro-jejunostomy using a circular stapler via trans-oral technique as described by Gagner.
- Gastrojejunal anastomosis can be ante colic as described or retrocolic.
- Pouch should be no more than 20–30mL in volume.
- Greater omentum can be divided to facilitate mobilization of omega loop, but this is not mandatory.
- There is no perceived benefit of making alimentary limb more than 100cm in patients with BMI <50kg/m^2, but for patients with a BMI >50kg/m^2 a limb of at least 150cm is advised.
- There is no general consensus with respect to closing mesenteric defects to avoid internal hernias.
- There is no need for the NGT to remain in situ nor to place an abdominal drain routinely.

Post-operative care
Immediate
- Nurse upright in recovery with oxygen.
- Allow sips as tolerates on the same day.
- Increase oral intake on the 1st post-operative day. Mobilize. Introduce soft diet.
- Home post-operative day 1–3.

Predicted weight loss
The predicted excess weight loss at 2 years is 60–80%.

Complications
Immediate
- Bleeding.
- Usually along the staple line. Can be controlled with ligaclips or sutures.

Early
- *Anastomotic leak:* this needs to be excluded as a matter of urgency if the patient is unwell and tachycardic post-operatively. Re-laparoscopy is preferable to imaging that will only delay a return to theatre.
- *Anastomotic strictures:* occur in about 5–10% of anastomosis and are more common when a circular stapler is used for the gastrojejeunal anastomosis size 21mm. Presents with retrosternal pain and vomiting to solid food. Can be treated with a series of balloon dilatations with good effect. A jejuno-jejunal anastomotic stricture may be diagnosed by the presence of a normal post-operative appearance at endoscopy and a contrast study/CT showing a dilated alimentary limb. Revisional surgery may be required.
- *Anastomotic bleeding:* usually self-limiting, but if continuous a combination of endoscopic injection therapy and laparoscopy may be required.
- *Dehydration and constipation:* a common problem as patients must get used to drinking on a regular basis. Re-education and occasional laxatives advised.
- *Dumping syndrome:* a carbohydrate load into the jejunum causes a shift of body fluids into lumen along with over-production of insulin. This leads to patients feeling very unwell and light headed, and sometimes is associated with passing of loose stool. Re-education of patient with avoidance of precipitating foods stuffs.
- *Anastomotic ulcers:* more common in smokers and patients who are *H. pylori* positive. If the ulcer is resistant to simple pharmacological measures then a fistula between the pouch and remaining stomach must be excluded. May require revisional surgery.

Late
- *Nutritional and vitamin deficiencies:* patient education, thorough preoperative work up and regular follow-up avoids most problems. Patient compliance is the biggest cause of such problems. Vitamin supplementation on a daily basis is essential and a B12 injection at maintenance dose usually suffices. Annual bloods including calcium, vitamin D, and trace elements allows for fine tuning of nutrients.
- *Internal hernia:*
  - More common with the laparoscopic compared to open approach and occur at three sites. Incidence is 0.2–9%.
  - Petersen's hernia is a hernia in the defect created between Roux limb anteriorly and transverse mesocolon posteriorly.
  - A hernia can occur behind biliopancreatic limb and Roux limb at jejunjenostomy.
  - If retrocolic route is used for Roux limb a defect can occur in transverse mesocolon.
  - High index of suspicion is required in all patients with abdominal pain with or without small bowel obstruction. Delayed diagnosis may lead to life-threatening complications. Closure of potential defects at time of 1° surgery is not, however, universal.
- *Hypersideroblastosis:* this uncommon problem is due to hyperplasia of the B cells of the pancreas as a result of excessive weight loss giving rise to a chronic hypoglycaemia picture. Pancreatic resection may be required.

Bilio-pancreatic diversion

Principle Combination of initial restrictive, but ultimately malabsorption.

Incisions See Fig. 10.9.

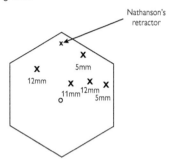

Fig. 10.9 Port sites for bilio-pancreatic diversion.

Procedure

- Ileum divided 260–360cm (depending on BMI) proximal to the ileocaecal junction.
- Jejunal-ileal anastomosis fashioned 60cm proximal to terminal ileum.
- Distal gastrectomy performed leaving a proximal stomach volume of 150–400mL.
- Gastro-jejunal anastomosis fashioned.
- Cholecystectomy performed.
- Resected stomach excised (Fig. 10.10).

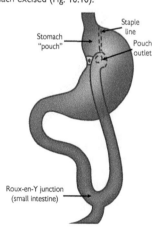

Fig. 10.10 Bilio-pancreatic diversion (Scopinaro)

Predicted weight loss 70–80% excess weight loss at 2 years.

Complications
- Anastomotic leak.
- Dumping syndrome.
- Anastomotic ulcers.
- Anastomotic strictures.
- Bone demineralization.
- Vitamin deficiency.
- Protein deficiency.
- Diarrhoea.
- Foul smelling stool.
- Anaemia.

Bilio-pancreatic diversion with duodenal switch
Principle
- Mildly restrictive and mainly malabsorption.
- A modification of the BPD incorporating a sleeve gastrectomy and longer common limb.

Incisions See Fig. 10.11.

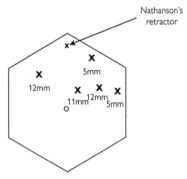

Fig. 10.11 Port sites for bilio-pancreatic diversion with duodenal switch

Procedure
- Sleeve gastrectomy fashioned.
- Duodenum divided 4cm distal to the pylorus.
- Small bowel divided at mid-point.
- Distal small bowel anastomosed to duodenum.
- Proximal small bowel anastomosed to ileum 100 proximal to terminal ileum.
- Cholecystectomy performed (Fig. 10.12).

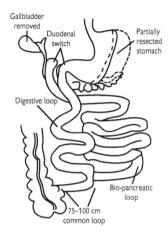

Fig. 10.12 Bilio-pancreatic diversion with duodenal switch.

Predicted weight loss 75–80 % excess weight loss at 2 years.

Complications
- Anastomotic leak.
- Dumping syndrome (less likely than a Scopinaro procedure).
- Anastomotic ulcers (less likely than a Scopinaro procedure).
- Anastomotic strictures.
- Bone demineralization.
- Vitamin deficiency.
- Protein deficiency.
- Diarrhoea.
- Foul smelling stool.
- Anaemia.

Gastric balloon
- A gastric balloon offers a non-surgical approach to weight management. It is a useful adjunct in the staged management of the super morbid obese (BMI >50kg/m^2) to aid weight loss before definitive surgical treatment. It has a license to be used with patients with a BMI >27kg/m^2, but this is a group not seen on the NHS. HH and previous gastric surgery contraindicate their placement.
- Procedure involves the placement of a soft silicone balloon filled with either saline or air inside the stomach. Inducing satiety. Fluid filled balloon systems are the commonest in the UK. The 15–20min procedure is performed as a day case in the endoscopy unit with sedation or pharyngeal local anaesthetic.

Steps
- A gastroscopy is performed to ensure no ulceration or large HH noting the position of GOJ.
- The gastroscope is removed.
- The deflated balloon is placed into the hypopharynx and patient asked to swallow balloon.
- A repeat gastroscopy is performed and balloon in filled with 400–700mL of methylene blue-stained saline under direct vision.
- Gastroscope is removed and inflation tubing pulled away from the self-sealing gastric balloon (Fig. 10.13).
- Patient is given an anti-emetic before procedure and is discharged with a week's supply of anti-emetic and PPI, continued for 6/12 until balloon is removed.
- Patients will feel nauseous and will vomit for first 3–4 days and must be made aware of this. This soon settles.
- Removal after 6 months involves a repeat gastroscopy with insertion of a needle on a suction tube. The balloon is deflated and removed. Very few people experience side effects.
- Expected mean weight loss is 15–18kg over 6 months. Rarely do the balloons rupture and patients are advised to report the passage of green/blue urine.
- Deflated balloon needs removal as it can be the cause of small bowel obstruction.

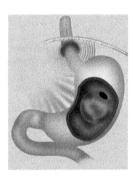

Fig. 10.13 Intragastric balloon.

Choice of procedure
Ultimately, it is the decision of the informed patient. Information should be made readily available in written form and by access to informative websites, e.g. British Obesity Surgical Patients Association and British Obesity (BOSPA) and British Obesity Metabolic Surgical Society (BOMSS).

Points to consider
- *Eating pattern:*
  - *Melt calorie consumers*—chocoholics, sweet eaters, and ice-cream relatively poor outcomes with pure restrictive procedures. Rapid transit through upper GI tract unrestricted in liquid form with all their associated calories and no sense of satiety.
  - Confirmed volume eaters may do well with a restrictive operation.
  - Emotional eaters better off with a bypass or malabsorbative procedure.
- *Age:*
  - Associated with co-morbidities and relatively poor performance status in obese patients.
  - Entrenched poor eating habits will be difficult to alter.
- *Sex:* Operation on males more demanding due to increased distribution of intra-abdominal fat.
- *High BMI:* consider a staged procedure, e.g. a balloon or sleeve gastrectomy before definitive surgery, e.g. a bypass of BPD.
- *Social isolation or rural home setting:* is a gastric band where regular follow-up and input from the bariatric team the best for patients from a rural setting?
- *Risk:* a parent with a dependent young family may not relish higher risk of BPD or gastric bypass, and opt for a lesser procedure. Many patients don't want to take the risk of a larger more complex procedure and opt for a lesser 'safer' operation.
- *Potential cancer risks:* little evidence; however, young patients with a history of a previous colonic malignancy or patients with pernicious anaemia are at a greater risk of upper GI malignancy hence avoid gastric bypass that excludes the majority of the stomach from endoscopy.
- *Previous small bowel resection and Crohns' disease:* may lead to significant malabsorption problem and vitamin deficiencies.
- *Patient medication with malabsorative procedures:* it is sometimes impossible to predict the pharmacodynamics of certain drugs following a gastric bypass. Changes in pH may either increase or decrease absorption with associated side effects. Certain drugs can be measured, e.g. lithium and anti-epileptics; many others cannot.

Relative contraindications
- Patient understanding.
- Poor motivation preoperatively.
- Poor attendance record at outpatients.

The only predictor of a patient's future behaviour is their past behaviour. If there is a history of non-attendance preoperatively, then there is a high risk of failure to follow-up.

Nutrition and dietetics

Role of the bariatric dietitian is essential in educating, advising, and supporting the obese patient at all stages of care.

Initial consultation

A comprehensive dietary history is taken with respect to:
- *Frequency of main meals:* many obese patients omit breakfast and shift workers have erratic eating patterns. The importance of regular meals is emphasized.
- *Pattern of eating:*
  - Volume eater vs. sweet-eater vs. grazer vs. combination of all three.
  - Helps to identify which operation most suitable, e.g. a restrictive procedure may be more beneficial in a volume eater compared with malabsorption.
- Healthy food choices.
- Calorific intake.
- Advising on a calorie controlled diet.
- Educating on importance of meal planning and basic cooking skills.
- *Portion size:* supply patients with an annotated plate that divides plate up into the major food groups and normal portion size.
- *Alcohol intake:* alcohol is calorie rich and consumption in excess is the cause of weight gain.

Preoperative liver reduction diet

Design a low carbohydrate and low fat diet to reduce glycogen storage of the liver to allow the likelihood of successful laparoscopic bariatric surgery. The diet starts 14 days prior to surgery.

Post-operative diet Initially all post-operative diets are similar with respect to liquids, followed by a pureed diet, then softer foods, then solids.

Gastric band/sleeve

- After a period of 4–6 weeks patients should be having 3 meals/day with no snacking between meals.
- Patients advised not to eat and drink at same time, to chew food well, not to rush their food and stop eating when they feel full.
- *Foods to avoid:* chocolate, ice cream, alcohol, and sweets that will easily pass through band/sleeve in a large volume without resulting satiety, but with all calories.
- Bread and large bolus of meat and fibrous vegetables should also be avoided, as they can cause bolus obstruction.

Gastric bypass

- Patients easily get dehydrated and constipated, and are advised to carry water with them at all times and sip continually. Ideally, patients should aim for 1.5–2L/day.
- *Highly restrictive gastric pouch:* patients advised to eat low volume meals frequently up to 6 times a day.
- A carbohydrate load can lead to dumping. Patients must take multivitamins with minerals and expect a B12 injection.

BPD and BPD with switch

Similar to a bypass, but requires a post-operative diet high in protein (60–80g) initially.

Revision bariatric surgery

- As the number of 1° bariatric procedures increases so does the rate of re-operations as a consequence of either a failed 1° procedure or complication.
- Redo bariatric surgery is associated with a higher mortality (2%) and morbidity (13% leak rate) compared with the 1° operation.
- Important to evaluate cause of failure.
- ? Technical failure or poor patient compliance?
- Discussion at the bariatric MDT is important in managing such patients with re-referral to both dietetics and psychology.

Anatomical assessment

- Plain radiography, contrast swallows, and contrast follow through studies are essential for a 'road map' of the surgically altered anatomy of the upper GI tract.
- Endoscopy useful adjunct looking at eroded bands, anastomotic strictures, ulcers, and assessing pouch sizes.
- Blood tests are needed for a full haematological and biochemical profile including trace elements and vitamin D.

Gastric band

Gastric bands are removable and the indications for removal are:
- Slippage.
- Infected system.
- Erosion.
- Damaged/leaking band.
- Intolerance.

Revision of the tubing and/or injection port is indicated for leakage from the tube and flipped port, respectively.

The surgical options once a band is removed are:
- Insertion of another band.
- Gastric bypass.
- Sleeve gastrectomy.

Sleeve gastrectomy

Surgical options following a sleeve gastrectomy are conversion to:
- Gastric bypass.
- BPD with switch.
- Banded sleeve.

Vertical banded gastroplasty

Surgical options following a VBG are conversion to:
- Sleeve gastrectomy.
- Gastric bypass.

Other revisional surgical approaches

- Reversal of jejunal-ileal bypasess (an operation now obsolete because of high incidence of malabsorption).
- Reversal/revision of Roux-en-Y gastric bypass and BPD/switch for malabsorption.
- Removal of eroded pre-anastomotic rings in Roux-en-Y bypass pouches (e.g. Fobi ring).
- Revision of gastric pouches, gastrojejunostomies, jejunal-jejunostomies, remnant gastrectomies for enlargements, strictures, and gastrogastric fistulae, respectively.

Upper gastrointestinal perforation

Oesophageal perforation

Traumatic injury to the oesophagus, in response to a variety of insults, is an unusual, but serious, potentially devastating event which can be hard to diagnose and extremely difficult to treat.

In an era of increasing use of endoscopy and therapeutic interventional techniques the majority of oesophageal injuries are iatrogenic more readily diagnosed than spontaneous perforation, but often occur in the presence of concomitant disease and can present equally difficult management dilemmas relative rarity of oesophageal injury means that wide experience of such problems is unusual. However, centralization of surgical services for oesophagogastric cancer does bring the potential for development of such experience and expertise.

Pathophysiology

Following a perforation, negative intrathoracic pressure leads to air, food, and fluids being drawn into the mediastinum and pleural cavity, causing to a chemical pleuromediastinitis. This leads to bacterial mediastinitis, septic shock, and multi-organ failure if adequate drainage is not performed:

- *If treated:* mortality 20–75%.
- Left untreated, condition has a mortality approaching 100%.

Spontaneous perforation (Boerhaave's syndrome)

Presentation and assessment

Aetiology There is a large increase in intra-abdominal pressure, generally due to pronounced vomiting parturition, defaecation, status epilepticus, and Heimlich manoeuvre.

Site of perforation Distal oesophagus on left side > mid-oesophagus on the right.

Clinical features

Mackler's Triad

- Vomiting or retching (90–100%), chest pain (90%), and sub-cutaneous emphysema (38%) on examination.
- Classic triad unusual as patients can also present with other respiratory or upper abdominal symptoms, or general signs of sepsis.
- Differential diagnosis encompasses a wide range of chest and abdominal disorders (Box 11.1) contributing to the difficulty in diagnosis. Patients often present late with severe sepsis in ITU with a diagnosis made on CT.
- A high degree of clinical suspicion is important as delay in diagnosis is likely to contribute to the high morbidity of the condition.

Box 11.1 Spontaneous perforation of the oesophagus: differential diagnosis
- Acute myocardial infarction.
- Pneumonia.
- Spontaneous pneumothorax.
- Pericarditis.
- Acute presentation of diaphragmatic hernia.
- Dissecting aortic aneurysm.
- Pancreatitis.
- Perforated duodenal/gastric ulcer.
- Gastric volvulus.
- Mesenteric ischaemia.

Assessment Detailed history of the presenting episode as well as relevant co-morbidities, especially as major surgery may be required.

Clinical examination
- Sepsis and/or shock, including sweating, tachycardia, and tachypnoea. Subcutaneous emphysema developing around the neck and upper torso.
- Systemic inflammatory response syndrome (SIRS) and multiple organ dysfunction syndrome (MODS) common.

Investigation
Radiology
- Chest X-ray signs often subtle or not evident at all, but include pneumo-mediastinum (43%), pleural effusion—unilateral (71%), bilateral (14%), sub-cutaneous emphysema, and hydro-pneumothorax.
- Re-inforces importance of maintaining high index of suspicion and if perforation is suspected then further investigation, water-soluble contrast swallow is required, which may well confirm diagnosis and give an indication of level, site, size of rupture, and extent to which this may be contained.
- *CT with oral and IV contrast:* delineates size of collections, presence of active leak, and information with regard to the disease process, such as respiratory problems or the presence of malignancy with metastatic disease (Fig. 11.1 and Fig. 11.2).

Endoscopy
Endoscopy is vital and in patients with confirmed perforation who are undergoing surgical treatment it may be performed as the first step in theatre following resuscitation and anaesthesia.

Performed carefully, it is safe and allows visualization of the site and size of the tear. It is more sensitive than radiology for small leaks and should be performed in patients with a high suspicion of diagnosis, but negative radiology, even if only to demonstrate a normal upper GI tract.

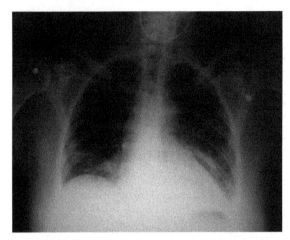

Fig. 11.1 Chest X-ray showing pneumomediastinum.

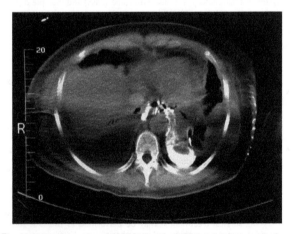

Fig. 11.2 CT scan demonstrating leak of oral contrast into left pleural cavity from lower oesophagus.

Management

The key to management is early vigorous resuscitation (concomitantly with investigation) early drainage, antibiotics, aggressive organ support, and response to 2° sepsis (Box 11.2).

Box 11.2 Initial resuscitation of patients with oesophageal perforation

- High flow oxygen.
- Wide bore cannulae and IV fluids.
- Broad-spectrum antibiotics.
- Anti-fungal agents.
- Analgesia.
- NBM.
- Wide bore chest drain.
- Close monitoring with urinary catheter arterial line and CVP.
- Early anaesthetic involvement.
- Cardiorespiratory support as required.

Operative or non-operative intervention

- Non-operative Rx feasible in patients with small leaks where mediastinal and pleural contamination minimal.
- Vast majority of patients are likely to require surgery if fit.
- Non-operative management patients require intense monitoring in critical care setting and close attention to nutrition, with team being prepared to resort to surgery should clinical course deem this necessary.

Surgery for perforated oesophagus

- Preferably within 24h, but even delayed surgery improves prognosis (100% mortality 14% for late presenting cases when operative intervention performed.
- Numerous techniques described; aim in all is debridement, lavage, and drainage of affected regions (mediastinal, pleural, or abdominal), and management of perforation, such to allow healing with reduced contiguous intrathoracic or abdominal sepsis.
- Endoscopy important as mucosal tear likely to be longer than the external muscular tear.

Thoracotomy

- Left for distal perforations or right for more proximal.
- Oesophagus can be mobilized from right to give access to left-sided surface.
- *Laparotomy still required:* allows insertion of a feeding jejunostomy for nutrition and placement of a gastrostomy for prolonged gastric drainage.

Primary laparotomy

- May be extended to a thoraco-abdominal approach as necessary.
- Hiatus mobilized and transhiatal access to perioesophageal mediastinal collection gained—drained as necessary. If evidence of minimal pleural contamination, transhiatal mediastinal drains placed prior to management of tear. If any evidence of significant contamination, pleural access widened, lavage, debridement, and drain placement bilaterally.

- Transhiatal approach associated with increased re-operation rate compared to thoracotomy, but does not translate into increased mortality or length of ITU stay overall.

Management of perforation

Influencing factors Time since presentation, degree of mediastinal and pleural soiling, and the general condition of the patient.

Primary repair
- Simple closure of perforation with drainage described for several decades.
- May be successful in those with little contamination and who are taken to theatre early, subsequent leak rate high associated with prolonged morbidity and high mortality.

Repair and re-inforcement
Use of intercostal muscle, pleura, and omentum described to re-inforce a 1° repair, but expertise in the use of the first two of these is limited and risk of leak is still high.

T-tube repair: creation of a controlled fistula
- This was initially described for late presentations, but it is equally useful in sick patients who present early.
- A large bore T-tube is placed into oesophagus via tear, which is sutured closed around tube, if feasible (oesophageal tissue likely to be very friable and may not hold sutures well).
- Aim of approach is to allow a controlled fistula to develop to minimize further sepsis. Wide bore drains are placed in mediastinum, pleural cavities, and upper abdominal cavity (Fig. 11.3).

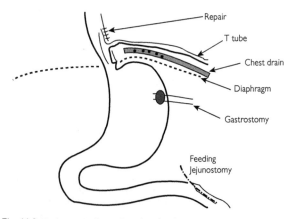

Fig. 11.3 T-tube repair of oesophageal perforation.

Resection
- Some advocate this as an approach as it rids patient of source of sepsis.
- In contaminated cases this involves creation of cervical oesophagostomy and delayed reconstruction when patient has recovered.
- May be mandated in presence of strictures, but should not be used indiscriminately due to morbidity of reconstruction procedure and poor HRQL associated with oesophagostomy.

Exclusion and diversion
- Cervical oesophagostomy, distal oesophageal transection.
- Useful in patients unfit to undergo a thoracotomy.
- Exclusion and diversion procedures are required in very rare circumstances. In conditions of persistent leak and continuing sepsis, or those patients not fit to undergo a major procedure they could be life-saving if performed early. As it is a relatively easy and quick procedure it should be considered early as a second line management option.
- Subsequent reconstruction complex.

Post-operative care
- Supportive in a critical care environment.
- Antibiotics and anti-fungal agents are prescribed and jejunal feeding instituted.
- It is important to maintain close observation for subsequent signs of sepsis or failure to improve, as mediastinitis may run a prolonged insidious course with development of further collections requiring radiological or surgical intervention.

Other techniques
- Covered SEMS.
- Advocated where minimal contamination present or in unfit elderly patients.
- Drainage of any associated sepsis is also important.
- Stent migration is a potential problem.
- *David, 2011 MD Anderson Centre USA:* 56/63 patients over 38/12 treated with covered SEMS—30 required thoracic intervention post-stent. 30-day mortality 10%. 23% failure to salvage oesophagus.

Minimally invasive approach
- VATS thoracoscopic lavage and debridement.
- T tube placed endoscopically into chest through defect and retrieved thoracoscopically.
- Hybrid radiological drainage and T tube insertion via guide wire introduced orally, and then retrieved via chest drain.

Iatrogenic perforation

This is more common than spontaneous perforation due to the high number of endoscopic procedures performed (Table 11.1). Although injury is often recognized at the time, this is not always the case and a high index of suspicion must be maintained in patients who do not recover quickly as expected after these procedures.

Table 11.1 Causes of iatrogenic perforation of the oesophagus

Rigid oesophagoscopy	Diagnostic
	Therapeutic: foreign body removal
Diagnostic flexible endoscopy	
Therapeutic endoscopy	Stricture dilatation
	Dilatation of achalasia
	Stent placement
	Laser and other endoscopic therapies
Radiological procedures	Stent placement
Surgery (open or laparoscopic/thoracoscopic)	Anti-reflux/HH surgery
	Cardio-myotomy for achalasia
	Bariatric surgery (placement of gastric band)
	Thoracic surgery
	Tracheostomy
	Spinal surgery

Site of injury
- Vast majority at site of pathology under investigation or treatment (see Table 11.1), largely distal oesophagus.
- Proximal injury to the cervical oesophagus can occur during difficult intubation in patients with neck problems or high strictures.

Presentation
- If not recognized at the time of injury patients may develop symptoms at any time over the next few minutes, hours, or days.
- Chest or abdominal pain, dyspnoea, fever.
- *Clinical signs:* surgical emphysema and general signs of sepsis.
- High index of suspicion essential in post procedure sepsis.

Investigation
- Water soluble contrast swallow and CT scan are key to determining the presence, site, and size of perforation together with extent of any leakage and whether such a leak is contained.

- If malignancy present or suspected CT assists staging and may influence decisions about the aggressiveness of management.
- Endoscopy useful depending on nature of the injury.

Management
Endoscopic Endoscopic closure using clips achievable where small perforations are immediately detected and local expertise exists.

Established perforations
Initial management
- Vigorous resuscitation with IV fluids, antibiotics, and anti-fungal agents, and cardiorespiratory support as necessary.
- Resuscitation should be performed in tandem with investigation as is deemed appropriate, given clinical condition of patient.
- A key decision will be whether to proceed with surgery or if non-operative treatment is appropriate.

Non-operative management
- Appropriate in patients who are clinically stable with no signs of sepsis and in whom the perforation appears contained.
- Localized collections may be drainable with radiological control. Broad-spectrum antibiotics and antifungal agents are required as is attention to nutrition.
- Placement of double or triple lumen NJ tube allowing gastric drainage, but enteral feeding is of use.
- High (cervical oesophageal) perforation usually heals spontaneously in absence of local pathology.
- In patients with malignant strictures placement of a stent may help seal iatrogenic perforations and deal with distal obstruction that is required for healing.
- All patients who do not undergo surgery should be closely monitored for signs of systemic sepsis as this may change the course of management.
- In advanced malignancy surgery is likely to be inappropriate regardless of degree of sepsis and this may be a terminal event.

Operative management
Indications for surgery include:
- *Clinical sepsis, gross leakage, and contamination:* underlying pathology (especially stricture) and failed non-operative treatment.
- Although principles of surgery are same as for spontaneous perforation, resection is far more likely to be considered in presence of stricture, malignant, or otherwise.
- Condition of patient, degree of soiling, and nature of pathology dictate whether a 1° reconstruction can be performed or if cervical oesophagostomy and delayed reconstruction is more appropriate.
- Evidence that dilatation (in itself) and perforation of a tumour lead to a worse outcome with regard to recurrence. However, decisions about surgery in the emergency setting should be made on an individual basis.

Traumatic perforation

Penetrating trauma
- Cervical oesophagus can be involved in stab injuries to neck where damage to any structures in vicinity of stab would be considered. Mortality 9–19%.
- Thoracic oesophagus relatively well protected and more likely to be damaged by gunshot injuries.
- Investigation and management is generally influenced by pattern of other injuries and priorities, but endoscopy is most valuable tool for assessing oesophageal integrity.

Blunt trauma
- Blunt traumatic perforation is rare as the oesophagus is generally well-protected in the chest.
- Severe neck flexion-extension injury may affect the cervical oesophagus and sudden deceleration may lead to damage at fixed points, such as the cricoid; a high index of suspicion is important in such cases.
- Major blunt chest injury is generally associated with more significant life-threatening injuries, which take immediate priority.

Ingestion injuries

Caustic injury
Injury due to strong acid or alkali generally follows two patterns:
- Children who sustain injury due to accidental ingestion.
- Adults in whom ingestion is often purposeful as a mode of attempted suicide.

Both lead to significant damage:
- *Acid:* coagulative necrosis.
- *Alkali potentially more harmful:* liquefactive necrosis, rapid damage, perforation, and mediastinitis.
- If perforation does not occur there is subsequent sloughing, granulation tissue formation, and late stricture.

Presentation
- A *history of ingestion:* nature, amount, and timing.
- Mouth burns may or may not be present agent often swallowed quickly and easily, especially in the case of alkalis.
- Pain, nausea, and retching are common; dyspnoea is a worrying sign indicating aspiration or airway oedema.

Investigation
- Investigations may yield little.
- *Chest X-ray:* pneumomediastinum in case of perforation.
- CT is also useful in such cases.
- Carefully endoscopy is important to determine the severity and extent of oesophageal damage.

Management
- Early resuscitation.
- Chemical neutralization and steroids both controversial and therefore cannot be recommended as routine.
- Most case will recover, but will require further endoscopic examination for the development of stricture.
- If evidence of full thickness oesophageal injury and perforation an emergency oesophagectomy will be required, with a decision about primary reconstruction or diversion and subsequent reconstruction.
- Patients who do recover have an increased risk of stricture formation which is likely to require repeated bougie dilatation.
- Long tight strictures require repeated dilatation which carries significant risk, surgical resection often required as an alternative.
- Patients with such caustic damage also have an increased risk of malignant change.

Foreign body ingestion
- Patients presenting to hospital due to problems with foreign body ingestion may be dealt with general or ear, nose, and throat surgeons or paediatricians.
- Children tend to swallow small objects such as toys or coins whereas adults generally present with problems due to food bolus—meat, bone, or fruit peel.
- *Those with dentures have a higher incidence due to reduced palate sensation:* patients may swallow their false teeth!
- The cervical oesophagus is a common site of impaction and such problems are generally dealt with by the ear, nose, and throat surgeons using a rigid oesophagoscope, which generally affords a better view of the pharynx and upper oesophagus despite its risk.

Presentation
- Often a clear history of ingestion or at least a good indication of what may have been ingested.
- Dysphagia and retching are common in cases with oesophageal impaction; foreign bodies in the stomach are generally asymptomatic unless there is perforation.
- Dyspnoea if impaction is near trachea or bronchi and if there is doubt about the site of impaction bronchoscopy may be necessary.
- Little abnormal on examination.

Investigation
- Plain radiography is the key investigation for radio-opaque objects and this is usually all that is required.
- Endoscopy generally therapeutic.
- Rigid oesophagoscopy is appropriate for upper oesophageal impaction, but for anything below this level then flexible endoscopy is preferable. Rigid oesophagoscopy of the lower oesophagus is associated with significant risk.

Management
- Endoscopic removal is treatment of choice for objects lodged within the oesophagus.
- Can be both difficult and dangerous, especially as some objects can erode through oesophageal wall and, in such cases, persistence with endoscopic technique can be dangerous.
- In some cases surgery may be necessary.
- Once objects reach stomach they generally pass through GI tract (except for long objects such as cutlery) and can be left.
- *Battery ingestion may cause:* gastric or intestinal erosion.
- Conservative approach appropriate if patient remains asymptomatic.

Gastric perforation

Spontaneous perforation

Causes
- Majority due to peptic ulcer disease although there are more unusual causes (Table 11.2).
- Gastric volvulus and strangulated HH can lead to perforation if all or part of stomach wall is rendered ischaemic.
- Although stomach has a good blood supply, on occasions severe foregut ischaemia can lead to gastric ischaemia and perforation, although such patients will usually be very unwell before the perforation is manifest.

Table 11.2 Causes of gastric perforation

Spontaneous	Peptic ulceration
	Perforated carcinoma
	Gastric volvulus
	Strangulated hiatus hernia
	Ischaemic disorders
Traumatic	Surgery
	Endoscopic/PEG complications
	Ventriculoperitoneal (VP) shunt
	VP shunt complication
	Sharp foreign body
	Erosion by battery
	Stab wound
	Blunt abdominal trauma (rare)

Presentation
- Peritonitis associated with varying degrees of shock.
- If perforation is in thorax in the case of strangulated HH, then patient is likely to have chest symptoms and general signs of severe sepsis, with little or no evidence of peritonitis.
- There are some instances where patients do not have abdominal symptoms or signs, but chest X-rays taken for other reasons indicate a pneumoperitoneum.
- *Perforated peptic ulcer is a common cause:* perforations frequently sealed by a plug of omentum or another viscus before significant soiling and peritonitis occurs.

Investigation
- Pneumo-peritoneum on erect chest X-ray absent in majority of cases.
- If generalized peritonitis diagnosis confirmed at laparotomy or laparoscopy.
- CT useful where diagnostic uncertainty in relatively well patient with sealed perforation.

Management
Operative or non-operative
- *Contributory factors:* general condition of patient, poor pre-morbid status, significant co-morbidities, and complicated pathology.
- Most cases within remit of general surgeon, but perforation due to strangulated HH in chest, better dealt with by dedicated upper GI surgeon.

Non-operative management
- Asymptomatic patients:
  - Pneumoperitoneum has co-incidentally been discovered.
  - CT to investigate pneumoperitoneum.
  - Early endoscopy is inadvisable because of the risk of insufflation disrupting the plug which has sealed any gastroduodenal perforation that may be present. Should be performed at some stage to exclude malignancy.
  - Treatment with antibiotics and PPIs is instituted, and in case of upper GI perforation a NBM policy is initially adopted.
  - Close observation as the development of sepsis or peritonitis may alter treatment radically and surgery may be required.
- Unfit patients:
  - Advanced peritonitis and sepsis in patients with significant co-morbidity and/or poor pre-morbid function as it may be deemed that they are unlikely to survive.
  - Important to discuss the implications with the patient and family.
  - Perforation of an advanced gastric cancer may be another indication for pursuing a conservative course.

Operative management
- Midline laparotomy:
  - Identify site and nature of the pathology.
  - Peritoneal washout with several litres of warm saline.
  - Tissue biopsies from the edge of ulcer because of risk of malignancy, even in benign-looking condition.

- May be possible to excise ulcer, which allows closure of 'healthy' gastric tissue, as well as providing histology.
- Consider distal gastrectomy if closure difficult.
- Closure with an omental patch, as in duodenal perforation, feasible in distal, or pre-pyloric ulceration.
- Management of a perforated gastric tumour at laparotomy is more difficult, especially with regard to decision-making. Even in cases of benign ulceration with perforation tissue can be oedematous and swollen and have appearances of a neoplasm.
- Decision to resect difficult, especially in unstable patients.
- If any doubt as to how to proceed, immediate patient safety must come first, with peritoneal lavage and drainage a priority.
- Perforated HH or gastric volvulus, when part or all of stomach may be in chest, present extremely difficult scenarios, even for specialized oesophagogastric surgeons.
- Surgery in this situation may require thoracotomy, resection, and then a decision to be made regarding primary or delayed reconstruction, as outlined in 📖 Spontaneous perforation (Boerhaave's syndrome), p. 328.
- *Operative management of the difficult perforated duodenal ulcer:*
  - Surgical management of a perforated duodenal ulcer (usually anterior D1) is generally straightforward, with an omental patch being fashioned after peritoneal lavage.
  - Large perforation may lead to the duodenum appearing to disintegrate and it may not be feasible to deal with it in usual way.
  - Various methods described to deal with difficult duodenum.
  - Finney pyloroplasty involves fully kocherizing duodenum and opening it longitudinally along most of its length. It is then closed transversely in similar fashion to simple pyloroplasty.
  - More often, however, it may be necessary to exclude or excise ulcer, close duodenum distally, and excise gastric antrum.

Traumatic perforation

Presentation and management

Major trauma

- Suspicion of gastric injury due to penetrating or blunt injury, management is along the lines of ATLS principles.
- Priority given to immediate life-threatening injuries.
- Gastric injury is likely to require surgery.
- Vital to inspect anterior and posterior gastric walls, GOJ, and to look for associated hepatic lacerations. Lesser sac must be entered with partial gastric mobilization.
- Primary closure generally achievable.
- *If not possible, i.e. in severe trauma:* damage limitation surgery approach—acute resection (stapling off) of damaged tissue, drainage, and delayed reconstruction at re-look laparotomy at 48h.

Further reading

Sutcliffe RP, Forshaw MJ, Datta G, et al. Surgical management of Boerhaave's syndrome in a tertiary oesophagogastric centre. *Ann Roy Coll Surg Engl* 2009; **91**(5): 374–80.

Index